T0177600

Otolaryngology and Head and Neck Surgery

Giles Warner
Consultant Otolaryngologist/Head and Neck Surgeon,
Hereford County Hospital & Worcestershire Royal Hospital

Andrea S. Burgess
Consultant ENT Surgeon,
Royal Hampshire County Hospital,
Hampshire, UK

Suresh Patel
Department of Otolaryngology/Head and Neck Surgery,
Bedford Hospital,
Bedford, UK

Pablo Martinez-Devesa
Department of Otolaryngology/Head and Neck Surgery,
Oxford

Rogan Corbridge
Department of Otolaryngology/Head and Neck Surgery,
Oxford and Royal Berkshire Hospital,
Reading, UK

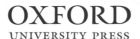

OXFORD
UNIVERSITY PRESS

OXFORD
UNIVERSITY PRESS

Great Clarendon Street, Oxford OX2 6DP

Oxford University Press is a department of the University of Oxford.
It furthers the University's objective of excellence in research, scholarship,
and education by publishing worldwide in

Oxford New York

Auckland Cape Town Dar es Salaam Hong Kong Karachi
Kuala Lumpur Madrid Melbourne Mexico City Nairobi
New Delhi Shanghai Taipei Toronto

With offices in

Argentina Austria Brazil Chile Czech Republic France Greece
Guatemala Hungary Italy Japan Poland Portugal Singapore
South Korea Switzerland Thailand Turkey Ukraine Vietnam

Oxford is a registered trade mark of Oxford University Press
in the UK and in certain other countries

Published in the United States
by Oxford University Press Inc., New York

© Oxford University Press, 2009

The moral rights of the authors have been asserted
Database right Oxford University Press (maker)

First published 2009, reprinted 2014, 2016, 2020

British Library Cataloguing in Publication Data
Data available

Library of Congress Cataloging in Publication Data
Data available

Typeset by Newgen Imaging Systems (P) Ltd., Chennai, India
Printed in China
on acid-free paper by
C&C Offset Printing Co., Ltd.

ISBN 978–0–19–923022–8 (flexicover: alk.paper)

10 9 8 7 6

Preface

This book is a natural progression from the introduction text 'The Oxford Handbook of ENT'. It will provide the ENT trainee with virtually all the information they will need to progress from their introduction to ENT practice through the hurdles of assessments and exams into independent practice in the field. The text covers all the major sub-specialist areas of ENT and will give the reader a solid knowledge base in each. The comprehensive index, 'key points' and bulleted text give the trainee rapid access to important information and advice when dealing with emergencies. This, unlike any other handbook, also covers all the common and important operative procedures in ENT and will give the reader a stepwise account of most of the operations they will need to learn to master. The blank sections within the text are ideal for making your own notes and individual key learning points from your personal experience and from your teaching. The ENT numbers section gives a review of wide areas and can also act as a useful revision aid. The Introduction section covers topics such as 'dealing with difficult patients and colleagues', 'Appraisal & Audit' as well as many other issues you will face on a daily basis in developing your medical practice. This book will become a trusted companion, valuable aid and 'study buddy' whether in clinic, on the ward, in the operating room or preparing for the next professional hurdle.

The authors of this book would like to pay a special acknowledgment to our senior colleague, mentor and friend Mr Andrew Freeland. Andrew has been a leader within our specialty and we all owe him a debt of gratitude for his influence on our careers. He continues to have an active interest in teaching and we hope that this book will be a fitting tribute to him. We wish him a long, healthy and happy retirement!

Contents

Detailed contents

Symbols and abbreviations

AAO-HNS	American Academy of Otolaryngology and Head & Neck Surgeons
BAHA	bone anchored hearing aid
BIPP	Bismuth Iodine Paraffin Paste
CPA	cerebello-pontine-angle
CPAP	continous positive airway pressure
EBV	Epstein-Barr virus
ECA	external carotid artery
ETT	endotracheal tube
GA	general anaesthesia
IAC	internal auditory canal
LA	local anaesthetic
LAUP	laser assisted uvulopalatoplasty
MRC	Medical Research Council
NGT	nasogastric tube
NPC	Nasopharyngeal carcinoma
OSA	obstructive sleep apnoea
PEG	percutaneous gastrostomy
RAST	Radio-allergosorbent test
SCM	sternocleidomastoid
SMAS	Superficial musculo-aponeurotic system
SPT	Skin Prick Test
URTI	upper respiratory tract infection
USS	ultrasound scan
UVPPP	uvulopalatopharyngoplasty

Introduction

Evidence-based medicine

Definition

The conscientious, explicit, and judicious use of best evidence in making decisions about the care of individual patients. This involves finding, critically appraising, and using this evidence in our clinical practice.

Simply put, evidence-based medicine is about reading the *right* papers, at the *right* time, and altering one's behaviour.

Steps for evidence-based practice

- Convert our information into answerable questions, i.e. formulate the problem.
- To track down the best evidence to answer these questions (evidence is usually from published literature searched via MEDLINE or Cochrane library: www.cochrane.org).
- To appraise the evidence critically (i.e. to weigh it up) to assess its validity (closeness to the truth) and its usefulness (clinical applicability).
- To use the results of this appraisal in our clinical practice.
- To evaluate our performance.

Levels or statements of evidence

Ia   Evidence from meta-analysis of prospective randomized controlled trials.

Ib   Evidence from at least one prospective randomized controlled trial.

II   Evidence from at least one well-designed controlled study (non-randomized), e.g. prospective cohort or retrospective case-control study.

III Evidence from well-designed non-experimental descriptive study, e.g. comparative or case studies.

IV   Evidence from expert committees or opinions and/or clinical experiences of respected authorities.

Evidence-based ENT practice

- 5000 papers are published each month of which >700 are clinical research papers.
- Only 10–15% have any scientific value.
- Positive studies are 20 times more frequently published than negative ones.
- 80% of ENT practice is based on descriptive case studies (Level 3 evidence).

Statistics for the non-statistician

Definition of statistics

Statistics can be broadly defined as the use of data from samples to draw inferences about the relevant larger population.

Key questions in data analysis

- What is the nature of data (type/properties)?
- How is it distributed?
- Which statistical tools do you use to make inferences about general population?

Types of data

- Parametric (quantative, numeric): where variables are related to each other and you can put a number to, e.g. height.
- Non- parametric (qualitative, categorical): where data are not related to each other, e.g. blood groups.
- Paired data: where two observations are performed on the same sample, e.g. lying and standing BP measurements on the same patients.
- Unpaired data: comparing two independent samples drawn from the same population, e.g. effect of drug A on study sample compared with placebo on controls.

Properties of data

- Mean is the cumulative total divided by the number of samples ('average').
- Mode is the most frequently occurring event.
- Median is the middle sample when the data is arranged in order.
- Variance, standard deviation, and standard error are all measures of spread of the data about the mean.

Distribution of data

- Normal (Gaussian) distribution: if a very large number of samples are plotted, this follows a bell-shaped curve with 95% of the data falling within 2 standard deviations of the mean.
- Skewed distribution: a non-normal distribution with the bulk of the data occurring on one side of the average.

Which statistical test is the most appropriate?

This depends on the nature of the data and its distribution. Some of the more common statistical tests are:

- Normally distributed parametric data: T-test, Pearson correlation test.
- Non-parametric tests: Wilcoxon test for paired data, Mann–Whitney test for unpaired data, Spearman rank correlation test.
- Categories: Chi-squared test.

Some important statistical terms

Probability: the way of describing how likely an event will happen (0 = never happens, 1 = always happens).

P-value: probability value, i.e. the result occurred by chance. Arbitrarily set at 0.05 (5%), which means that 5% of the time the result we have on the samples is not representative of the whole population. If a P-value is less than 0.05(5%), results are described as statistically significant and unlikely to have occurred by chance.

H0 = null hypothesis: there is no real difference between the populations.

H1 = alternative hypothesis: there is a real difference between the populations.

Type 1 error: a false-positive result, i.e. rejecting the null hypothesis when in fact we should not.

Type 2 error: a false-negative result, i.e. failure to reject the null hypothesis when in fact we should.

Power of a study: probability we will make a type 2 error, i.e. fail to detect a difference when one exists. Usually because of the sample numbers are too small.

Standard deviation: indicator of the spread of the data about the mean.

Confidence intervals: usually set at 95%. We are 95% certain that the population mean lies in the given range. If the range crosses zero, the results may not be statistically significant.

Bias: the result we have is different to what it should be. This can be due to sampling error, unfair exclusions, incomplete response to questionnaire studies, incomplete blinding, not using matching controls, non-randomization, not including all the data in the analysis, analysing the data too early in the study, and using the wrong statistical test for the data.

Confounding: when part of the observed relationship between two variables is due to action of a third, e.g. alcohol consumption and lung cancer are both more common in smokers and if you are not aware of this, your analysis may indicate alcohol causes lung cancer.

Critical appraisal of papers

Definition of critical appraisal

The practice of systematically examining research evidence to assess the validity of methodology and results, and the relevance to our clinical work.

Standard appraisal questions

- Are the objectives of the paper clearly stated? Is the question worth asking?
- Do the authors or their institution have expertise in the subject area? Do the authors have bias?
- Did the authors have the right type of study to address the research question (see below)?
- Was the sample size justified? Was a power calculation performed?
- Are the measurements likely to be valid and reliable?
- Are the statistical methods described?
- Did untoward events occur during the study?
- Was the basic data adequately described?
- Do the numbers add up? Were patients excluded, lost to follow up, or die?
- Was statistical significance assessed?
- What do the main findings mean? What were the outcome measures?
- How are the null findings interpreted?
- Are important effects overlooked?
- How do the results compare with previous reports?
- Were the aims fulfilled in the discussion?
- What implications does the study have for your practice? Are the patients similar to your unit?

Additional questions for specific studies

Surveys

- Who was studied?
- How was the sample obtained?
- What was the response rate?

Cohort studies (for papers addressing prognosis)

- Who exactly was studied?
- Was a control group used or should one have been used?
- How adequate was the follow-up?

Clinical trials (for papers addressing effectiveness of drug treatment)

- How were the treatments randomly allocated?
- Were all patients accounted for?
- Was analysis performed on an intention-to-treat basis (i.e. according to the groups they were initially randomized to?)
- Were the outcomes assessed blind?

Case controls (for papers addressing causation)
- How were the cases obtained?
- Is the control group appropriate?
- Was data collected in the same way for cases and controls?

Review papers
- How were the papers identified?
- How was the quality of the papers assessed?
- How was the result summarized?

Medico-legal issues in clinical practice

The most important issues facing a doctor in their everyday work are:
- Capacity of a patient.
- Principles of consent (see 📖 p10).
- Issues of patient confidentiality.
- Notification to coroners court.
- Access to medical records.
- Clinical negligence.

Capacity of patient

Definition

'Mental competency of patient to make a decision'.[1]

The patient has to be able to comprehend what is being said to him and be able to weigh up this information to make an informed decision.

Basic principles

- Adult is competent until proved otherwise.
- Once proved incompetent, the patient remains so until proved otherwise.
- Burden of proof lies with the doctor in changing mental capacity.

A mentally competent adult can make an unwise decision against good advice, e.g a patient on hunger strike may not be force fed but a patient with anorexia, in certain circumstances, may be.

A doctor may have to assess capacity before providing medical treatment or before witnessing a legal document, e.g. a will (patient must understand what making a will means and the value of the property to be disposed of).

Confidentiality

Doctors have an ethical duty not to disclose personal information about patients to third parties. Written permission is required from patients before disclosure is permitted. Confidentiality does not end with the death of the patient and permission should be sought from the next of kin.

Important exceptions

- Sharing information with registered medical practitioners involved with the patient's clinical management.
- If disclosure is in the patient's best medical interest and the patient is incapable of giving consent or if seeking consent may be harmful to the patient.
- Notification of certain infectious diseases.
- Where children are at risk, e.g. suspected child abuse.
- Where public safety is at risk.

Notification to coroner's court

The purpose of an inquest is to determine who died, where, when, and how. The following deaths should be reported:
- Any deaths occurring during operation or before recovery from anaesthetic (within 24h of surgery).
- Suspected ill treatment or neglect.

---

1 Mental Capacity Act 2005. Department of Health Website.

- Crime-related deaths.
- Death from septicaemia.
- Poisoning of any type, including food poisoning.
- Death of patients detained under the Mental Heath Act.

If in doubt, discuss the case with the coroner.

Access to medical records

Courts have the absolute power to order the disclosure of medical records. Patients also have the right to access their medical records, unless information about another patient will be revealed from their records.

As medical records may be used as part of a legal action, they must be legible, dated (possibly timed), and signed. Do not write anything that you would not be prepared to show the patient and never make unfounded or unprofessional observations.

Clinical negligence

This occurs when:

1. a person is owed a duty of care by a health care provider, i.e. he/she is a patient.
2. there is a breach of that duty.
3. the patient suffered harm as a result.

Breach of duty is usually judged by the Bolam test, i.e. care must be provided with accepted medical practice as determined by experts in the field. Nowadays, many units have protocols or care pathways in keeping with best practice.

Medical defence organizations have no role in litigation against NHS employees because, from 1990, NHS hospitals began indemnifying their employees against patients' allegations of medical negligence. Therefore doctors are not sued directly. Trusts became defendants in legal proceedings and the NHS accepted financial responsibility for claims.

However, NHS indemnity does not cover you for:

- Disciplinary procedures by your trust or GMC.
- Good Samaritan acts outside your hospital.

Consent

Definition

'Patient authorizes the doctor to initiate a medical plan'.[2]
It is more than just a signature. For consent to be legally valid:
- The patient has to be properly informed.
- The patient has to be competent (have the capacity) to give consent.
- The patient has to give consent voluntarily and without coercion.

Consent and the law

Two main areas of relevant law are:
- Battery: if one person touches another without consent, this may constitute battery even though no-one suffered harm as a result of the incident.
- Negligence: patients need information when choosing whether or not to accept a treatment, e.g. nature of treatment, benefits, risks, and alternative. If a doctor does not provide this information prior to consent, then he or she may be negligent.

Types of consent

Implied

Patient consent is needed before an examination. However, we don't obtain specific consent for these procedures as the courts recognize the concept of 'implied consent', e.g. 'I would like to examine your throat' and patient opens his mouth. However, if a competent patient refuses to be examined and the doctor ignores this and proceeds to examine him, this constitutes battery. The fact that the patient came to see the doctor or is admitted to hospital does not imply consent to examination, investigation or treatment.

Expressed

Whereby specific written consent is obtained, e.g. prior to surgery.

Surgical consent form

The patient has to sign a consent form before surgery because:
- Legally, it provides evidence that the patient has given permission for a procedure.
- It communicates the patient's wishes to other members of the healthcare team.

For consent to be legally valid, the patient needs to understand the requirement for treatment and the consequences of not having it, its risks, success rates, and other alternatives. The patient should be informed of all life-threatening or life-changing risks, no matter how unlikely.

Ideally, the consent should be obtained by the consultant or the person carrying out the procedure. A competent patient can withdraw consent at any time.

---

2 Reference Guide to Consent for Examination or Treatment. Department of Health Website.

Decision-making for incompetent patients

- Best interests: doctor makes a decision in 'best interests' of patient, e.g. life-saving surgery. Doctor is legally accountable and this may be assessed by the Bolam test.
- Proxy: a proxy, e.g. next of kin, takes the place of an incompetent patient and makes decisions for the patient.
- Substituted judgement: 'If the patient was competent, what treatment would he chose?' The doctor uses evidence from patient's past, by knowing the values of the patient and from the experience of relatives.
- Advance directives ('living will'): statement written by patients when fully competent, making decisions about their medical care and what they want and don't want in the future, if they become incompetent.

Minors and consent

The law is complex here. In general, do not deny urgent life-saving treatment to a child under 18 years of age because of lack of consent from the minor or parents.

Child age 16–17 years

Presumed to have capacity to consent until proved otherwise. If patient refuses consent, parents or courts can over-ride decision and can give consent in child's best interests.

Child aged <16 years

Presumed not to have capacity to consent unless they satisfy health professionals that they do have such capacity. Tested by 'Gillick competency' whereby a child <16 years is deemed to have sufficient mental maturity to understand need for treatment and come to a reasoned decision. If child refuses consent for life-saving treatment, parents or courts can over-ride it.

Child who is not competent

Parents should give consent. However, if parents refuse and the doctor feels it is not in the child's best interest, then the courts should be involved. In an emergency, when there is no time for consent or to involve the courts, the doctor should treat the child to preserve the child's life.

Consent for photos and videos

BMA, GMC, and the Institute of Medical Illustrators all publish guidelines indicating that the patient has the right to be given as much information as possible on where an image might be used. Specific consent should be obtained for all images, especially if the patient can be identified.

Breaking bad news

Most doctors feel uncomfortable breaking bad news to patients and relatives. It requires expertise, knowledge, and skill, as well as compassion. In the past, doctors avoided telling patients bad news as they may have felt the patient did not want to know or they were trying to protect the patient in some way, but these attitudes have now, quite rightly, changed.

Patient and family reaction to bad news
Five stages of dying are:
- denial.
- anger.
- bargaining.
- depression.
- acceptance.

If the doctor breaking bad news is aware of these reactions and which stage the patient may be in, he can be more thoughtful and prepared, and the overall experience of being told bad news can be less traumatic.

Approaches to giving bad news
- Allow ample time for consultation and take precautions to avoid unnecessary interruptions whilst with the patient, e.g. switch off phones, place 'Do Not Disturb sign' outside room.
- Use a suitable private room, furniture arranged appropriately and tissues to hand.
- Ensure you have a member of staff with you, to help you and support the relatives.
- Check case notes in detail beforehand to ensure you have all the information you need. Take notes with you to the consultation.
- During the consultation, give the patient a warning that they are about to receive significant information so that they prepare themselves, e.g. 'I have some important news'.
- Allow the patient to have somebody with them for support and to help absorb the information during the consultation.
- Use appropriate body language, eye contact, and voice tone.
- Determine what the patient already knows or believes about their illness, e.g. 'What have you been told about your illness?'.
- Determine what the patient and their family want to know before you tell them, e.g. 'Would you like me to tell you the full details of the diagnosis/results?'.
- Most patients only remember approximately 40% of what they are told and it is likely the information will need repeating or writing down. Consider drawing diagrams to explain what you are saying more clearly.
- Respond to the patient's concerns and hopes as accurately as possible without being unrealistic or falsely reassuring. Be honest—if you don't know something, say so and find out the information for them.
- Avoid using medical jargon when talking to patients, e.g. use blockage rather than stricture.

- Some patients may be too shocked or bewildered to make informed decisions about their treatment.
- Arrange for a follow-up appointment to discuss further patients' questions and plan management. Specifically, patients will often want to know the size of the tumour, the different treatment options, and their side-effects.
- Make sure all people being told the bad news are given the same information with the same options, including the offer of a second opinion.
- Provide patients with sources of information, e.g. Cancerlink, Macmillan, and hospice support, written information about their condition and its treatment, internet links, relevant social support.
- Inform the patient's GP promptly of the discussion so that he/she can deal effectively with the patient. Make sure the medical records are fully updated with the notes of your discussion to set a baseline for future explanations.

Dealing with relatives when a terminally ill patient dies
- Most of the above points are also relevant when dealing with bereaved relatives.
- If possible, collect all family members for one meeting. This will avoid repetition.
- Use clear, unambiguous language, e.g. 'died' rather than 'lost'.
- Help the bereaved obtain the information they need to understand why their loved ones died and to say goodbye to the body of the deceased, if they so wish. Viewing the body enables the bereaved to begin to accept that death has happened.

Communicating with patients and colleagues

With patients

Because of changes in the NHS, the care of the patient is often fragmented. Patients are often placed wherever a bed is available, not necessarily on an ENT ward, and often looked after by nurses not familiar with their specific clinical needs. Also, with the reduction in junior doctor hours, it is less likely a familiar doctor will be available to talk to relatives. Attitudes and expectations of the public to doctors have also changed.

The key to this problem is good communication between medical and nursing colleagues, as well as with patients and relatives.

Tips for a good outpatient consultation

- Stand up and greet the patient. Use handshake, if appropriate, as well as the correct eye contact.
- Listen carefully to what the patient has to say, and try and answer all their concerns in turn.
- Avoid using medical jargon. Use terms and analogies the patient will understand.
- Consider writing things down and drawing clear diagrams for patients to look at after the consultation.
- When discussing treatments, give the pros and cons of each option. If the patient is included in the discussion, they are more likely to comply with the final treatment choice.
- Never hurry a consultation. Switch off phones and make the patient feel your time is solely for them.
- Try and supplement the consultation by giving the patient and relatives the appropriate information leaflets.
- At the end of the consultation, stand up and escort the patient to the door. Ensure follow-up arrangements are understood.

With colleagues

To be 'successful' as a doctor, one has to be perceived as such by your colleagues.

Tips on what makes a good colleague

- Most doctors prefer a friendly, affable, optimistic colleague rather than a taciturn, abrasive, and pessimistic one.
- First impressions are very important, e.g. shaking hands, eye contact, being well-dressed, and remembering the name of a new acquaintance.
- You must communicate effectively on clinical, academic, and management matters. Communication can be verbally or, more commonly, by letters and emails.

Dealing with difficult patients and colleagues

Tips on handling difficult patients

- Have a third independent person present, if only to corroborate your version of events at a subsequent enquiry.
- Try to be on the same level with the other person. Avoid looking down on them, as they will feel threatened.
- Keep your own voice as level as possible. Communicate calmly with the person.
- Allow them plenty of personal space, as getting too close may make them feel threatened.
- Acknowledge the patient's feelings with an empathetic statement. The irate patient, when realizing that you understand, will no longer have to prove their anger.
- Indicate you are paying attention by reflective listening and repeating back a summary of what was said.
- Try turning difficult questions back on the patient, e.g. you can ask them, 'What makes you ask that question?'.
- If you are unsure how to respond to an angry patient, it is best to stay quiet. Faced with silence, most people run out of steam and begin to feel foolish.
- Avoid questioning an angry patient.
- If you are in a closed space or room, check you are well positioned for leaving quickly, or at least ensure that a large piece of furniture separates you from the complainant.
- If the patient is abusive, terminate the interview as soon as possible. Document the occurrence and inform the risk manager of the hospital, possibly with corroboration from the independent witness. Report the patient to their GP and ask the GP to refer the patient elsewhere.
- If the patient threatens violence, never lose your temper as this only makes things worse. If the person needs restraining, always involve hospital security staff or police, who are trained in the proper techniques. Remember your job is to treat the patient.
- If the patient is making an informal complaint, give them an explanation of what went on and, if necessary, an apology. Remember an apology is not necessarily an admission of guilt. Try and put a human face on the problem. Reassure the patient that steps will be taken to stop the problem happening again. It is vital the whole team learn from any mistakes.
- Try and remain polite, honest, caring, and dignified at all times.
- If you feel the patient does not believe your professional opinion, consider referring them to a colleague for a second opinion.

Tips on handling difficult colleagues

Many so-called 'difficult colleagues' are simply people we would not choose to associate with socially. A truly difficult colleague may continue to act this way because no one has ever discussed their inappropriate behaviour with them.

Reasons for talking to a colleague about their conduct include:
- Excessive alcohol consumption.
- Drug abuse.
- Actions that affect the health and safety of other.
- Behaviour that may be offensive or embarrassing to others,
  e.g. workplace bullying.

Usually the best course of action, after establishing the facts, is to confront the individual, bringing your concerns to their attention and then attempting to address the issues. Try and resolve the situation with a sympathetic discussion.

If a colleague's behaviour continues to be a problem, especially if substance abuse is involved or patients are at risk, then the clinical or medical director should be informed. It is better to act and stand by a colleague as a friend than to feel that the best way to support them is not to report the issue. Remember, your primary duty of care is to your patients and you should report your colleagues for any such professional breach of conduct at work.

Clinical governance

Definition

'A framework through which all NHS organizations are accountable for continuously improving the quality of their services and safeguarding high standards of care by creating an environment in which excellence in clinical care will flourish.'[3]

Essential principles

- Setting of realistic and evidence-based standards of care.
- Monitoring of performances against these standards.
- Implementation of change to ensure that these standards are reached and, if possible, exceeded.

Five pillars of clinical governance

- Multidisciplinary clinical audit.
- Clinical effectiveness.
- Clinical risk management.
- Quality assurance.
- Staff development/continual professional development.

Clinical governance focuses on a team approach to patient management and addresses the whole patient journey (rather than just the patient's treatment).

Clinical audit

The monitoring of performances within a given area with comparisons with others' performances; reasons that account for that difference are identified and then changes are put in place to improve performance. Reassessment should confirm that a better outcome has been achieved. All steps of the patient journey can be audited with the goal of improving the quality of care. The results of audit have to be open and accountable to outsiders.

Clinical effectiveness

The evaluation of effectiveness of a particular therapy, e.g. by monitoring morbidity and mortality, cure rate, etc. Also involves the use of evidence-based medicine in clinical practice, i.e. there is no point providing a treatment that is ineffective. Evaluating clinical effectiveness ensures that ineffective treatments are identified and discontinued, and effective treatments are administered to the highest possible standards. Often, 'care pathways' are used to ensure consistently high quality care.

Clinical risk management

The near misses, device-related incidences, drug reactions, discussion of medical negligence cases. By recognizing and reviewing adverse events that occur, we can identify ways to prevent them. Goal of risk management is to reduce occurrences and consequences of adverse events. Adverse events can be reported by any healthcare worker. Near misses are much more common than minor or major injuries and as such constitute important 'free lessons' by which more serious incidents can be avoided.

3 A First Class Service. Quality in the New NHS, Department of Health, 1998.

Quality assurance

The monitoring and measuring of performances against standards. There is some overlap between quality assurance and clinical audit. Quality assurance programmes are important in screening, e.g. radiology (breast screening). Also review of formal patient complaints may identify failings in service and problems in the patient pathway.

Staff development/continual professional development

In the past, staff development in the NHS was a passive process. However, appraisal and assessment have been introduced and all staff must provide evidence of continual medical education to demonstrate they are keeping abreast of recent developments.

Principals of clinical audit

Definition
'The systematic critical analysis of the quality of medical care which includes the procedures used for the diagnosis and treatment and the use of resources and the resulting outcome and quality of life for the patient.'[4]

An alternative definition is:

'A system whereby a process/outcome is analysed with respect to targets/standards, change is instigated and the process/outcome is re-evaluated to ensure improvement.'[5]

Aims
- Improve the delivery of healthcare to patients by identifying opportunities to raise the standards of clinical practice by implementing change.
- Secondary benefits are improved knowledge and work satisfaction, publication opportunities, and better communication with colleagues and managers.

Audit is an essential part of clinical governance. It is now a contractual requirement for doctors in the hospital and community services and this is supported by the Royal Colleges.

Building-blocks of audit (by Auedis Donabedian)
- Structure (resources and facilities available for care).
- Process (activities of care).
- Outcome (resultant effect on patients).

Each of these building blocks can be analysed as part of the audit process. At least two loops of the audit spiral should be completed to ensure any changes have resulted in improvement to the services. Guidance and practical support from the clinical effectiveness and audit department can be invaluable when setting up an audit design and during data collection and analysis.

---

4 White Paper. Working for Patients, Department of Health, 1989.
5 National Institute for Clinical Excellence 2002.

Preparing for the consultant interview

Before the interview

- Anticipate everything and be prepared for all possible situations! There may be traffic jams delaying your arrival, difficulty finding the interview venue, and tricky questions during the interview. If you arrive late, you may have difficulty regaining composure and also it gives a bad first impression to the interviewers.
- Dress to reassure the members of the panel that they are looking at a young consultant and a future colleague.
- Go into the interview room positively, smiling and determined to enjoy it!

During the interview

- Your main aim is to convince the panel you will make a delightful colleague and achieve your goals.
- Remember, it's normal to feel nervous and the opening question from the interviewers is usually to relax you and settle you into the rest of the interview. Also, not all members of the panel will know each other, so they may feel nervous too.
- Be relaxed but business-like, sit upright and look at the chairperson initially, who should ask you the first question.
- Be friendly and smile with a degree of authority. Show enthusiasm for the job.
- Address your answers to the questioner but do look around to try and engage all the panel with your answers.
- If you don't understand a tricky question, say so. Make sure you answer the question asked. Take your time to formulate your answer rather than saying something quickly and ill-considered.

Specific interview questions

- Opening questions are usually concerned with a review of your CV and asking you about any unusual features or gaps in your training.
- There will be questions to try and get you to talk about yourself. Do so with confidence, intelligence, charm, honesty, maturity, and occasional humour.
- Inevitably, there will be a question of your research and audit experience.
- There may be questions on recent government reports and agendas, and the implications on your proposed service.
- Questions on your strengths and weakness are always worth thinking about beforehand.
  - What can you do to improve on your weaknesses and past mistakes? (this tests your virtues, intellectual honesty, maturity, and self awareness).
  - What are your strengths and greatest achievements? (this tests your standards, leadership style and ability).
- What are your relationships like with your colleagues? (this tests your personality: social or self contained, conforming or independent, extrovert or sensitive).

- Why do you want this job? This is an opportunity to show you have researched the hospital. Have you identified any challenges that the institute faces? What visions do you have for the future of the department and hospital?
- Where do you see your career going?

At the end of the interview

- Usually you are invited by the panel to ask any questions you may have. As you will have researched the job beforehand, it is acceptable not to ask anything.
- You should remain in the hospital grounds until all the interviews are over. Leave your contact details with the personnel officer.

Appraisal

Why participate in appraisal?

- It helps the trainee to reflect on experience and assists in the acquisition and development of understanding of new concepts. It is done by a senior colleague whose opinion is important to the trainee.
- It is part of the revalidation process.

Types of appraisal

Formative

Formative appraisal attempts to measure skills, behaviour, attitudes, and knowledge, and encourages the trainee to identify and fix weaknesses. Appraisal is usually conducted through a series of meetings by an experienced consultant. The first meeting is at the beginning of the job and sets up a training agreement and defines goals. The second meeting is halfway through the attachment and reviews progress and revises the learning goals. The final meeting is at the end of the job and reviews the trainee's experience and assists the trainee to reflect on experience gained. The records of formative appraisal are usually confidential.

Summative

Summative appraisal measures the ability of the trainee in order to permit progress over a performance hurdle, e.g. RITA assessment. Summative assessment also tests skills, behaviours, and attitudes but is regulatory (i.e. tests to certain standards). The methods and criteria are set by examiners on behalf of an assessing body. Examiners themselves will have been trained in summative assessment methods. The aim of summative assessment is to identify trainees not ready for independent practice. Its outcome will enhance or impede career progression. The results of summative assessment are not confidential.

Aims of appraisal

- To help identify educational needs at an early stage.
- To assist in the skills of self-reflection and self-appraisal that will be needed throughout a trainee's career.
- To provide a mechanism for reviewing progress and to identify problems in time for remedial action to be taken.
- To provide a method for giving feedback of the quality of training provided.

What is discussed at an appraisal?

- Preparation for exams. What courses to go on.
- Advice on research projects.
- Clinical experience and skills.
- Appropriate knowledge level.
- Organization and planning ability.
- Teaching skills of trainee.
- Career pathway.
- Personal skills and attributes (interpersonal communication, decisiveness, teamworking, flexibility and resilience, thoroughness, drive and enthusiasm, probity).

ENT history and examination

History and examination of the ear

Key points
- Hearing loss (progressive or sudden, uni- or bilateral).
- Tinnitus (type of noise, frequency, central or uni-/bilateral).
- Otalgia (severe or ache, deep or superficial, constant or intermittent).
- Otorrhoea (scanty debris or mucopurulent, clear or infected).
- Dizziness/vertigo (true rotatory vertigo: onset, duration, symptoms associated, repetition of episodes; imbalance/dizziness: first and further episodes, impact on daily life).

Examination of the ear
- Start by examining the better-hearing ear.
- Examine the pinna, in front and behind, looking for skin inflammation, discharge, scars, (Fig. 2.1) or skin lesions (pre-auricular sinus, skin tumours) .
- Examine the external ear canal with a speculum and head light or an otoscope. Pull the ear backwards (and upwards for an adult). Notice inflammation, oedema, presence of wax and debris.
- Visualize the tympanic membrane entirely in quadrants starting from the attic at 12 o'clock (so as not to miss any pathology). Notice the status of the tympanic membrane (normal or dull, thin or tympanoscle-rotic), any possible perforation or retraction pockets, the state of the ossicles and the middle ear.
- Perform a pneumatic otoscopy with a Siegle's speculum or similar (Fig. 2.2), to assess middle-ear function, alternatively ask the patient to do a Valsalva manoeuvre while examining the tympanic membrane.
- If a mastoid cavity is seen, notice the shape, size, height of the facial ridge, remnant tympanic membrane, and ossicles, as well as size of meatoplasty.
- A fistula test can be carried out by applying intermittent pressure in the tragus with the finger, and observing for nystagmus (if there is reported dizziness/vertigo in the history).
- Tuning fork tests (Rinne and Weber at least, see 📖 p284).
- Free field hearing test (see 📖 p28).
- Check facial nerve function (see 📖 p36).
- Examine the post-nasal space with endoscope (especially if unilateral middle ear effusion to exclude malignancy).
- Examination of the cranial nerves (see 📖 p36).

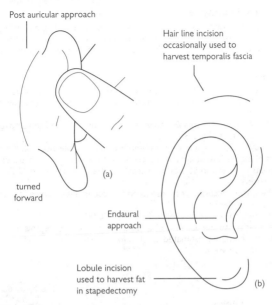

Post auricular approach

turned
forward

(a)

Hair line incision
occasionally used to
harvest temporalis fascia

Endaural
approach

Lobule incision
used to harvest fat
in stapedectomy

(b)

Fig. 2.1 Common surgical scars.

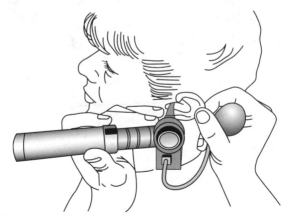

Fig. 2.2 Pneumatic otoscopy.

Free field hearing test

Most patients will usually have a formal pure-tone audiogram (PTA) to assess their hearing; however, there are some situations in which it may be not possible to perform a PTA, such as at the bedside of the patient, or an outreach clinic with no audiological facilities.

Procedure

- During this test the examiner's voice is used as a sound stimulus, while the patient's non-test ear is masked by rubbing the finger over the tragus.
- The patient's eyes are shielded with the examiner's hand to remove any visual clues (Fig. 2.3).
- Start by whispering a two-digit number or a bisyllable word (at the end of expiration) at approximately 60cm from the ear. If the patient repeats correctly in 50% of the occasions, the thresholds are 12dB or better.
- If there is no accurate response, then use conversation voice at that distance (= 48dB).
- If there is no response, use loud voice (= 76dB).
- Move closer to the ear (15cm) and repeat the procedure, this time the thresholds are estimated at 34dB for a whisper and 56dB for a conversation voice.

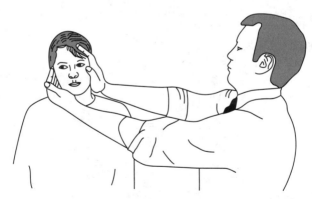

Fig. 2.3 Free field testing.

History and examination of the nose

Key points
- Nasal obstruction (or congestion).
- Rhinorrhoea and post-nasal drip.
- Facial pain and headaches.
- Anosmia.

Examination of the nose
- Examine the nose externally from the front and side views, looking at the skin type and thickness, scars and lesions.
- Look and feel the nasal bones and nasal cartilages (septum, upper and lower lateral), looking for any asymmetry and deformity.
- Tilt the head of the patient backwards to examine the columella and the vestibule.
- Check the patency of the nasal airway on each side with a metallic tongue depressor or by occluding the nostril with the thumb and asking the patient to sniff through the nose.
- Perform Cottle's test to check for obstruction of the nasal flow at the anterior nasal valve area. This is done by asking the patient to sniff when applying upward and lateral traction to the skin lateral to the nose (and in turn the lower lateral nasal cartilage) opening the anterior nasal valve area (Fig. 2.4). This manoeuvre tests for collapse of the lower lateral cartilage as cause of nasal obstruction.
- Inspect nasal cavities using thudichum speculum and assess the nasal septum for deviation, perforation, vessels, mucosal lesions, inferior turbinates (hypertrophy, mucosal changes), nasal masses (polyps, lesions).
- Perform a rigid naso-endoscopy (see below) to inspect the rest of the nasal cavity and post-nasal space.
- In the absence of endoscopes, the post-nasal space can also be seen with a Sinclair–Thompson mirror (Fig. 2.5).
- Examine the neck for lymphadenopathy.

Rigid naso-endoscopy
This is regarded as the standard technique for assessing the nose. It may be performed with the patient seated or laying supine on an examination couch.

Procedure
- Before starting, warn the patient that the nasal spray tastes dreadful, that their throat will be numb, and that hot food or drink should not be consumed for an hour to avoid burns.
- Prepare the patient's nose with co-phenylcaine spray (lidocaine with ephedrine)—usually upto five sprays to each nostril. The anaesthetic and vasoconstrictive effect of the spray takes 6min to work, so it is essential to wait 6min before starting the procedure. A diluted solution of the co-phenylcaine can be given to children.
- Use a 4mm 0° and 30° endoscope. A 2.7mm scope can be helpful in a narrow nose.
- Use the standard three-pass technique; Fig. 2.6 shows the endoscopic views.

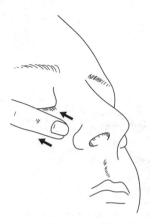

Fig. 2.4 Cottle's test.

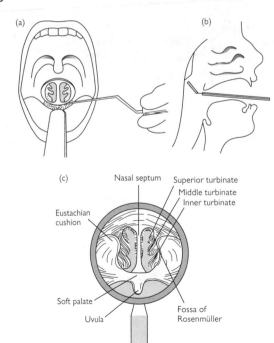

Fig. 2.5 Mirror examination of the post-nasal space.

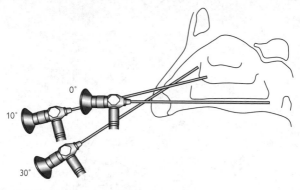

Fig. 2.6 The 3 pass technique used in endoscopic examination of the nasal cavity. Note the differing endoscopes used to gain a good view of all areas.

History and examination of the throat and neck

Key points

- Pain (in the mouth, throat and/or radiated to the ears).
- Dysphagia (and odynophagia).
- Dysphonia.
- Dyspnoea and stridor.
- Weight loss, malaise.
- Haemoptysis, cough, aspiration.
- Gastro-esophageal reflux (GOR), post-nasal drip (PND).
- Neck lump/s (onset, change in size, pain).

Examination of the oral cavity, pharynx, and larynx

- Ask the patient to remove any dentures, and open the mouth wide to assess for trismus.
- Inspect in order the tongue (dorsum, lateral edges, and ventral aspect), floor of the mouth, teeth, gums (including retromolar trigones), and parotid duct opening opposite the upper second molar teeth.
- Then inspect the hard and soft palate, palatine tonsils, and posterior pharyngeal wall. Ask the patient to say 'aahh' to assess palatal elevation.
- Feel with a gloved finger any pathological areas and perform bi-manual examination of the submandibular gland with a finger of one hand in the floor of the mouth and the other hand on the neck.
- Examine next the hypopharynx and larynx with a flexible naso-endoscope (or a laryngeal mirror).

Flexible naso-endoscopy

- Use topical anaesthetic and decongestant as per rigid naso-endoscopy (see 📖 p30).
- The endoscope is passed through the nose either between middle and inferior turbinates or under the inferior turbinate, along the floor of the nasal cavity into the post-nasal space, where the Eustachian tube and adenoids can be seen. The soft palate can also be assessed for elevation and velopharyngeal competence.
- By advancing over the superior aspect of the soft palate, the tongue base, vallecula, laryngeal inlet and piriform fossa can be seen. Visualization of these areas can be improved by asking the patient to stick out their tongue, and performing a Valsalva manoeuvre.
- Asking the patient to say 'eeee' and to speak helps to assess vocal cord movement.

Stroboscopy

- Fine movements of the vocal cords ('mucosal wave') require stroboscopic examination. Most often performed in a specialist voice clinic.
- The endoscope used is usually a rigid endoscope through the patient's mouth, but some flexible naso-endoscopes can also been used.
- A microphone is placed on the patient's neck and the frequency of cord vibration ('fundamental frequency') is matched to the frequency of a strobe light flashing.

- The resulting images shown in effect a slow motion recording of the vocal cords and allows detailed assessment during phonation.

Indirect laryngoscopy

- Place the patient sitting up and leaning forward with the head slightly extended.
- An appropriate size laryngeal mirror is selected.
- The mirror surface is gently warmed.
- Ask the patient to open their mouth and put out their tongue as far as they can.
- Gently wrap the tongue in gauze and hold it between finger and thumb.
- Introduce the warmed mirror into the mouth, gently pushing the soft palate and uvula upwards. If there is a strong gag reflex, local anaesthetic spray (i.e. xylocaine) may be helpful.
- Ask the patient to concentrate on their breathing; sometimes asking them to pant improves the view.
- Once a view of the larynx is obtained ask the patient to say 'eeee' and note the movement of the vocal cords.

Examination of the neck

- Start by inspecting the neck from the front, looking for scars or masses, deformity or asymmetry.
- Ask the patient to swallow and look for any possible thyroid mass rising on swallowing.
- After enquiring if there are any areas of pain or tenderness in the neck, move behind the patient and feel, in a systematic and comprehensive way, all levels of the neck (Fig. 2.7).
- If a neck lump or other abnormality is found, describe it adequately and its relation to the anatomical structures in the neck: site, size, shape, consistency, fixity, pulsation, overlying skin. The position of the neck lump will give clues as to the likely diagnosis (Fig. 2.8).

Examination of the thyroid

Full neck examination is required, plus some additional important points:

- Start by examining the patient's hands and looking at their face; note cold or hot and sweaty hand, which may indicate hypo- or hyperthyroidism. Look at the skin of the face and hair quality, in particular for loss of the hair in the lateral part of the eyebrow, which may occur in hypothyroidism.
- Look at the neck at the front and ask the patient to swallow.
- Ask the patient also to speak and to cough, listening for a breathy voice or a weak cough, which may represent a vocal cord palsy due to infiltration of the recurrent laryngeal nerve.
- Move behind the patient and feel the midline from the chin to the sternal notch. Feel for any midline lumps, in particular thyroglossal cysts, which will elevate on protrusion of the tongue, so distinguishing them from thyroid lumps in the isthmus.
- The normal thyroid gland is impalpable, if there is a palpable lump, try to ascertain if this is solitary or if there are multiple nodules. Localize it in either lobe or isthmus. Remember to ask the patient to swallow again to check the lump rises during swallowing.

- If a thyroid mass is present, feel above and below it. Assess retrosternal extension by percussion on the sternum and assess vascularity by auscultation.

Examination of the cranial nerves

This is carried out at any part of the examination of the ear, nose, throat, and neck when there is clinical suspicion of cranial nerve affectation by the pathology (i.e. otorrhoea with facial palsy, nasopharyngeal mass and dysphonia, parotid lump and facial palsy, etc.).

- Test for smell sensation (I).
- Test visual acuity (II), pupilary reaction (II, III), and extra-ocular muscle movements: superior oblique muscle—downward and outward gaze (IV); lateral rectus—lateral gaze (VI); and the rest of the extra-ocular muscles (III).
- Test corneal reflex and facial sensation (V).
- Test facial motor function (VII): raise the eyebrows (frontal branch), close the eyes (zygomatic), blow up the cheeks (buccal), smile or show teeth (marginal mandibular).
- Test hearing (VIII) with tuning fork, free field test and/or audiometry.
- Test palatal sensation (IX) and elevation (X), vocal cord movement (X, on laryngoscopy).
- Finally test sternomastoid contraction and shoulder elevation (XI).
- Tongue movement and protrusion (XII).

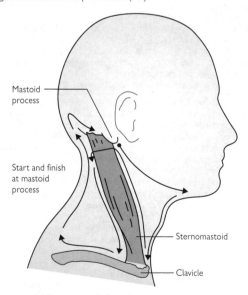

Mastoid process

Start and finish at mastoid process

Sternomastoid

Clavicle

Fig. 2.7 Systematic examination of the neck.

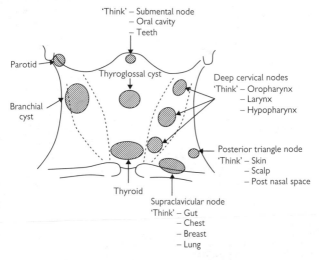

Fig. 2.8 Diagram of the neck lumps by position and likely diagnosis.

Common methods of presentation

Patients present with symptoms (e.g. a hoarse voice) rather than diagnosis
(e.g. laryngitis or vocal cord cancer). The following pages will help the
inexperienced ENT Surgeon to arrive at a sensible differential diagnosis
when presented with a patient's symptoms. Further reading is then
referenced to the appropriate page in this handbook.

Hoarse voice

History	Examination		Diagnosis	Page no
Lasted less than 2 weeks + pyrexia + a sore throat + URTI symptoms		→	Acute laryngitis	
Lasted more than 3 weeks Constant Progressive Patient is a smoker dysphagia pain otalgia a neck lump	→ Vocal cord lesion	→ Unilateral	Laryngeal cancer Vocal polyp Vocal granuloma Papillomata	p.146 p.171 p.170 p.710
		↗ Bilateral	Reinkes oedema Papillomata Vocal nodules	p.171 p.710 p.171
		↗ Immobile	Vocal cord palsy	
Variable + voice abuse Comes and goes GORD	→ No vocal cord lesion		Muscle tension dysphonia	p.182

Epistaxis (nosebleed)

History	Examination	Diagnosis/treatment	Page no
Trauma or injury has occured	Anterior bleed → Blood vessels on Little's area → First aid	First aid	📖 p.522
Hypertension		Nasal cautery	📖 p.523
Anticoagulation	Posterior bleed	Nasal packing	📖 p.523
Bleeding tendency			
+ nasal obstruction	Nasal mass/polyp → Sinonasal tumours	Sinonasal tumours	📖 p.616
+ serosanguinous discharge			
+ facial swelling			
+ proptosis			
+ facial paraesthesia			
+ a neck lump			
Adolescent boys	→ Angiofibroma	Angiofibroma	📖 p.560

Dysphagia (swallowing difficulty)

History	Examination	Diagnosis	Page no
Constant	a neck lump	Carcinoma	📖 p.216
Progressive	Endoscopy—lesion seen	Post-cricoid web	📖 p.211
Solids worse than liquids	Endoscopy—pooling of saliva	Achalasia	📖 p.212
Pain			
Otalgia			
Neck lump			
Constant			
Progressive			
Regurgitation	→	Pharyngeal pouch	📖 p.213
Halitosis			
Liquids worse than solids	→ + neurology/cranial nerve palsies	→ Neurological dysphagia	📖 p.210
Intermittent			
Saliva worse than solids or liquids			
Variable	→ Normal	→ Globus'	
With or without variable voice problems		GORD	📖 p.208
Heartburn			
Feeling of a lump in the throat			
Mucus in the throat			

A feeling of a lump in the throat

History	Examination	Diagnosis	Page no
Constant			
Same site			
Worse with solids	→ Lesion seen on examination	Carcinoma of pharynx	📖 p.169
Unilateral	Palpable neck lump	Carcinoma of oesophagus	📖 p.100
pain			
otalgia			
neck lump			
hoarse voice			
Patient is a smoker			
Variable site			
Comes and goes			
Worse with saliva	→ Examination normal	Globus	📖 p.208
No true dysphagia			
Central in the neck			
Variable voice problems			
Anxiety			
Patient has a cancer phobia			
Heartburn/GORD			

A lump in the neck

All of the below may apply to children, but the majority of neck masses in children are benign and most are reactive lymph nodes. Parotid lumps in children are more frequently malignant than in adults.

History	Examination	Diagnosis	Page no
Short history (weeks/months)	Laterally placed	Malignant lymphadenopathy	p.260
Lump is enlarging	Firm/hard	ENT primary	p.264
Unilateral nasal obstruction	Single/multiple		
Otalgia			
Sore throat			
Patient is a smoker			
Hoarse voice			
Swallowing problems			
Weight loss	Multiple	Malignant lymphoma	p.260
Night sweats	Rubbery		
Anorexia	Groin/axillary nodes	Glandular fever/toxoplasma	p.255
Fever			
Foreign travel		Tuberculosis	p.267
Previous/recent URTI	Multiple/single	Reactive lymphadenopathy	p.255
			p.258

Long history (months/years) No associated symptoms	Single and lateral ──────────►	Branchial cyst	p.256
	Single and midline		
	Rises on swallowing ──────────►	Thyroid lump	p.240
	Rises on tongue protrusion ────►	Thyroglossal cyst	p.255
		Dermoid cyst	p.255
	No relation to swallowing ─────►	Lymph node	p.260
	Parotid region		
	No facial weakness ────────────►	Benign parotid tumour	p.116
	Facial weakness and pain ──────►	Malignant parotid tumour	p.118
	Submandibular region ──────────►	Submandibular gland tumour	p.122
Changes with eating	Parotid ───────────────────────►	Parotid stone/parotitis	p.130
	Submandibular ─────────────────►	Submandibular stone/sialadenitis	p.130

Mouth or tongue ulcer

History	Examination	Diagnosis	Page no
Trauma or injury	Lateral tongue		
Poor fitting denture	Buccal mucosa →	Traumatic ulcer	
Sharp tooth			
Pain			
			📖 p.90
Patient is a smoker	Lateral tongue		
Alcohol	Floor of mouth		
Betel nut chewer	Tonsil →	Malignant ulcer (SCC)	
Progressive	Firm/hard ulcer		
Pain	Neck nodes		
Neck mass			
Otalgia			
			📖 p.86
Normal immune function	Multiple ulcers		
Recurrent →	Tongue tip/lateral border →	Aphthous ulcers	
Dietary insufficiency →	Angular stomatitis →	Dietary/blood disorders	
	Skin lesions		

Stridor

History	Examination	Diagnosis	Page no
Neonate			
Feeding problems		Laryngomalacia	p.688
Failure to thrive	Positional	Tracheomalacia	p.704
Abnormal cry		Vocal cord lesion/palsy	p.694
	Biphasic stridor	Subglottic stenosis	p.706
Child			
Preceding URTI			
Rapid onset	Drooling	Croup	p.710
Malaise	Pyrexia	Epiglottitis	p.710
Voice muffled/changed	Toxic		
Short history	Inspiratory/mixed stridor	Foreign body	p.682
Previously well child	Expiratory wheeze		p.785
Short lived coughing fit			

Adult

Normal voice
Recent surgery (thyroid/chest) —————⟶ Inspiratory stridor —————⟶ Bilateral cord palsy   📖 p.167

Preceding URTI
Malaise —————⟶ Inspiratory stridor ⟶ Supraglottitis   📖 p.134
Swallowing difficulty   Pyrexia
Sore throat   Drooling

Long standing hoarse voice —————⟶ Inspiratory stridor ⟶ Laryngeal carcinoma   📖 p.146
Pain   Neck node
Patient is a smoker

Facial nerve palsy

History	Examination	Diagnosis	Page no
Recent trauma Haemotympanum	Head injury Trauma to ear canal/drum CSF from ear/nose	Fractured Temporal bone	📖 p.494
Rapid onset Other weakness	Forehead unaffected Abnormal neurological exam	Cerebro Vascular Accident(CVA)	
Rapid onset Isolated weakness	Forehead affected	Bell's palsy	📖 p.444
Otalgia	Vesicles in ear	Ramsay Hunt	📖 p.444
Gradual onset Other weakness	Abnormal neurological exam	Multiple Sclerosis (MS) Motor neurone disease	
Gradual onset Facial pain	Parotid lump	Parotid carcinoma	📖 p.118
Hearing loss Balance disturbance	Sensorineural hearing loss ataxia	Cerebello Pontine Angle (CPA) tumour	📖 p.502
Ear discharge	Conductive hearing loss	Cholesteatoma	📖 p.388

Nasal obstruction

Careful examination of the nasal anatomy will reveal what is responsible for nasal obstruction. Always remember that several anatomical problems can co-exist. Symptoms can vary, especially for mucosal problems, so ascertain the severity of the problem when you examine the patient's nose.

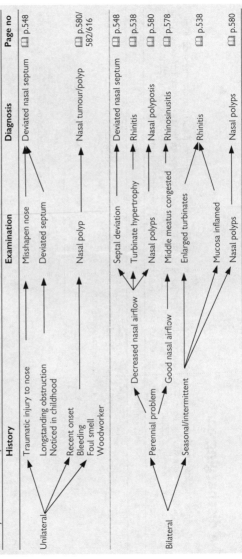

History	Examination	Diagnosis	Page no
Unilateral			
Traumatic injury to nose	Misshapen nose	Deviated nasal septum	🕮 p.548
Longstanding obstruction	Deviated septum		
Noticed in childhood			
Recent onset	Nasal polyp	Nasal tumour/polyp	🕮 p.580/ 582/616
Bleeding			
Foul smell			
Woodworker			
Bilateral			
Perennial problem	Decreased nasal airflow	Septal deviation	🕮 p.548
		Turbinate hypertrophy → Rhinitis	🕮 p.538
		Nasal polyps → Nasal polyposis	🕮 p.580
	Good nasal airflow	Middle meatus congested → Rhinosinusitis	🕮 p.578
Seasonal/intermittent		Enlarged turbinates	
		Mucosa inflamed → Rhinitis	🕮 p.538
		Nasal polyps → Nasal polyps	🕮 p.580

The discharging ear

The timing of the onset of discharge in relation to any pain often helps with diagnosis. Otitis externa in particular can be secondary to infection spreading from the middle ear. Microsuction, or dry mopping, is often necessary to visualize the tympanic membrane. A final diagnosis is sometimes not possible until the ear has been cleaned and the local infection has been treated. It is important to visualize the ear-drum after treatment in order to exclude serious pathology at the level of tympanic membrane.

History	Examination	Diagnosis	Page no
No pain	External Auditory Canal (EAC) appears normal and the Tympasnic membrane (TM) appears to have attic retraction/keratin	Cholesteatoma	📖 p.388
	External Auditory Canal (EAC) appears normal and the TM is perforated or has grommets	Chronic Supurative Otitis Media(CSOM)/infected grommet	📖 p.380
Pain before discharge	Normal External Auditory Canal (EAC) with a bulging TM	Acute otitis media	📖 p.360
	Granulations in floor of External Auditory Canal (EAC) with a normal TM	Necrotising otitis externa	📖 p.337
Pain after discharge	Narrow oedematous External Auditory Canal (EAC) when the TM is normal or not seen	Otitis externa	📖 p.334

Dizziness and vertigo

The most important aspect here is the patient's history. Take great care to elicit the character of the dizziness and its time course to establish if this is dizziness or true vertigo.

History	Examination	Diagnosis	Page no
Lasts for **seconds** Positional	Hallpike test +ve	Benign Paroxysimal Positional Vertigo	📖 p.480
Lasts for **hours** Aural fullness Fluctuating hearing loss Recurrent episodes	PTA fluctuating sensorineural loss (sometimes low tone affected)	Menieres	📖 p.484
Lasts for **days** Single severe attack Unwell for 1 week	PTA normal Unte-berger's test +ve	Vestibulitis Cerebrovascular (older risk factors)	📖 p.478
Constant Elderly patient Intermittent Previous severe attack of vertigo	PTA normal Vestibular function tests normal PTA normal	Multifactorial causes Decompensation of vestibular function	📖 p.476

True Vertigo

Disequilibrium

Otalgia (earache)

Patients who present with otalgia can present a challenging problem. A careful history can help distinguish many conditions. Beware the red reflex—a reflex dilatation of the blood vessels on the handle of the malleus caused by the otoscope speculum touching the bony ear canal. This is often misdiagnosed as early acute otitis media, and the true cause of otalgia is missed. Always consider if the otalgia is referred pain.

History		Examination (using an otoscope)	Diagnosis	Page no
Severe pain Child/preceding URTI Very painful	→	Erythema—a bulging drum A high temperature Distressed patient	Acute otitis media	📖 p.360
Severe pain Preceding itch Longstanding Surfer/swimmer	→ Not diabetic	Narrow EAC Mucopus	Otitis externa	📖 p.334
Severe pain Elderly	→ Diabetic	EAC floor granulated Patient unwell Cranial nerve palsies	Necrotising otitis externa	📖 p.337
Intermittent severe pain At night time Known glue ear	→	Middle ear effusion	Glue ear	📖 p.372
Severe pain Anterior to tragus Worse with eating	→	Normal TM Tender over TMJ Malaligned bite	TMJ dysfunction	
Moderate/severe pain	→	Normal TM Tumour head and neck region	Referred pain	📖 p.148

Hearing loss

A diagnosis of hearing loss in children and adults depends on combining the information from the patient's history, the examination and any special investigations. An audiogram, or a tympanogram with tuning fork tests will help to distinguish conductive from sensorineural hearing loss and will determine if the problem is bilateral or affects only one ear.
Sudden hearing loss is an emergency.

History	Examination (otoscopy)	Type of loss (unusual features)	Diagnosis	Page no
Sudden onset after URTI	→ Middle ear effusion	→ Conductive	→ Effusion	□ p.372
Sudden onset after trauma	→ Disrupted TM annulus	→ Conductive Type Ad tympanogram	→ Ossicular discontinuity	□ p.428
Gradual onset Hong Kong/Southern Chinese Neck nodes, epistaxis	→ Middle ear effusion	→ Conductive	→ Nasopharyngeal Carcinoma	□ p.556
Gradual onset Family history Female/pregnancy	→ Flamingo pink blush or normal TM	→ Conductive Carhart's Notch on audiogram	→ Otosclerosis	□ p.406
Sudden onset	→ Normal TM	→ Sensorineural	→ Vascular/Auto immune	□ p.470
Gradual onset Tinnitus	→ Normal TM	→ Sensorineural High frequency	→ Acoustic Neuroma	□ p.502

Unilateral

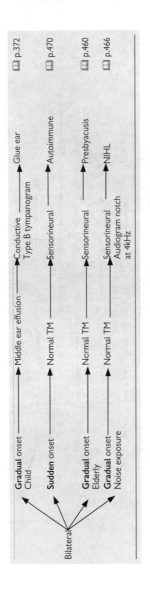

Bilateral

Gradual onset → Middle ear effusion → Conductive → Glue ear   📖 p.372
Child   Type B tympanogram

Sudden onset → Normal TM → Sensorineural → Autoimmune   📖 p.470

Gradual onset → Normal TM → Sensorineural → Presbyacusis   📖 p.460
Elderly

Gradual onset → Normal TM → Sensorineural → NIHL   📖 p.466
Noise exposure   Audiogram notch
                            at 4kHz

Tinnitus

It is important to distinguish between objective tinnitus (which the examiner can hear) and subjective tinnitus (which only the patient can hear). The character of the tinnitus is also important. A thorough otoneurological examination—of the ears, cranial nerves, and central nervous system—is essential. Auscultate the ear, eye, and carotids.
Remember that tinnitus can be caused by medication or other drugs

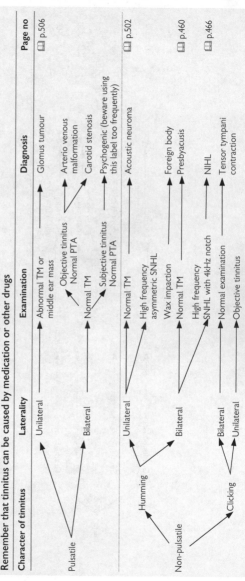

Character of tinnitus	Laterality	Examination	Diagnosis	Page no
Pulsatile	Unilateral	Abnormal TM or middle ear mass	Glomus tumour	📖 p.506
	Bilateral	Objective tinnitus Normal PTA	Arterio venous malformation / Carotid stenosis	
		Subjective tinnitus Normal PTA	Psychogenic (beware using this label too frequently)	
Non-pulsatile (Humming)	Unilateral	Normal TM	Acoustic neuroma	📖 p.502
		High frequency asymmetric SNHL		
	Bilateral	Wax impaction	Foreign body	
		Normal TM	Presbyacusis	📖 p.460
		High frequency SNHL with 4kHz notch	NIHL	📖 p.466
(Clicking)	Bilateral	Normal examination	Tensor tympani contraction	
	Unilateral	Objective tinnitus		

Facial pain

Patients with this problem may present to a variety of specialties for an opinion e.g. ENT, neurology or maxillofacial surgery. It is important to have a broad mind to avoid a misdiagnosis. Never be afraid to ask for another specialist's opinion.

History	Examination	Diagnosis	Page no
Severe acute pain Pain periorbital/cheeks Provoked by URTI Nasal obstruction Temperature	Pus/polyps in middle meatus	→ Acute sinusitis	📖 p.573
Chronic fullness Worse bending over Nasal obstruction	Middle meatus occluded/narrowed	→ Chronic sinusitis	📖 p.578
Severe pain Localized to specific site No nasal obstruction No rhinitic symptoms	Normal nasal examination Normal nasendoscopy	→ Atypical facial pain	
Intermittent pain Worse on eating Radiates to ear	Normal nasal examination Normal nasendoscopy Tenderness over TMJ	→ TMJ dysfunction	

Imaging in head and neck

Introduction

- The aim of imaging is to give the surgeon precise information on the anatomical relationship of pathology in the head and neck as it relates to normal structures.
- Imaging will often provide a 'roadmap' for surgical intervention.
- May suggest the diagnosis and in some cases may be diagnostic.
- Useful in staging of head and neck tumours and nodal metastasis.
- Develop a good relationship with your radiologist—their help will be invaluable!
- Become familiar with the scans yourself—don't just read the report.
- Be aware of techniques available in interventional radiology.
- Give good information on request cards in order to get sensible reports.
- Ensure you let the radiologist know what you want to know!
- Plain X-rays are now obsolete except for soft tissue neck and CXR.

Computerized Tomography (CT)

- CT uses a highly collimated X-ray beam that is differentially absorbed by various body tissues.
- The degree of attenuation of X-ray photons is assigned a numeric readout called the Hounsfield Unit (HU). Water has a HU of 0.
- Complex mathematical reconstruction algorithms are used to create images.
- The range of densities above and below the window level (the midpoint of the densities chosen to display) define the window width (WW).
- Window width and levels can be altered to better define different tissues, e.g. soft-tissue WW 250–400 HU, bone WW 2000–4000 HU.
- Slice thickness is usually 1–1.5mm.
- Spiral CT allows continuous acquisition of data permitting high speed examinations.
- One breath hold is sufficient to scan the whole of the head and neck.
- Temporal bone imaging requires at least two projections (axial and coronal) for full examination of the temporal bone.
- Coronal and sagittal images can be obtained with electronic reconstruction techniques but may loose some image definition.
- 3D surface reconstruction of bone or soft tissue is possible from axial slices.
- Contrast is not routinely used in examination of the temporal bone but may be indicated in vascular anomalies, tumours, and intracranial pathology.

Magnetic Resonance Imaging (MRI)

- MRI produces high-resolution cross-sectional images in any plane without having to reposition the patient or reconstruct images and without exposure to ionizing radiation.
- The theory is based on proton imaging because hydrogen ions are present in all parts of the body in high concentrations.
- When placed in a strong magnetic field and stimulated with electromagnetic energy, protons absorb and release energy at specific radio frequencies.
- Detection and spatial encoding of emitted energy allows reconstruction of an image.
- MRI is superior in soft-tissue contrast to CT because the image is a composite of at least four factors:
  - proton concentration.
  - T1 relaxation time.
  - T2 relaxation time.
  - flow.
- T1 relaxation time is the time taken by a proton deflected away from the main magnetic field lines to return to its original position. This is dependant on the physical state of the protein-bearing material, i.e. fat has a high signal intensity on T1, water has a low signal intensity.
- T2 relaxation time is the time taken for a proton deflected into a plane transverse to the magnetic field lines to lose its coherence.
- Signal intensity of different tissues is directly proportional to the amount of free proton in the tissue. Pathological processes are recognized when the proton density and relaxation times of abnormal tissue differ from normal surrounding tissues.
- The appearances and ∴ the information obtained from the images can be varied by changing the relative contributions of T1 and T2 relaxation times.

MRI sequences

T1-weighted imaging produces excellent soft-tissue contrast and anatomical delineation. Fat looses its signal intensity with increased T2 weighting. Most head and neck masses are higher signal intensity on T2 compared with T1. Paramagnetic gadolinium compound is used for lesion enhancement in conjunction with T1 sequence. Various fat-suppression techniques give better contrast between high signal fat and high signal gadolinium enhancing lesions. The advantages are that it provides increased lesion enhancement and delineation of margins of a mass relative to the lower signal muscle, bone, vessels, and eye. Gradient echo techniques take advantage of phenomenon of flow related enhancement—any rapidly flowing blood will appear extremely bright. These are useful for localizing normal vessels, detecting obstruction of flow in compressed or thrombosed vessels, or for showing vascular lesions that have areas of rapid blood flow. (See Box 4.1).

Box 4.1 Quick-identification table

T1-weighted image:
- Fat = white.
- CSF/vitreous = black.
- Normal mucosa/muscle = intermediate.

T2-weighted image:
- Fat/muscle = low/intermediate.
- CSF/vitreous = white.
- Air, bone, calcium, rapid vascular flow, haemosiderin = black.

Fast spin echo image:
- Fat = white but less than T1.
- CSF/vitreous = intermediate.
- Air/bone = black.
- Muscle, fluid filled structures = intermediate.

Gadolinium enhancement:
- Fat = white.
- CSF/vitreous = black.
- Nasal/pharyngeal muscosa, lymphoid tissue of Waldeyer's ring, extra-ocular muscles, slow flowing venous blood = white.

Magnetic Resonance Angiography (MRA)

- Selectively produces images of structures with rapid blood flow.
- 2D and 3D images of normal vessels, vascular lesions, and vascularity of tumours can be generated.
- Can distinguish between arterial and venous phases of bolus injections.
- Not yet equivalent to spatial resolution of conventional angiography.
- Useful in the head and neck for evaluating vascular compression, vessel patency, and characteristics of vascular masses and malformations.

Positron Emission Tomography (PET)

- Provides functional views of tissues rather than simply depicting anatomy.
- 18F-fluorodeoxyglucose (FDG) is taken up into tissues in proportion to the metabolic rate, which is geneally increased in neoplastic processes.
- Focal asymmetric uptake is suggestive of a tumour but is non-specific, as FDG is also concentrated in areas of inflammation.
- Useful in the following scenarios:
  - Search for an unknown primary lesion.
  - Assessment for residual or recurrent disease following primary therapy.
  - Search for synchronous or metachronous primary lesions or distant metastases.

USS

- Useful technique for the assessment of masses in the neck, thyroid goitres, and for suspected salivary gland pathology.
- Particulary useful in determining whether a lesion is cystic or solid.
- Ultrasound appearance of medullary cell carcinoma is virtually pathognomonic.
- No radiation exposure and can be linked to fine-needle aspiration cytology.
- A high-frequency (7.5–10mHz) hand-held probe is placed directly on the neck and the needle can be seen directly entering the mass.
- Operator dependant but in specialist hands lymph node ultrasound, in combination with FNAC, has a sensitivity of over 90%, with a specificity of over 85%.
- Ultrasound (US) wave does not penetrate bone, cartilage, or gas, making it an inappropriate technique for staging many primary head and neck cancers,
- The US beam is also attenuated (weakened) as it passes through tissues, making examination of fat necks and deep structures (e.g. deep lobe of the parotid gland) more difficult.
- Information can be gained on the margins and texture of neck masses, which may give information about the nature of the neck mass.
- Loss of normal contours and architecture may be helpful in identifying pathological neck nodes.
- Doppler US is flow-sensitive and can be used to evaluate the neck vessels and relationship of masses to important vascular structures, or the vascularity of neck masses. Arterial injury following penetrating neck trauma can also be assessed.

Angiography and embolization

- Angiography shows the typical finding of a splayed bifurcation of the carotid artery with vascular blush in carotid body tumours.
- Vascularity of skull base paragangliomas can be ascertained with the benefit of pre-operative embolization.
- Angiography is the gold standard for evaluating vascular injury (particularly when the injury involves zones I and III) and is therapeutic when used with interventional neuroradiology embolization.
- The evaluation of potential tracheal injuries should be coordinated with the assessment of adjacent structures, with angiography of the aortic arch and thoracic outlet vessels usually taking precedence.
- Pre-operative embolization of large vascular tumours e.g. angiofibromas.
- Identifaction and embolization of vessels in patients with intractable epistaxis who are too unfit for surgical intervention.
- Angiography should be considered in the investigation of parapharyngeal space lesions if the initial CT and MRI suggest a vascular tumour or if there is suspected carotid artery involvement. The precise vessels supplying the tumour can be embolized prior to surgery. It may be necessary to perform a carotid occlusion study to determine if a patient can tolerate the loss of the carotid artery.

Skull base radiology

Radiological assessment of skull-base lesions
- Where is the lesion?
  - Central, anterolateral, or posterior skull base
- What lesions occur there?
  - Site-specific lesions (p. 71).
  - Lesions that occur anywhere (p. 72).
- Will the radiology change the surgical approach?

CT techniques

Advantages
- Good anatomical localization.
- Shows patterns of bony change.
  - Smooth erosion, i.e. benign lesions.
  - Splintering destruction, i.e. malignant lesions.
  - Sclerotic change, i.e. malignant lesions.
- High-resolution CT shows 1–1.5mm slices and reconstruction on bony algorithms shows sharp bony–soft tissue interface.
- Quicker than MRI.

Disadvantages
- Highly contrasting densities between skull base and surrounding soft tissues can cause difficulty in differentiating contiguous soft tissue structures.
- Based on one variable (electron density of the tissues) versus MRI, which is based on multiple variables.

Magnetic resonance imaging (MRI)

Advantages
- Good anatomical localization.
- Better tissue characterization in any image plane.
- Can give specific information:
  - Venous outflow, sinus occlusion (MRV).
  - Investigation of tinnitus, e.g. dural AVM (artetio-venous malformation) (MRA).
  - Relationship to other soft-tissue structures, i.e. the ICA.
  - Perinerural spread.
  - Post-gadolinium soft-tissue differentiation.
- >100 times greater resolution than CT.
- Fat suppression important in the skull base as it seems similar to contrast-enhancing skull-base lesions.
- No radiation.

Disadvantages
- Expensive.
- Slow, uncomfortable, claustrophobic, noisy.
- Motion susceptible.
- Contraindicated in some patients (cochlear implants, cardiac pacemakers).

Site-specific lesions

1) Posterior skull-base

- Hypoglossal schwannoma.
    - Denervation changes in the tongue seen on MRI.
- Jugular fossa lesions:
    - MRV valuable to establish patency of tranverse sinus and presence of cross-flow across the torcula to document dominance of right- versus left-sided jugular flow in one-sided lesions.
- Glomus tumours:
    - Irregular bony lytic destruction on CT.
    - Post-contrast enhancement on CT and MRI.
    - Flow voids on MRI.
- Schwannoma:
    - CT shows a smooth, scalloped bony enlargement of the passage/foramen with fusiform soft-tissue mass. Enhance with contrast.
    - MRI shows uniform intensity to brain, but enhance especially with T2.

2) Petrous apex

(See Table 4.1.)

3) Clival lesions

- Chondrosarcoma:
    - CT shows a varied appearance. Calcification of the matrix is characteristic, but not always present. No sclerosis of tumour-bone margin. Small calcified ringlets.
    - MRI—high signal intensity on T2.
- Chordomas:
    - CT shows a destructive midline clival lesion. No evidence of calcified ringlets as in chondrosarcomas.

4) Anterolateral skull-base

- Juvenile andiofibroma:
    - CT shows anterior displacement of the posterior wall of the maxillary sinus and remodeling of the pterygoid plates posteriorly.
    - CT and MRI (T1 with contrast) show high enhancement due the high vascularity, but MRI (T1 without contrast) shows flow voids from larger high-flow vessels.

Lesions that can occur anywhere

1) Fibrous dysplasia

- CT shows thickened, sclerotic bone, which may be uniform density or with cystic lesions if early in disease process.
- MRI shows expanded and thickened areas of bone.

2) Meningioma

- CT shows soft-tissue enhancement, calcifications, and hyperostosis.
- MRI shows the lesion to be isointense with brain but enhances with Gadolidium, revealing a dural tail at the margin of the tumour.

3) Metastases

- From lung, kidney, breast, prostate.
- Lytic destruction.
- May get sclerotic change in prostate metastases or SCC.

4) Paget's disease

- CT shows expanded skull-base bone associated with calvarial involvement.
- T1 shows high signal foci of fat collections; T2 shows high signals from fibrovascular marrow in active disease.

5) Histiocytosis X

- Single or multiple areas of pure osteolysis in skull base and calvarium.

Table 4.1 Radiological appearances of the common lesions of the petrous apex/CPA

Lesions	CT	T1	T1 with gadolinium	T2
Cholesterol granuloma	Smooth margin, expansile lesion, density similar to brain, no enhancement with contrast	Hyperintense	Hyperintense, no further enhancement with contrast	Hyperintense
Cholestea-toma	Smooth margin, expansile with thinning and elevation of superior petrous ridge	Hypo heterointense	No further enhancement	Hyperintense
Schwan-noma	Expansion of IAC, fallopian canal or jugular fossa depending on the etiology	Hypointense	Hyperintense	Hyperintense
Lipoma	Smooth margin, expansile	Hyperintense	No further enhancement	Hypointense
Meningioma	Isodense with brain	Hypointense	Hyperintense	Hyperintense
Arachnoid cyst	Multicystic mass	Hypointense	Hyperintense	Hyper-variable
Petrous apicitis	Expansile with irregular margins, ring enhancement with contrast if abscess forms	Hypointense	Hyperintense	Hyperintense
Cavernous Angioma	Expansile mass	Hyperintense with flow voids	Hyperintense with flow voids	Hyperintense with flow voids
Metastastic adenocarci-noma	Mass with irregular margins	Hypointense	Hyperintense	Hyper-variable
Lymphoma	Mass	Hyperintense	Hyperintense	Hyperintense

Ward care

Pre-operative care

Pre-assessment

The process of pre-assessment has become established. In many units, nurse-led pre-assessment clinics can identify problems ahead of the planned surgery date, thus avoiding costly delays in the operating schedule. These clinics can only run efficiently if there is good communication between the doctor, nurse, and the anaesthetist.

Protocols have been developed to ensure that only appropriate investigations are ordered, to avoid unnecessary expense.

Clerking

- Effective documentation is important for improved care and to fulfil medico-legal requirements.
- The minimum standard is a confirmation of the need for the surgery or investigation, an ENT examination, a list of medications with known allergies, and a list of the results from any investigations ordered.
- Documentation of the consent process is usually provided by the consent form, which is kept in the patient's notes.

Investigations

- Any investigations ordered should be based on the protocol and discussed with the anaesthetist.
- The first step is ordering investigations; but most important is finding and documenting the results of the investigations.

Special considerations

Deep vein thrombosis (DVT) prophylaxis

The risk of DVT for all surgical patients should be classified as low/medium/high (Box 5.1 + 5.2). This is determined by the length of surgery, the patient's underlying condition, and their past thrombo-embolic history.

Antibiotic prophylaxis

Antibiotics may be given to patients with pre-existing cardiac problems, such as valve problems, or for patients who have had major head and neck surgery, to reduce the risk of post-operative infection and fistula formation.

- Cefuroxime 1.5g every 8h for 5 days.
- Metronidazole 500mg PR every 8h 5 days.

Diabetic patients

Diabetic patients should be placed first on the operating list. Take regular BM-stix to monitor sugar level. Use a sliding scale insulin regime until eating, if insulin dependent.

Box 5.1 DVT Prophylaxis-Management

Low	Compression stockings
Medium	Compression stockings + LMW heparin + intra-operative compression boots
High	Stockings + LMW heparin/pneumatic + intra-operative compression boots.
Low	Compression stockings

Box 5.2 Low molecular weight (LMW) heparin e.g. dalteparin sodium

Medium risk	2500 units 1–2h pre-op
	2500 units every 24h until ambulatory
High risk	2500 units 1–2h pre-op
	5000 units every 24h

Post-operative care

Documentation

It is important to document the patient's daily progress and ward-round instructions. Any important changes during the day should also be documented. Use a system approach for major head and neck patients, e.g. CVS/RS/nutrition, etc.

Drain care

Monitor drainage for a 24-h period. Remove when it has drained less than 30ml in a 24-h period. If the drain loses its vacuum or becomes 'devacced' (loss of vacuum pressure), examine drain position, change the drain bottle for a new one, and consider pressure to the wound or connect the drain to continuous low pressure wall suction.

Nutrition/fluid balance

Involve dietician for long-term feeding requirements.

Fluid and electrolytes

Calculate 24-h maintenance fluid requirements by the patient's weight:
- 0–10kg: 100ml/kg/24h.
- 11–20kg: 1000ml + 50ml/kg/24h.
- 20kg>: 1500ml + 20ml/kg/24h.

This volume of fluid requires a composition of 1–2Eq of Na^+ and 0.5 mEq K^+ per kg/24h:
- 1L N/saline contains 154mEq of Na^+.
- 1L D/saline contains 77mEq of Na^+.

Maintenance is best undertaken with dextrose/saline to avoid sodium overload, plus addition of 20mmol/L of K^+.
- Properly kept fluid balance charts are essential in order to monitor the patient's fluid input and output.

Calories

Post-operative patients require between 40 and 70kcal/kg per day. Most ENT patients will be able to be fed either via the mouth or via a nasogastric tube—enteral feeding.

Monitoring intake of calories and other vital substances
- Check weight daily.
- Keep a food record chart.
- Do regular urinalysis for glucose.
- Check levels of FBC, calcium, magnesium, phosphate, zinc, LFTs, U + Es, as required.
- Vitamins trace elements screen, e.g. Zn, Mg^{2+}.

How to unblock a blocked nasogastric tube
- Flush with water.
- Flush with soda water.
- Flush with a 5% sodium bicarbonate solution.
- Aspirate tube with empty syringe.
- Flush tube with smaller syringe.
- Use Creon powder with sodium bicarbonate to flush the tube.

Care of myocutaneous flaps

It is very important to monitor the viability of these flaps accurately. Often patients are nursed on wards with limited plastic surgery expertise.

- Ask your local plastic surgeon about the post-operative protocol for the care of free flaps.

General principles

- Maintain intravascular volume.
- Maintain oxygen carrying haematocrit but not polycythaemia.
- Monitor flap appearance by using a flap chart.
- Monitor blood supp, e.g. Doppler flow.

Protocol example

- Keep pulse <100.
- Maintain systolic BP >100mmHg.
- Keep urine output >35ml/h.
- Aim for haemoglobin level of 8.5–10.5g/dl.
- If haematocrit <25 give blood.
- If haematocrit >35 give colloid.

Flap observations

- Doppler and colour observations.
- Every 30 min for the first 4h, then …
- Every hour for the next 48h, then …
- Every 2h for the next 48h.

Tracheostomy care

The formation of a tracheostomy causes some physiological problems, mainly because it bypasses the nose. The initial requirements of inspired air are: humidification, warming, and filtering. After 48h the mucous glands in the trachea hypertrophy and help in this process.

Irritation caused by the tube

- The presence of the tube can cause coughing and excess secretion from the bronchopulmonary tree.
- Regular suction and inner-tube cleaning may be needed as often as every 30min in the initial stages.

Securing the tube

The first tube is usually sutured to the skin to prevent dislodgement. Tapes are then applied, unless there is a free flap where the feeding vessels may be occluded.

In the first week after a tracheostomy, the tube should be treated very carefully to prevent dislodgement. The tract between the skin and the trachea is poorly developed and tube displacement during this time could be catastrophic.

▶ Always keep a spare tracheostomy tube and tracheal dilators by the bedside of tracheostomy patients.

Discharge planning

- There is always pressure to discharge patients from the ward with the greatest of haste. Prior planning, often before surgery, can help with this process.
- Nursing staff have good protocols—so liaise with them and seek their advice.

General points

Consideration of the following questions will help in planning effective discharge:

- Is the patient fit to leave—are they orientated, mobile, and pain free?
- Is the patient's nutritional support catered for?
- Is their wound satisfactory?
- Does the patient need transport?
- Do they have enough medication—both that prescribed in hospital and their regular medication?
- Do any medications need monitoring—such as warfarin?
- Does the patient's GP need to know that the patient is leaving hospital before the discharge letter arrives?
- Is a district nurse required?
- Is outpatient follow up organized?

Mouth, tonsils, and adenoids

Anatomy

Oral cavity
- Extends from the lips to the anterior pillar of the tonsil.
- Includes the buccal mucosa, upper and lower alveolus and gingiva, floor of mouth, anterior two-thirds of the tongue, and the hard palate.
- The mouth is lined by a mucous membrane covered with stratified squamous epithelium and is adherent to the deeper structures. On the lips, cheek, and tongue, the mucous membranes are attached to the underlying musculature, and on the hard palate and alveolus to the periosteum, thus creating a mucuperiosteum. Small mucous glands are scattered throughout the mouth, especially the lower lip.
- The floor of the mouth contains two sublingual glands lying beneath the oral mucosa, anterior to the border of hyoglossus. They are in contact with the lingual fossa, a smooth depression on the lingual aspect of the mandible (Fig. 6.1).
- Medially the submandibular duct and lingual nerve separate the lingual gland from the genioglossus.
- The hard palate is composed of the palatal processes of the maxilla, with the horizontal plate of the palatine bone posteriorly and a small anterior contribution from the premaxilla. This is covered by a mucous membrane attached firmly to the periosteum anteriorly and more loosely posteriorly, where the connective tissue contains numerous mucous and salivary glands.
- The nasopalatine foramen lies in the midline, posterior to the incisor teeth, between the maxilla and premaxilla. The greater palatine foramen lies between the maxilla and the crest of the palatine bone, medial to the second or third molar tooth. There are two or three lesser palatine foramen just posterior to this.
- Blood supply of hard palate is the greater palatine artery (a branch of the maxillary artery).
- Nerve supply of hard palate is the branches of the maxillary nerve via the pterygopalatine ganglion, the anterior palatine nerve emerging through the greater palatine foramen to supply the palate as far forward as the nasopalatine foramen, from which the nasopalatine nerves emerge to supply the area behind the incisor teeth.

Oropharynx
- Extends from the anterior tonsillar pillar to the posterior pharyngeal wall and from the level of the hard palate to the plane of the hyoid or the apex of the vallecula.
- It contains the tonsils, base of the tongue, soft palate, and posterior pharyngeal wall.

Nasopharynx
- Located above the hard palate and posterior to the posterior choanae.
- The Eustachian tubes open laterally into the nasopharynx, which contains the adenoids.

The tongue

- The anterior two-thirds and the posterior two-thirds of the tongue have different embryological origins and therefore different nerve supplies.
- Sensation to the anterior two-thirds of the tongue is via the lingual nerve.
- The posterior third is supplied by the glossopharyngeal nerve.
- Motor supply to the tongue is via the hypoglossal nerve.
- Special taste fibres pass with the facial nerve to the middle ear. From here they separate—as the chorda tympani—and pass forwards. As they exit the middle ear they merge with the mandibular division of the trigeminal nerve to eventually run with the lingual nerve.
- Marginal lymphatics drain unilaterally while central vessels drain bilaterally.

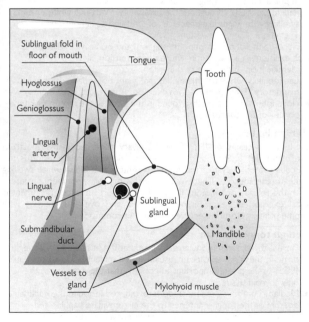

Fig. 6.1 Coronal cross section to show the anatomy of the floor of mouth.

Benign lesions of the oral cavity

A great variety of benign lesions can be found arising from, or beneath, the oral mucosa, most of which are hyperplasias and granulomas. However, surgical excision is crucial if malignancy is expected.

Buccal, alveolar, and gingival lesions

- Epiludes: inflammatory overgrowth of the gingiva containing immature vascular granulation tissue. Treat by conservative local excision.
- Denture granuloma: seen in the buccal sulcus in relation to the flange of an overextended denture.
- Diffuse gingival enlargements: seen with certain drugs such as phenytoin.
- Leaf polyp (fibro-epithelial polyp): found flattened between an upper denture and palate, this lesion is easily concealed and stresses the importance of removing dentures when examining the oral cavity.
- Papilloma: found throughout the oral cavity. Wart-like white or pink swelling with finger like processes of stratified squamous epithelium. Tretament is simple excision.
- Fibro-epithelial polyp: found throughout the oral cavity. Treatment is excision via a transfixion suture under tension, allowing easy identification of the base of the lesion.
- Leukoplakia (white patch): implies malignant potential ∴ biopsy is mandatory. Treatment involves excision or repeated laser therapy with close follow-up, especially if found in the floor of the mouth or lateral border of the tongue.

Benign lip lesions

Lip lesions account for 15% of minor salivary gland neoplasms (mostly in the upper lip) ∴ excision is mandatory. The commonest lesion is the mucous retention cyst or mucocele presenting as a bluish-white swelling beneath the mucosa. There is often a history of spontaneous rupture with the release of a viscous fluid, followed by recurrence. Treatment is local excision of lesion, associated gland, and overlying mucosa with simple primary closure. Recurrence is not uncommon.

Benign tongue lesions

- Lingual thyroid: rare nodular mass found at the base of the tongue, in or near, the foramen caecum, usually in the midline. Ultrasound scan (USS) of the neck is important to confirm that the mass is not the only thyroid tissue.
- Median rhomboid glossitis: smooth, ovoid, red lesion in the midline dorsum of the tongue, anterior to the circumvillate papillae and foramen caecum, which is said to represent a persistent tuberculum impar. It has been linked to reflux and candida infection but usually reassurance is all that is required.

Floor of mouth lesions

Dermoid cysts: true cysts lined by squamous epithelium containing keratin and squamous material. Thought to be due to epithelial cell rests left after fusion of the hyoid and mandibular arches. Usually present in the midline in the floor of the mouth. Treatment is simple surgical excision.

Ranulas

See salivary gland 📖 p124.

Palatal lesions

- Minor salivary gland tumours: 60% occur on the palate, pleomorphic being the most common. They do not occur anterior to the line between the first upper molars. Usually well circumscribed and encapsulated, making excision easy. Occasionally large defects may require closure with a flap or obturator.
- Torus palatinus: presents as a bony hard swelling of the hard palate. Present in 20% of people but size very variable. Increased risk in mongoloid and Inuit peoples. Presents before the age of 30. Represents an overgrowth of the palatal processes of the maxilla— a true exostosis composed of compact lamella bone. Treatment is reassurance, unless interfering with the fitment of a dental plate.

Excision of torus palatinus

Preparation
- Direct infiltration with local anaesthetic (LA).
- Greater palatine nerve block (especially if posterior): infiltrate just medial to the 2nd molar tooth, halfway between the gingival margin and the midline of the palate.

Incision
Gingival palatal.

Procedure
- Raise a full thickness mucoperiosteal flap preserving the greater palatine nerves.
- Take care raising the flap over the midline, since it is very thin here.
- With a burr.
- Irrigate wound.
- Replace flap and suture interdentally.
- A previously prepared acrylic plate can help prevent haematoma formation.

Other lesions
Pleomorphic adenomas may require sacrifice of the mucosa, in which case a Whitehead's varnish on ribbon-gauze pack can be sutured to the defect and left in-situ for 7–10 days, at which point it is removed to reveal a freshly granulating area.

Palateal fenestrations can be closed with an obturator or covered using a posterioly based, full thickness, palatal rotation flap supplied by the contralateral greater palatine artery. The secondary defect is dealt with as above.

Oral cancer

Risk factors
- Smoking (especially pipe smoking).
- Alcohol (particularly spirits).
- Chewing tobacco and betel nut.
- Poor dentition; mechanical irritation from poorly fitting dentures has also been implicated, but not proven.

Demographics
- Peak incidence is 50–60y.
- ♂ : ♀, 2 : 1.

Signs and symptoms
- Raised or indurated ulcer on lateral border of tongue, the floor of the mouth, or gingiva.
- Malignant lesions may be exophytic.

Assessment
- Take a full history, including an assessment of co-morbidity and fitness for surgery.
- The size and extent of the tumour should be measured by palpation, together with assessment of tongue mobility and dental hygiene.
- Note the presence of trismus, implying fixity to bone.
- Check for nodal metastases, paying particular attention to levels I–III. FNA any palpable nodes.
- General ENT examination should be completed, including flexible nasendoscopy.
- Investigations include an OPG and CXR plus spiral CT or MRI scan to confirm the extent of the tumour and check for local spread.

Management
- Urgent EUA and biopsy plus panendoscopy within 2 weeks to exclude a second primary, and complete clinical TNM staging (Box 6.1) Depth is the most important prognostic indicator in tongue cancer ∴ the biopsy must be deep.
- Referral to a joint head and neck clinic for treatment decisions.
- Some patients will require an anaesthetic assessment, as well as consideration of a feeding gastrostomy for patients who have large tumours and require prolonged swallowing rehabilitation.

Treatment
- Surgery is the mainstay of treatment unless the tumour is obviously incurable.
- For T3 and T4, surgery is combined with post operative radiotherapy
- The N0 neck should be treated for any T stage > 1 because of the increased risk of micrometastases.

- N+ necks should be treated with either functional or radical neck dissection.
- If the tumour crosses the midline, the clinically negative contralateral neck should undergo a supraomohyoid neck dissection.

Box 6.1 T-staging for tumours of the lip and oral cavity

TX Primary tumour cannot be assessed.

T0 No evidence of primary tumour.

Tis Carcinoma *in situ*.

T1 Tumour 2cm or < in greatest dimension.

T2 Tumour >2cm but not >4cm in greatest dimension.

T3 Tumour >4cm in greatest dimension.

T4a Lip: tumour invades through cortical bone, inferior alveolar nerve, floor of mouth, or skin of face (i.e. chin or nose).

T4a Oral cavity: tumour invades through cortical bone, into deep extrinsic muscle of tongue (genioglossus, hyoglossus, palatoglossus, and styloglossus), maxillary sinus, or skin of face.

T4b Tumour involves masticator space, pterygoid plates, or skull base and/or encases internal carotid artery.

Surgery for malignant lesions of the tongue and floor of mouth

General preparation

- General anaesthetic (GA).
- Prophylactic antibiotics for inta-oral lesions that will be in continuity with a neck dissection.
- Head ring and shoulder bag, if a neck dissection is to be performed.
- Good headlight.
- Tracheostomy for all cases, except a hemiglossectomy without neck dissection when nasal intubation is acceptable.
- Cutting diathermy or CO_2 laser should be used to excise tongue lesions with a 2cm margin.

Hemiglossectomy (Fig. 6.2)

- Indicated for T1 and T2 tumours.
- Peroral approach.
- Insulated cheek retractors.
- Stay sutures to tip of tongue.
- Mark excision line with diathermy preferably with a 2cm margin (frozen section should be used to confirm clear margins).
- Divide tongue from tip back to circumvillate papillae.
- Divide along floor of mouth just medial to the submandidular duct.
- Continue incision posterior-laterally to anterior faucal pillar.
- Suture ligate the lingual artery.
- Vicryl sutures can be placed anteriorly but the rest of the raw surface can be left to granulate (furthur closure results in significant tethering of the tongue and long-term problems with articulation).
- Free mucosal grafts can be raised from the inner cheek which may help prevent scar formation and aids tumour surveillance post-operatively.

Anterior mandibulotomy (Fig. 6.3)

- Indicated for T3 and T4 oral tumours.
- Provides excellent access for large lesions involving the tongue and floor of the mouth; the incision can be incorporated into that used for the neck dissection.
- The lip is split in the midline controlling the inferior labial arteries.
- Expose the mentum of the jaw 1.5cm either side of the midline.
- Holes are drilled either side for fixing the appropriate plate.
- Stepped mandibular osteotomy using the osscilating saw.
- Having split the jaw, the floor of the mouth is exposed by retracting the two halves laterally using Langenbeck retractors.
- The excision is then performed as above.
- The adjacent tissues of the floor of the mouth may have to be resected for large tumours, resulting in a defect into the neck.
- Preservation of the contralateral hypoglossal nerve and lingual artery is essential.

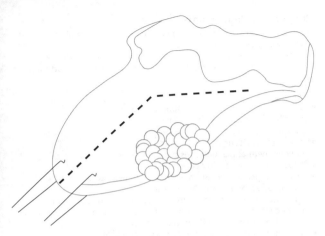

Fig. 6.2 Lines of resection for a standard hemiglossectomy.

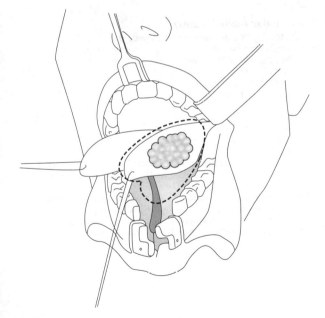

Fig. 6.3 Resection of an extensive tumour of the tongue via an anterior-mandibulotomy approach.

Marginal mandibulectomy

- For tumours that are fixed to the mandible, where there is no clinical or radiological evidence of invasion.
- Care must be taken to preserve adjacent periosteum, since it is through the periosteal vessel that the bone receives its blood supply.

Approach

- Per oral approach for an upper alveolectomy (Fig. 6.4a).
- Combined intra-oral/external approach for an inner table mandibulectomy (Fig. 6.4b and c).
- Mark incision lines.
- Stay sutures to tongue.
- Remove teeth at planned sites of osteotomies.
- Mucosal and mucoperiosteal incisions.
- Raise mucoperiosteum 3mm either side of planned osteotomy.
- Fashion osteotomies with fissure burr.
- Malleable copper retractors prevent damage to adjacent tissue.
- Bony edges are cut back, providing a free edge of intact mucoperiosteum to which a skin or mucosal flap can be sutured.
- Soft tissue work is performed per orally and kept in continuity.
- Small defects are best reconstructed using a nasolabial or local tongue flaps.

Segmental mandibulectomy

- Indicated for T3 and 4 tumours that invade the mandible.
- A visor flap can be utilized if the mental nerves are going to be sacrificed as part of the resection (Fig. 6.5). Otherwise a lateral approach is used after raising the upper cervical flap and clearance of the submandibular triangle.
- Adjacent teeth to the mandibulotomy are removed.
- Incise mucosa.
- Expose lateral aspect of mandible down to periosteum along length of planned resection.
- The lingual surface is only exposed where the osteotomies are to be performed.
- Incise periostium and perform osteotomies using an osscilating saw.
- Preserve as much of the buccal-alveolar membrane as possible.
- Complete the intra-oral part of the resection.
- Large defects are reconstructed using a pedicled myocutaneous flap (e.g. pectoralis major, which allows the jaw to swing freely) or a free flap (e.g. radial forearm, which can be combined with a segment of vasculised radius for reconstruction of the segmental defect).

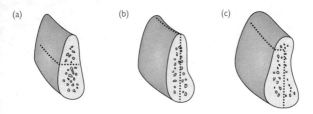

Fig. 6.4 (a) Upper alveolectomy. (b) Inner-table mandibulectomy, (c) Modified inner-table mandibulectomy.

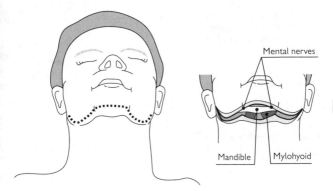

Fig. 6.5 Visor flap used for a segmental mandibulectomy.

Total glossectomy

This still remains a controversial operation. Proponents argue that these large tumours can be resected oncologically and with appropriate reconstruction good functional outcome can be achieved. However, many patients require extensive post-operative swallowing rehabilitation and are percutaneous gastrostomy (PEG) fed for many months to maintain nutrition. A subsequent laryngectomy may be required for intractable aspiration. Some units therefore prefer to treat advanced tumours with chemoradiotherapy as an alternative.

Approach

- Covering tracheostomy.
- Anterior mandibulotomy.
- Incise around floor of mouth leaving a good rim of mucosa around the lingual plate of the mandible to facilitate flap insertion.
- Commence excision anteriorly.
- Preserve tongue base/vallecullae if possible (reduces chance of aspiration).
- Reconstruct with a pedicled or free latissimus dorsi myocutaneous flap.
- The larynx maybe suspended from the mandible with wires or nylon.
- Close wound with interrupted Vicryl.
- Pass nasogastric tube if the patient has not had a pre-operative gastrostomy.

Post operatively

- Cork tracheostomy at 48–72h.
- Leave in situ until oral feeding has commenced and there is no problem with aspiration.
- Start oral feeding at 7 days.

Specific complications

- Orocutaneous fistula. Predisposing factors:
  - Previous radiotherapy.
  - Poor preoperative nutritional status.
  - Wound dehiscence.
  - Reconstructive flap necrosis.
- Management of orocutaneous fistula
  - Small fistula with no tissue loss—conservative, nil by mouth, nasogastric feed, IV antibiotics.
  - Large fistula with tissue loss—re-explore neck and excise dead tissue. Repair with a pectoralis major or latissimus dorsi flap, with or without a skin paddle. The external surface can be split skin grafted if necessary.

Brachytherapy

- Interstitial brachytherapy involves the loading of iridium[192] wires into a tumour. Suitable lesions are T1/T2 lesions located in the anterior mobile tongue.
- Advantages: maintenance of good oromandibular function with superior speech and swallowing compared to surgery and very precise high dose radiation compared to external beam radiotherapy resulting in less side effects.
- Disadvantages: haemorrhage/haematoma from the wire insertion, soft tissue radionecrosis, osteoradionecrosis, local fibrosis and the nature of the treatment (requires isolation in a lead room for several days with minimal human contact).

Oropharyngeal cancer

Sites
- Tonsil.
- Tongue base.
- Soft palate.
- Posterior pharyngeal wall.

Tonsil carcinoma
Symptoms and signs
- Presents as an ulcero-proliferative lesion of the tonsil.
- Progressive sore throat.
- Pain radiating to the ear.
- Change in voice.
- Dyspagia.
- Odynophagia.
- Neck lump.

Aetiological factors
- Tobacco and alcohol intake.
- Dental sepsis.
- Iron-deficiency anaemia.
- Human papilloma virus infection.
- Betel-nut chewing.

Investigation
- CT chest—higher incidence of distant metastases and second primary tumours in oropharyngeal index tumours than in any other primary site.
- MRI neck—to assess the size and extent of primary tumour and nodal enlargement in neck and retropharyngeal area.
- Orthopantomogram.
- Panendoscopy and biopsy under general anaesthetic (GA)—palpation is of vital importance to assess tongue base and palate involvement.
- Fine-needle aspiration cytology of neck nodes.

Box 6.2 T-staging of oropharyngeal tumours

T1 Tumour 2cm or < in greatest dimension.
T2 Tumour >2cm but not >4cm in greatest dimension.
T3 Tumour >4cm in greatest dimension.
T4a Tumour invades the larynx, deep/extrinsic muscle of tongue, medial pterygoid, hard palate, or mandible.
T4b Tumour invades lateral pterygoid muscle, pterygoid plates, lateral nasopharynx, or skull base, or encases carotid artery.

Management of the primary tumour
- T1 and T2 with limited nodal disease are treated as effectively with radiotherapy as with surgery.
- T3 and T4 and with lymph nodes greater than 2cm, surgery followed by radiotherapy or primary chemoradiotherapy.
- High volume T2/T3 lesions: combined therapy, i.e. radical excision via a midline mandibulotomy and reconstruction with microvascular free flap or pedicled flap, followed by post-operative radiotherapy.

Management of the neck
- 50% of patients with tonsillar carcinoma have palpable metastatic nodes at initial presentation and another 25% have occult disease in clinically NO neck.
- NO neck: selective neck dissection (levels I–IV).
- N+ neck: modified or radical neck dissection.

Surgery for cancer of the oropharynx

Oropharyngeal resection with ascending ramus of mandible

Preparation

- GA.
- Tracheostomy.
- Broad-spectrum IV antibiotics.
- Reverse trendelemburg.
- Head ring and shoulder bag.
- Prep and drape to allow access to the whole and the neck and mouth, as well as the donor site.

Incision

- Apron with vertical limb extension to split the lower lip in the midline.
- Perform neck dissection first.
- Tumour resection is approached both perorally and from the neck.
- Resection is with a 2cm cuff of normal tissue.
- Mark mucosal incisions with methylene blue or point diathermy.
- The anterior osteotomy will be placed 1cm anterior to the anterior mucosal margin.
- The mandible is approached from the neck.
- Elevate periosteum and soft tissues from the lateral aspect of the mandible from the site of the planned osteotomy.
- Elevate mandibular attachment medially and perform an osteotomy with an osscilating saw. The coronoid process and condyle of the mandible can be left attached to the soft tissue.
- Rotate acscending ramus laterally to enter oral cavity at the anterior limit of the resection and extend these incisions superiorly and inferiorly to visualise the tumour.
- The excision can also be performed per-orally using a head light.
- Part of the soft palate and tongue base may need to be excised for adequate clearance.
- Be aware of the carotid arteries that need to be protected.
- Identify and preserve the lingual and hypoglossal nerves.
- Complete the excision by dividing the mucosa and musculature of the posterior pharyngeal wall with curved scissors.
- Reconstruction is with a pedicled myocutaneous flap with the skin sutured to the mucosa and muscle to muscle.

Closure

- Flap 3/0 vicryl.
- 2 large Blake's drains (do not cross the pedicle).
- 2-layer closure to neck.
- Suture tracheostomy rather than tapes.

Post-operatively

- NBM 7 days.
- Start feeding via NGT day 1.
- Deflate tracheostomy tube cuff day 1 or 2. Remove tube when patient able to tolerate occlusion for 24h.

Alternative approaches
- Lateral mandibulotomy for access followed by a lateral pharyngotomy to access the tumour. Particulary useful for tongue-base tumours that do not involve the mandible.
- Anterior mandibulotomy combined with a lip-splitting incision is useful for tongue-base tumours that extend into the floor of mouth.
- Transhyoid pharyngotomy. Useful for small tumours of the tongue base. The muscular attachments from the superior surface of the hyoid are detached and the tongue base pulled anteriorly to expose the tumour, which is excised and the defect closed primarily.

Tonsils and adenoids

Anatomy and physiology (Fig. 6.6a + b)

- Components of the Waldeyer lymphoid ring in association with the lingual tonsils.
- Involved in inducing secretory immunity and regulating immunoglobulin production.
- These tissues are most active from the ages of 4–10 and tend to involute after puberty.
- The palatine tonsils contain crypts that extend deeply into the tissue and are lined by stratified squamous epithelium. Although this gives extra exposure of tissue to surface antigen, it may also be the reason why tonsils are so commonly infected.
- The pharyngobasilar fascia forms a distinct capsule, which binds the deep surface of the tonsil. Between this and the superior constrictor forming the floor of the fossa there is a plane that is utilized in tonsillectomy and is also the site of a peritonsillar abcess.
- Deep to the superior constrictor lies the glossopharyngeal nerve; the neurovascular bundle of the carotid sheath is found deeper.
- The palatoglossus muscle forms the anterior pillar, while the palatopharyngeus forms the posterior pillar.
- Blood supply: based primarily at the inferior pole—tonsillar branch of the doral lingual artery, ascending branch of the palatine artery and the tonsillar branch of the facial artery; superior pole—ascending pharyngeal artery.
- Nerve supply: glossopharyngeal nerve (this also has a tympanic branch thus severe tonsillitis often presents with referred pain to the ear).
- The adenoids are located on the superior and posterior wall of the nasopharynx. When enlarged they can obstruct this space. However, they normally regress by the age of 5y.

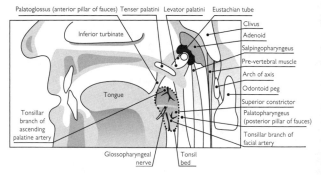

Fig. 6.6 a Sagittal section showing relations of the tonsil and adenoid. The tonsil has been removed to reveal structures on its deep aspect.

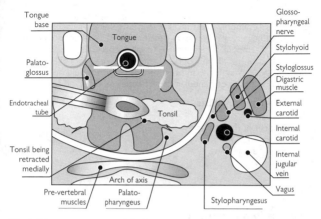

Fig. 6.6 b Axial section showing relations of the tonsil.

Tonsillitis

Tonsillitis is commonly seen in ENT and in general practice. Common bacterial pathogens are group A beta-haemolytic streptococcus, pneumococcus, haemophilus influenzae, staphylococcus and actinomyces. Treatment consists of appropriate antibiotics (e.g. penicillin), regular simple analgesia, oral fluids, and bed rest. Ampicillin should be avoided if there is any question of glandular fever, because of the florid skin rash.

Signs of acute tonsillitis
- Sore throat.
- Enlargement of the tonsils.
- Exudate on the tonsils.
- Difficulty in swallowing.
- Pyrexia.
- Malaise.
- Bad breath.
- Ear ache.

Complications of tonsillitis
Suppurative
- Airway obstruction: rare, but may occur in association with glandular fever. Treatment is insertion of a nasopharyngeal airway or intubation.
- Quinsy (paratonsillar abscess): this appears as a swelling of the soft palate and tissues lateral to the tonsil, with displacement of the uvula towards the opposite side. The patient is usually toxic with fetor, trismus, and drooling. Needle aspiration or incision and drainage is required, along with antibiotics, which are usually administered intravenously.
- Parapharyngeal abscess: see Deep neck space infections 📖 p270.
- Chronic adenotonsillar hypertrophy.

Non-suppurative
- Scarlet fever.
- Acute rheumatic fever.
- Post-streptococcal glomerulonephritis.

Glandular fever
- Epstein–Barr virus causes acute pharyngitis as part of the infectious mononucleosis syndrome.
- It is common in teenagers and young adults.
- Transmission is by oral contact, the 'kissing disease'.
- Patients with glandular fever may present a similar picture to patients with acute bacterial tonsillitis, but with a slightly longer history of symptoms.
- Diagnosis relies upon a positive monospot or Paul–Bunnell blood test.

Signs and symptoms
- Sore throat.
- Pyrexia.
- Cervical lymphadenopathy.

- White slough on tonsils.
- Petechial haemorrhages on the palate.
- Marked widespread lymphadenopathy.
- Hepatosplenomegaly.

Treatment
Largely supportive with analgesia, IV fluids, and a short course of corticosteroids.

Complications
Patients should be advised to refrain from contact sports for 6 weeks because of the risk of splenic rupture.

Other tonsil infections

- Viral: adenovirus, rhinovirus, respiratory syncytial virus.
- Fungal: oropharyngeal candidiasis (particulary in immunocompromised patients.
- Vincents angina: due to infection with *treponema vincentii* and *spirchaeta denticulate*, seen in conditions of overcrowding.

Tonsillectomy (Fig. 6.7)

- GA.
- Neck extended with shoulder bag.
- Insert Boyle–Davis gag.
- Suspend on Draffin bipod.
- Pull superior pole of tonsil medially with a Denis–Browne forceps.
- Incise mucosa from apex of the anterior faucal pillar inferiorly towards the tongue base, and then over the top of the upper pole.
- Blunt dissect the tonsil capsule to expose the plane between the tonsil and pharyngeal musculature.
- Introduce the forceps into this plane and retract medially.
- Blunt dissection continues with a Gwynne–Evans tonsil dissector from the upper pole and towards the tongue base.
- Clamp the junction between the inferior pole and tongue base with a negus clamp and remove the tonsil.
- The lower pole is tied to avoid haemorrhage.
- 2.0 linen ties are placed around the clamp and tied using a Negus knot pusher.
- Place a swab in the fossa and proceed to the second side.
- Haemostasis is with either bipolar diathermy or a ligature.
- Clear the post-nasal space and pharynx of blood.
- Release the Boyle–Davis gag and remove slowly, taking care not to displace the ETT.
- Alternatives include bipolar dissection, coblation, laser, and monopolar scissors. Most of these have a higher incidence of secondary haemorrhage as compared with cold steel.

Complications
- Primary, reactionary, and secondary haemorrhage.
- Infection.

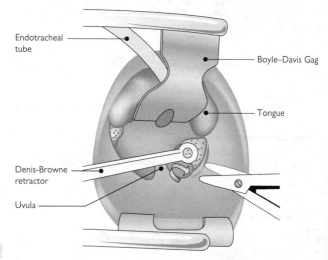

Fig. 6.7 Surgeons view of tonsillectomy showing incision of mucosa with scissors.

Simple snoring

- Very common—60% of men over 60 snore!
- Snoring occurs because of a partially obstructed airway. The mechanism involves the Bernoulli effect, causing collapse and vibration of the pharyngeal tissues.
- Obstructive sleep apnoea occurs when there is no airflow, despite respiratory effort. The apnoea index (AI) is the number of apnoeas occurring per hour.
- Hypopnoea implies a reduction in respiratory flow sufficient to cause a reduction in ventilation by 50%. The apnoea–hypopnoea index (AHI) is the number of episodes of apnoea and hypopnoea occurring in 1h.
- The key to managing such patients is an accurate assessment and relevant investigations.
- The aim of the assessment is to differentiate between simple snoring and obstructive sleep apnoea.

Assessment

History

- Sex, age.
- Collar size.
- Length of time the patient has been snoring.
- Improvement with weight loss?
- Is the partner still sleeping in the same room?
- Daytime somnelesce?
- Nasal symptoms?
- Relevant past medical, surgical and drug history.
- Smoking and alcohol intake.

Examination

- Body mass index related to height and weight.
- Any retrognatia, mircognathia?
- Macroglossia occurs in Down's syndrome and acromegaly.
- Rhinitis, deviated nasal septum, polyps.
- Size of tonsils and uvula. Relative crowding of the oropharynx leading to narrow airway at this level.
- Examine neck for any masses, including a goitre.
- Perform a flexible nasendoscopy to assess the posterior nasal cavity, postnasal space, tongue base, position of the epiglottis, and to exclude any laryngeal lesion.
- It is also worthwhile performing Muller's manoeuvre and a jaw thrust manoeuvre to check the effect on the airway.

Investigations

- Epworth sleepiness score.
- If the patient has recently put on weight and has symptoms of daytime somnelesce, thyroid function tests should be performed to exclude hypothyroidism.
- Sleep nasendoscopy is advocated by some units but most authorities now regard snoring induced by anaesthetic agents as poorly representing habitual snoring.
- Sleep study to exclude OSA if suspected.

Treatment
Conservative treatment
- A thorough explanation is given to the patient and his/her partner about the nature of the snoring and possible causes.
- Emphasize that simple snoring is a socially inconvenient problem and does not predispose to any medical sequelae.
- The partner may wish to use ear-plugs or leave the radio on at night.
- If the BMI is still high, further loss of weight and exercise should be advised.
- Exercise will also increase tone in the pharyngeal dilators preventing collapse.
- Altering the sleeping position at night also may help, e.g. avoid sleeping on their back, a tennis ball in the pyjamas.
- The patient should be advised to reduce smoking as this causes rhinitis and nasal obstruction.
- Treat rhinitis with nasal steroid sprays.
- Alcohol, especially at night, sedatives and hypothyroidism reduce tone of the pharyngeal dilators and predispose to airway collapse and snoring.

Surgical treatment
- If the patient has a symptomatic septal deviation or polyps, this should be corrected first and this will alleviate snoring in about 50% of patients. Tonsillectomy in patients with large tonsils can reduce pharyngeal obstruction.
- UVPPP (uvulopalatopharyngoplasty) or LAUP (laser assisted uvulopalatoplasty) (See p.110).
- Palatal surgery is effective in up to 90% of selected patients initially but the effects are not maintained, with only 45% still having relief at 1 year.

Non-surgical treatment
- If the patient has retrognathia, a large tongue base, or significant improvement of their airway on jaw thrust manoeuvre whilst observing with the nasendoscope, a mandibular advancement device is advised.
- Nasal CPAP (continous positive airway pressure) is very effective in abolishing snoring and OSA but is poorly tolerated by the patients.

Uvulopalatopharyngoplasty (UVPPP)

Technique
- GA.
- ETT.
- IV antibiotics.
- Head ring and shoulder bag.
- Boyle–Davies gag.
- Tonsillectomy.
- Push palate back until it meets the posterior pharyngeal wall and note point of contact.
- The palatal incision is made below this horizontally to the anterior pillars, part of which are resected.
- Preserve most of the posterior pillar.
- Resection of the palate is made easier if it is held under tension by an assistant.
- Beware two arteries found in the uvula that can retract into the soft tissues and cause troublesome bleeding.
- The posterior pillar is pulled forward and sewn to the anterior pillar with 3/0 vicryl sutures.
- The sutures should be placed through the muscle layer, as well as through the leading edge of the soft palate.
- Inject 0.5% marcaine into the surgical margins.

Post-operatively
- Adequate analgesia—effervescent diclofenac, paracetamol, and local anaesthetic lozenges, opiates PRN.
- Soft diet should be started as soon as possible.

Complications
- Airway obstruction.
- Primary haemorrhage.
- Temporary velopharyngeal insufficiency.
- Hypernasal speech.
- Nasopharyngeal stenosis.

Alternative procedures
- Simple tonsillectomy.
- Palatal stiffening.
- Laser-assisted uvulopalatoplasty (LAUP). Performed under L.A, a special CO_2 laser handpiece with a backstop to protect the posterior pharyngeal wall is used. Vertical incisions are made through the palate on each side of the uvula. The uvula is then reshaped and shortened.

111

The salivary glands

Anatomy

- Three main pairs of salivary glands—the parotid, the submandibular, and the sublingual.
- Minor salivary glands are scattered throughout the mucosa of the nose, oral cavity, oro-pharynx, and larynx.
- Saliva is needed for digestion and for lubricating the food bolus.

The parotid gland (Fig. 7.1)

- This gland lies on the side of the face and upper neck behind the angle of the mandible and anterior to the tragus.
- The gland is pyramid-shaped and covered in thick fibrous tissue formed from the continuation of the deep cervical fascia.
- It produces watery, serous saliva.
- The parotid duct opens into the mouth opposite the second upper molar tooth.
- The external carotid artery, retro-mandibular vein, and lymph nodes all lie within the parotid gland.
- The facial nerve traverses the skull base and exits at the stylomastoid foramen. It then passes through the parotid gland (creating the division between deep and superficial) splitting into its five main divisions as it does so:
    - temporal.
    - zygomatic.
    - buccal.
    - mandibular.
    - cervical.

The submandibular gland (Fig. 7.2)

- This gland lies just below the jaw in front of the angle of the mandible.
- It produces thick, mucoid saliva.
- The submandibular duct runs from the deep lobe and ends as a papilla at the front of the floor of the mouth.
- The lingual nerve, which gives sensation to the anterior two-thirds of the tongue, and the hypoglossal nerve, which provides the motor supply to the intrinsic muscles of the tongue, lie in close apposition to the deep surface of the gland. The hypoglossal nerve runs inferior to the lingual nerve, from a postero-inferior position to antero-superior.
- The marginal mandibular branch of the facial nerve runs just deep to the platysma close under the skin, which overlies the gland. It leaves the parotid gland at variable distances below the angle of the mandible, usually 1–2cm, and courses anteriorly below the lower border of the mandible to the area of the mandibular notch and facial vessels.
- The gland wraps around the free edge of the mylohyoid muscle, which runs obliquely from the hyoid to the mandible.
- The submandibular duct is 'double crossed' by the lingual nerve. Posteriorly the nerve loops down, crossing superficial/lateral to the duct; it courses anteriorly below then deep/medial to the duct.
- Lymph nodes lie close to or even within the capsule of the submandibular gland.

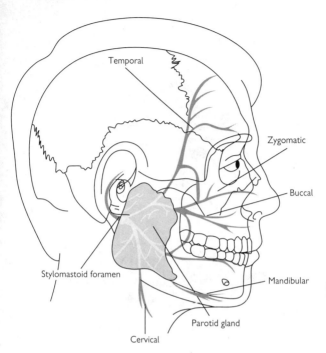

Fig. 7.1 Relationship of the parotid gland to the facial nerve.

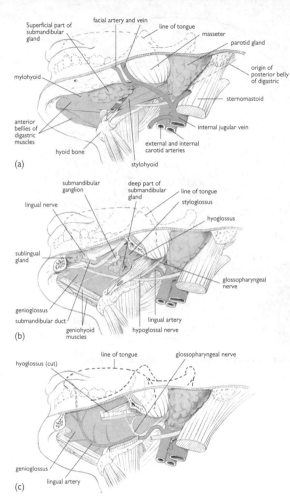

Fig. 7.2 Progressively deeper dissections (a), (b), and (c) of the side of the floor of the mouth; viewed from below and to the left. Reproduced from Oxford Textbook of Functional Anatomy Volume Three (second edition), (2005), by Pamela McKinnnon and John Morris (Oxford; Oxford University Press).

The sublingual gland

- This is the smallest of the major salivary glands. It can be felt in the floor of the mouth, running along the submandibular duct, into which it opens via 10–15 tiny ducts.

Parasympathetic secretor motor supply to the salivary glands (Fig. 7.3)

Often this is learnt the week before the intercollegiate exam, and then forgotton!

- Pre-ganglionic secretor motor fibres to the submandibular gland arise in the superior salivary nucleus, travel via the facial nerve, chorda tympani and lingual nerve to synapse peripherally in the submandibular ganglion.
- Post-ganglionic fibres then pass straight to the gland.
- The chorda tympani can be damaged during middle-ear surgery and although patients may complain of an altered taste, overall salivary function is unimpaired.
- Pre-ganglioic secretor motor fibres to the parotid gland arise in the inferior salivary nucleus and travel via the glossopharyngeal nerve, Jacobson's nerve, the lesser petrosal nerve, and the mandibular nerve to synapse in the otic ganglion.
- Post-ganglionic fibres travel via the auriculotemporal branch of the lingual nerve to reach the gland.

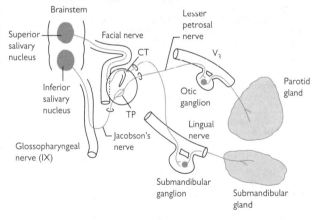

Fig. 7.3 Parasympathetic secretor motor supply to the salivary glands.

Benign salivary gland tumours

- 80% of salivary tumours occur in the parotid gland of which 80% are benign.
- In the submandibular gland, 50% are benign.
- In the minor salivary glands, 35% are benign.

Pleomorphic adenomas

- Pleomorphic adenomas, or benign-mixed tumours are the most common salivary tumour.
- ♀ > ♂.
- 3rd to 6th decades.
- Deep-lobe tumours may present as parapharyngeal space masses with medial displacement of the tonsil and distortion of the soft palate.
- Malignant transformation to carcinoma ex-pleomorphic adenoma is rare.
- Often present as an asymptomatic lump behind the angle of the mandible.
- Weakness of the facial nerve suggests a malignant infiltration.
- Arise from the distal portions of the salivary ducts, including intercalated ducts and acini.
- Mixture of myoepithelial, epithelial, and stromal elements.
- Diagnosis is usually made via fine-needle aspirate.
- FNA has an 85% accuracy rate in determining between benign and malignant.
- MRI can be useful, particularly in deep-lobe tumours.
- Treatment is surgical excision with clear margins.
- Prognosis is excellent, with a 4% rate of recurrence.

Warthin's tumour/adenolymphoma

- Also known as a papillary cystadenoma lymphomatosum.
- Found almost exclusively in the parotid gland.
- Arises from ectopic ductal epithelium.
- ♂ > ♀.
- 5th to 7th decade.
- 10% bilateral.
- Usually arises in the tail of the parotid.
- Surgical excision is curative.

Other benign swellings in the saliva glands include:
- lipoma.
- cysts.
- haemangioma.
- monomorphic adenomas (oncocytoma, basal cell adenoma, canalicular adenoma, myoepithelioma).

Malignant salivary gland tumours

- 3–4% of head and neck malignant disorders.
- Aetiology poorly understood but viral infections, radiation, and environmental factors may contribute.
- 20% of parotid, 50% of submandibular, and >70% of minor salivary gland tumours are malignant, with a ratio of 1 : 10 : 40, respectively.
- Malignant salivary gland neoplasms are divided histologically into low, intermediate, and high grade.
- Mucoepidermoid is most frequent in the parotid and half of malignant tumours of the submandibular gland are adenoid cystic.
- The prognosis varies according to histologic type, stage and primary site.

See Table 7.1 for the WHO classification of malignant salivary gland tumours, Table 7.2 for frequency of occurrence, and Box 7.1 for staging.

Presentation

- Neck mass.
- Pain.
- Facial or other nerve weakness.
- Skin involvement, such as ulceration or fixation of the overlying skin.
- Bloodstained discharge into the mouth.
- Local lymph node enlargement suggesting metastasis.

Investigations

FNA and CT or MRI are mandatory.

Mucoepidermoid

- Most commom.
- 90% occur in the parotid gland.
- ♀ > ♂.
- 5th decade.
- Histologically a mixed population of cells: mucin-producing cells, epithelial cells, and intermediate cells.
- Local invasion, lymph node involvement, and clinical aggressiveness are all more common in high-grade tumours.
- High-grade mucoepidermoid is distinguished from squamous cell carcinoma by the presence of intracellular mucin.
- 5-y survival: low grade is 70%, high grade only 47%.

Table 7.1 WHO classification of malignant salivary gland tumours

Carcinomas
Mucoepidermoid carcinoma
Adenoid cystic carcinoma
Acinic cell carcinoma
Malignant mixed tumor
Carcinoma in pleomorphic adenoma
Carcinosarcoma
Polymorphous low-grade adenocarcinoma (Terminal duct adenocarcinoma)
Epithelial-myoepithelial carcinoma
Salivary duct carcinoma
Basal cell adenocarcinoma
Mucinous adenocarcinoma
Papillary cystadenocarcinoma
Adenocarcinoma, not otherwise specified (NOS)
Clear cell carcinoma
Sebaceous carcinoma and lymphadenocarcinoma
Oncocytic carcinoma
Malignant myoepithelioma (Myoepithelial carcinoma)
Squamous cell carcinoma
Adenosquamous carcinoma
Lymphoepithelial carcinoma
Small cell carcinoma
Undifferentiated carcinoma
Other carcinomas

Tumors
Sarcoma

Malignant Lymphomas

Secondary Tumors
Melanoma
Squamous cell carcinoma
Renal cell carcinoma
Thyroid carcinoma

Unclassified Tumours

Table 7.2 Frequency of salivary gland malignant neoplasm by histologic type

Histological Type	Frequency of Occurrence
Mucoepidermoid carcinoma	34%
Adenoid cyctic carcinoma	22%
Adenocarcinoma	18%
Malignant mixed tumor	13%
Acinic cell carcinoma	7%
Squamous cell carcinoma	4%
Other	<3%

Box 7.1 Staging of malignant salivary gland neoplasms

- TX Primary tumour cannot be assessed.
- T0 No evidence of primary tumour.
- T1 Tumour 2cm or < in greatest dimension without extra-parenchymal extension.*
- T2 Tumour >2cm but not >4cm in greatest dimension without extra-parenchymal extension.*
- T3 Tumour >4cm and/or tumour having extra-parenchymal extension.*
- T4a Tumour invades skin, mandible, ear canal, and/or facial nerve.
- T4b Tumour invades skull base and/or pterygoid plates and/or encases carotid artery.

* Extra-parenchymal extension is clinical or macroscopic evidence of invasion of soft tissues. Microscopic evidence alone does not constitute extra-parenchymal extension for classification purposes.

Adenoid cystic

- 10% of malignant salivary gland neoplasms.
- 70% arise in the minor salivary glands.
- ♀ = ♂.
- Usually presents as an asymptomatic mass.
- Histologically three subtypes: tubular, cribiform (characterized by a 'Swiss cheese' pattern), and solid. Best prognosis tubular, worst prognosis solid.
- Indolent and protracted clinical course.
- Perineural spread in up to 80%, ∴ adjuvant radiotherapy is often recommended.
- Good 5-yr survival rate; poor 20-yr survival rate.
- Distant metastases can occur up to 20 yrs post-treatment.
- Disease-specific survival continues to decline for >20y after the initial treatment.

Acinic cell carcinoma

- Low-grade malignant tumours.
- 15% of malignant parotid disease.
- 80% occur in the parotid.
- ♀ > ♂.
- 5th decade.
- Histologically two cell types: serous acinar and clear cytoplasm.
- Four histological patterns: solid, microcystic, papillary, and follicular.
- 5-yr survival rate 78%.

Malignant-mixed tumours

- Arise in benign pleomorphic tumours.
- Carcinoma ex-pleomorphic is the most common.
- Histologically distinguishing feature is that the malignant component is purely epithelial.
- Other types include carcinosarcoma.
- All are classified as high grade, with a 5-yr survival rate <10%.

Others

- Metastasis to the salivary gland (usually from skin cancer ∴ in all parotid lumps make a careful check of the skin of the scalp/pinna/face/forehead.
- Adenocarcinoma.
- Epithelial–myoepithelia cell carcinoma.
- Salivary duct adenocarcinoma.
- Clear cell carcinoma.
- Squamous cell carcinoma.
- Lymphoma.

Minor salivary gland tumours

- Tumours are usually painless swellings anywhere in the upper aero-digestive tract and may be present for years or months.
- Pain is associated with adenoid cystic.
- Tumours involving the oral cavity are usually amenable to incisional biopsy for management planning.
- Tumours are excised with wide margins including periosteum but the bony palate should be preserved where possible, unless bone erosion has occurred.
- Frozen section should be used introperatively.
- Combined radiotherapy should be considered in all cases except low-grade mucoepidermoid carcinoma.

Submandibular gland excision (benign conditions)

Indications
- Recurrent sialadenitis.
- Chronic sialadenitis.
- Ranula.
- Submandibular duct obstruction.

Consent
- Scar.
- Drain.
- Marginal mandibular palsy 1–5%.
- Haematoma.
- Rarely hypoglossal and lingual nerve damage.

Preparation
- GA.
- Supine.
- Neck flexed, head extended and turned away from the side of surgery.

Incision
- Bupivicaine and adrenaline infiltration unless using nerve monitor.
- Mark out curvilinear incision two finger-widths below the mandible extending from the posterior aspect of the gland to a point 1–2cm beyond the anterior border.

Procedure
- Incise down onto gland and raise a subcapsular flap (do not raise a subplatysmal flap) (Fig. 7.4).
- The facial vein lies medial to the marginal mandibular nerve. Thus identification and low division will help protect the nerve.
- Grasp gland and retract posteriorly.
- Identify posterior margin of mylohyoid and retract this anteriorly to reveal the deep aspect of the gland.
- Identify the lingual nerve, hypoglossal nerve and submandibular ganglion.
- Divide the attachments of the gland from the ganglion.
- Ligate and transect the duct.
- The facial vessels may need to be ligated at the posterior aspect of the gland, or can be dissected free with cautery to the branches to the gland.

Closure
- 3mm Readivac drain.
- 4/0 vicryl in layers.
- 5/0 ethilon to skin.

For malignant submandibular conditions:
- The incision is continued to the mastoid tip, ± an inferior limb, to allow a composite neck dissection.
- Raise a subplatysmal flap and identify the nerve at the mandibular notch and dissect it free.
- Most neck dissections will involve clearing all node-bearing structure from level 1—the submandibular gland will be removed as part of this procedure. Patients should be warned of the risk of damage to nerves in this area.

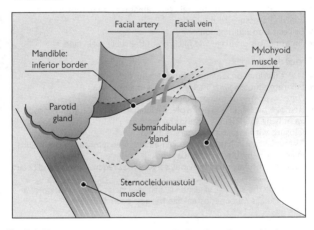

Fig. 7.4 The marginal mandibular nerve may be found anywhere within the shaded area (i.e. upto 2 fingers breath below the angle of the mandible) therefore a subcapsular flap is raised, i.e. deep to the plane of the nerve.

Ranula

This is a mucous extravasation cyst occurring in the floor of the mouth seconday to obstruction to the duct of a lingual salivary gland.

- Latin diminutive meaning 'small frog'.
- Bluish, cystic appearance arising from the floor of the mouth lateral to the submandibular duct.
- A 'plunging ranula' extends through or behind the mylohyoid muscle and presents as a neck swelling.
- Communication with the oral component may be demonstrated by applying pressure to the neck.
- Brilliant transillumination.
- Treatment is drainage and excision of the sublingual gland.

Procedure

- Insert lacrimal probe into submandibular duct.
- Infiltrate mucosa with 1% lignocaine and adrenaline.
- Anterio-posterior mucosal incision lateral to probe.
- Remove tissue (including involved sublingual gland) lateral to probe identifying the lingual nerve in the process.
- Closure with interrupted Vicryl sutures.
- Marsupialization has been recommended as an alternative but results in an unacceptable recurrence rate.
- Patients who have had previous surgery may require a submandibular approach.
- Access to the sublingual gland via a gingival incision and creation of a full-thickness mucoperiosteal flap has also been described.

Parotidectomy

Types
- Superficial conservative parotidectomy.
- Total conservative parotidectomy.
- Total radical parotidectomy.
- Extended total parotidectomy.

Superficial conservative/partial parotidectomy
Indications
- Benign neoplasms affecting the superficial lobe.
- Chronic siadenitis and chronic suppurative parotiditis (rare).
- As part of a total parotidectomy or infratemporal resection.

Preparation
- GA without muscle relaxant.
- Supine with shoulder bag.
- Head turned to opposite side.
- Reverse trendelemburg.
- Facial nerve electrodes.
- Leave ipsilateral eye and corner of mouth exposed.

Incision
- 1 : 300 000 adrenaline is used to hyrdrodissect the face and neck flap, and aids in haemostasis.
- Cervico-mastoid-facial incision (Fig. 7.5a).

Procedure
- Raise skin flap deep to platysma and superficial to the superficial musculo-aponeurotic system.
- Hold flap forward with stay sutures and retract ear lobe back.
- Identify and divide the greater auricular nerve.
- Separate gland from tragal cartilage and mastoid process by blunt dissection. Identify the tragal pointer.
- Devide fascia over SCM and peel this forward off the muscle.
- Expose the posterior belly of digastric, which determines the depth of the facial nerve.
- Using a haemostat, expose the tympanomastoid suture to identify the nerve. The facial nerve bisects the apex of this groove 5mm below the bony meatal edge. In addition, the facial nerve lies just superior to the posterior belly of digastric and 1cm deep and inferior to the tragal pointer (Conley's pointer), (Fig. 7.5b). In difficult cases, identification of a peripheral branch and retrograde dissection or a cortical mastoidectomy may be required.
- If there is any doubt, stimulate the structure with the monitor.
- Insert haemostat along the superficial axis of the main nerve trunk to identify the bifurcation.
- Dissection can proceed in a superior or inferior direction.
- The haemostat is advanced, blades opened, and tissue lifted laterally.
- Parotid tissue is divided by sharp dissection only cutting tissue superficial to the nerve, which is exposed and on view at all times.

- This technique is repeated to excise the entire superficial lobe being careful to avoid inadvertently entering the tumour.
- Stimulate the facial nerve to confirm that the nerve is in continuity.

Top tips
- Use 'ligaclips' or tie small vessels with fine Vicryl. Only use bipolar cautery and with caution.
- Loops or an operating microscope may be useful to trace branches peripherally.

Closure
- Vacuum drain.
- Close platysma with 4/0 vicryl.
- Clips or interrupted nylon to skin.

Complications
- Haematoma.
- Facial weakness: 10% temporary or 1% permanent.
- Anaethesia of lower half of pinna.
- Salivary fistula.
- Frey's syndrome: gustatory sweating is due to neo-innervation of parasympathetic secretomotor fibres into sympathetic sweat fibres of the face.

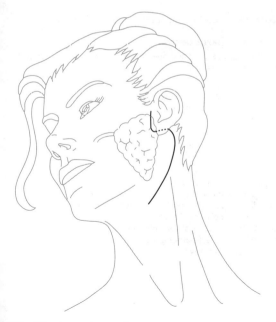

Fig. 7.5 a Incision for parotidectomy.

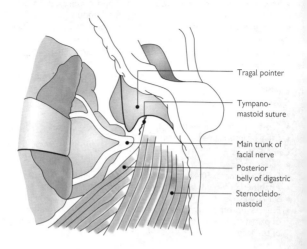

Fig. 7.5 b Identification of facial nerve (Left side).

Total conservative parotidectomy

Removal of both the superficial and deep lobes of the parotid gland with preservation of the facial nerve.

Indication
- Benign neoplasms affecting the deep lobe.
- Recurrent pleomorphic adenoma.
- Malignant tumours.
- Chronic sialectasis.
- Chronic parotoditis.
- First-arch branchial abnormality.

Operative approach
- Superficial parotidectomy, as above.
- Mobilize the facial nerve and elevate with a nerve hook.
- Mobilize the deep lobe from the styloid process, ascending ramus of the mandible, and temporomadibular joint.
- Ligate ECA and posterior facial vein inferiorly, superiorly ligate the posterior facial vein, superficial temporal artery, and maxillary artery to allow deep lobe to be removed.

Total radical parotidectomy

- High-grade carcinomas of the parotid gland invading the facial nerve.
- A total parotidectomy is performed with sacrifice of the facial nerve.
- Clearance of the tumour with the nerve should be confirmed by frozen section in cases of adenoid cystic carcinoma.
- The distal branches of the nerve are marked with silk and a primary cable graft (either sural or great auricular) is used for re-anastomosis.
- If the nerve if not re-anastomosed or is unsuccessful, facial slings, pedicled muscle transposition or free muscle transfer maybe required.

Inflammatory salivary gland conditions

Acute sialadenitis

- Rapid inflammation of the gland.
- Usually due to *Staphylcoccus aureus* infection.
- Erythema, pain, tenderness, swelling, and purulent discharge from affected duct.
- Associated with elderly, debilitated, dehydrated patients, trauma, major surgery, radiation therapy, immunosuppression, chemotherapy, or Sjögren's syndrome.

Treatment

- Rehydration.
- Warm compress.
- Antibiotics.
- Sialogogues.
- Oral irrigations.

Chronic recurrent sialadenitis

- Recurrent discomfort/pain and enlargement of the gland, especially noted on eating, caused by decreased salivary flow, stasis, and alteration in composition.
- Treatment as for acute, plus massage or radiological salivary duct dilation.

Sialolithiasis

- 80% of cases affect the submandibular gland.
- Calculi composed of hydroxyapatite.
- Multiple in 25% of cases.
- 35% parotid calculi and 65% of submandibular calculi are radiopaque.
- Pain and swelling of gland, particulary at meal times.

Treatment

- Transoral sialodochoplasty or sialolithectomy.
- If the stone is situated at the hilum of the submandibular duct, a submandibular gland excision is appropriate.

Sjögren's syndrome

- Autoimmune disorder.
- Keratoconjunctivitis sicca, xerostomia, abnormal taste, unilateral or bilateral salivary gland enlargement.
- Associated with connective tissue disorders, e.g. rheumatoid arthritis, SLE, polyarteritis nodosa.
- Menopausal women.
- May progress to lymphoma and rarely Waldenstrom's macroglobulinaemia.

Diagnosis

- Sublabial minor salivary gland biopsy demonstrating a lymphocytic infiltrate.
- Autoantibosies SS-A and SS-B.

The larynx and trachea

Anatomy

The larynx not only produces voice but also protects the respiratory tract from the digestive tract. The larynx consists of a framework of cartilages connected by ligaments, membranes, and muscles covered by a respiratory and stratified squamous mucosal epithelium (Fig. 8.1). Fibroelastic membranes (conus elasticus, quadrangular, and thyrohyoid membranes) and ligaments further divide the larynx and act as barriers to the spread of tumours. The supraglottis has a rich, bilateral lymphatic drainage in comparison to the glottis, where there is paucity of lymphatics. Thus glottic cancers have a lower incidence of both occult and clinical lymphatic metastasis in the neck.

Anatomical divisions of the larynx
- The supraglottis extends from the tip of epiglottis (lingual and laryngeal surfaces) superiorly to the glottic ventricle inferiorly and includes the arytenoid cartilages, aryepiglottic folds, false cords, and the epiglottis.
- The glottis extends from the ventricle to 0.5cm below the free edge of the true cords.
- The subglottis extends from the inferior extent of the glottis to the inferior edge of the cricoid cartilage.

Muscles of the larynx
- The muscles of the larynx are divided into intrinsic and extrinsic groups.
- The intrinsic muscles are those of the vocal cords and cartilages contained within the larynx; they are all supplied by the recurrent laryngeal nerve, apart from crycothyroid, which is supplied by the external branch of the superior laryngeal nerve.
- The extrinsic muscles, the strap muscle, and constrictors, help with laryngeal elevation and pharyngeal constriction.

The vocal cords
- The true vocal folds are comprised of three layers:
  - the epithelium.
  - the lamina propria.
  - the vocalis muscle (thyroarytenoid).
- The lamina propria is devided into three:
  - the superficial layer (this is Reinke's space).
  - the intermediate layer.
  - the deep layer.

The later two form the vocal ligament (Fig. 8.2).

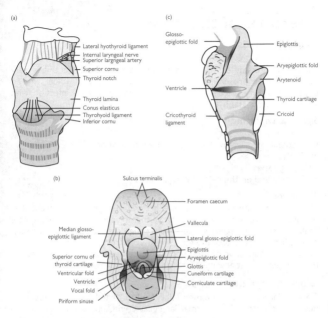

Fig. 8.1 Anterolateral (a), posterior (b) and sagittal (c) view of larynx.

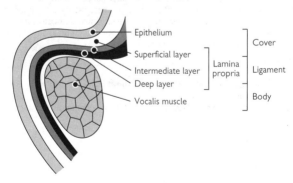

Fig. 8.2 Layered structure of the vocal fold.

Infections of the larynx

Acute laryngitis

Inflammation of the larynx may occur in isolation or as part of a general infective process, affecting the whole of the respiratory tract. It is very common, often presenting as a sore throat and loss of voice with an upper respiratory tract infection. There maybe secondary infection with streptococci and staphylococci.

Signs and symptoms
- Dysphonia.
- Hypopharyngeal pain, dysphagia, pain on phonation.
- Malaise.
- Slight pyrexia.
- Oedema and erythema of the vocal cords.

Treatment
Most patients with acute laryngitis either self-medicate or are treated in the primary care setting with supportive therapy such as voice rest, simple analgesia, steam inhalations, and simple cough suppressants. If necessary, give penicillin V 500mg/6h PO for 1 week. Voice rest is especially important for any professional voice-user, since haemorrhage into the vocal cord can produce permanent adverse effects on the voice.

Chronic laryngitis

Chronic laryngitis is a common inflammation of the larynx caused by a number of factors. The normal laryngeal epithelium is non-keratinizing stratified squamous epithelium. In chronic laryngitis there is oedema and keratinization of the vocal cords, with an abundance of lymphocytes and macrophages. It often begins after an upper respiratory-tract infection. Smoking, vocal abuse, chronic lung disease, sinusitis, post-nasal drip, reflux, alcohol fumes, and environmental pollutants may all conspire together to maintain the inflammation.

Signs and symptoms
- Dysphonia.
- Globus symptoms (feeling of a lump in the throat).
- Throat clearing or coughing.
- Laryngoscopy reveals thickened, erythematous, oedematous vocal cords.

Treatment
- The patient should be referred for a laryngeal examination if their symptoms fail to settle within 4 weeks.
- If any concern remains, the patient should undergo microlaryngoscopy and biopsy under general anaesthesic to exclude laryngeal malignancy.
- The agents that are causing the chronic laryngitis should be removed.
- Cessation of smoking.
- Voice rest.
- Laryngitis secondary to reflux is treated with antacid medication, sleeping with the head of their bed elevated and waiting 3–4hrs after eating before going to bed.
- Speech therapy.
- Patients will also respond well to explanation and reassurance that they do not have a more serious condition.

Supraglottitis and epiglottitis
See 📖 p. 184.

Rigid endoscopy 1: direct pharyngo-laryngoscopy

Indications
- Diagnosis and biopsy of laryngeal lesions.
- Removal of foreign bodies.
- Check cricoarytenoid mobility.
- Treatment of laryngeal lesions, e.g. laser, injection of vocal cords.

Pre-operative check
- Dentition.
- Neck mobility.
- Possibility of airway obstruction during intubation or post-operatively requiring tracheostomy.
- Close liaison with anaesthetist.

Preparation
- GA.
- Small-bore ETT (metal if laser required) or jet ventilation.
- Check correct scopes, light cables, instruments, and connections.
- Supine position on table with head extended at the atlas, with the neck flexed 'sniffing the morning air' (Fig. 8.3).

Method
- Teeth guard or damp swab if edentulous.
- Open mouth with free hand.
- Place laryngoscope on tongue, identify uvula, slide over base of tongue.
- Aspirate saliva.
- Identify tip of epiglottis then advance scope under the epiglottis to visualize larynx.
- Following the ETT can be helpful.
- Access all parts of larynx and pharynx prior to biopsy, which may require changing scopes.
- Inspect lateral and posterior pharyngeal wall, laryngeal surface of epiglottis, piriform fossa, aryepiglottic fold, posterior part of larynx, post-cricoid, upper oesophagus, anterior commissure and the subglottis.
- Consider using an anterior commissure scope if access to the anterior commissure is difficult.
- Examine the neck.

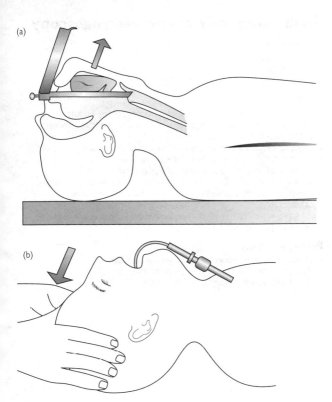

Fig. 8.3 (a) 'Sniffing the morning air' position for pharyngolaryngoscopy, with alignment of the oral, pharyngeal and laryngeal axis. The dark arrow shows the correct direction of scope elevation for compression of the tongue base (redrawn after kleinsasser, 1992). (b) Manoeuvre to achieve head extension with simultaneous neck flexion. This position may be maintained with the left hand or with a small 'neck-roll' pillow.

Rigid endoscopy 2: microlaryngoscopy

Advantages
- Magnification.
- Laser mountable.
- Two free hands for laryngeal procedures.

Method
- Ask your anaesthetist to insert a Microlaryngoscopy Endotracheal Tube or consider supraglottic jet ventillation in order to allow an unobstructed view of the larynx.
- Mayo table for support of suspension arm of laryngoscope.
- Select a 400mm objective lens for magnification.
- Insertion of scope as per pharyngolaryngoscopy.
- Connect camera to microscope for teaching and recording images.
- Microlaryngeal instruments are used for manipulation, biopsy, or excision.
- A Hopkins' rod (30 or 70 degrees) passed via the scope is useful to examine the subglottis and laryngeal ventricle.

Post-operatively
- LA (4% xylocaine) spray to prevent laryngospasm.
- Voice rest for 48h, if intervention performed.
- OPA to review histology.

Rigid bronchoscopy

Preparation

- For children, choose an age-appropriate bronchoscope (Table 8.1).
- Ensure correct fittings to attach to the anaesthetic circuit (particularly important if the bronchoscopy is required in an emergency situation) (Fig. 8.4).
- GA.
- Patient set up as per laryngoscopy.

Method

- Negus laryngoscope maybe required to identify larynx.
- Introduce bronchoscope through the right side of the mouth, rotating the tip through 90 degrees as the glottis is approached, allowing a view of the left vocal cord. Gentle rotate through 90 degrees once the scope has passed between the vocal cords.
- Fit the anaesthetic system once in the trachea.
- Attach glass lens to proximal end of bronchoscope—this prevents gas escape.
- Advance scope slowly, viewing tracheal walls.
- Position the scope in the right corner of the mouth to enter the left main bronchus, and the left corner for the right main bronchus.
- Use a 70-degrees Hopkin's rigid telescope for inspecting segmental bronchi.
- Telescopic forceps can be used for removal of foreign body.

Table 8.1 Paediatric bronchoscope sizes

Size marked on bronchoscope (mm)	External diameter (mm)	Age range
2.5	4.0	Premature/neonate
3.0	5.0	Neonate–3 months
3.5	5.7	4–12 months
4.0	7.0	13–36 months
5.0	7.8	3–9 years
6.0	8.2	Over 9 years

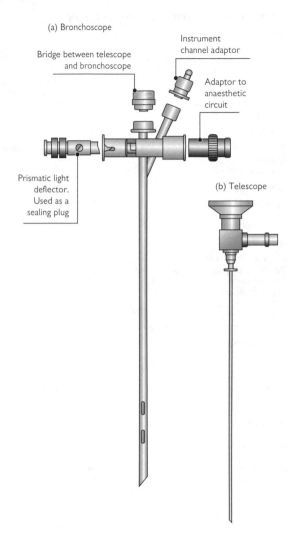

(a) Bronchoscope

Instrument channel adaptor

Bridge between telescope and bronchoscope

Adaptor to anaesthetic circuit

Prismatic light deflector. Used as a sealing plug

(b) Telescope

Fig. 8.4 (a) Ventilating bronchoscope and (b) telescope.

Microscopic laser laryngoscopy surgery (CO_2)

The addition of a laser component to a procedure automatically increases the complexity of the process. Resources are expended for additional instrumentation, added safety measures, and an extra 'laser nurse' in the operating room. As a result, the choice to use laser surgery should be based on a clearly identified advantage over alternative procedures that do not employ the laser.

Advantages
- Accurate incisions with improved haemostasis in a region with limited exposure.
- Capacity to vaporize tissue.

Disadvantages
- Concern over thermal injury with scarring of adjacent normal tissue.
- Added cost, time, use of personnel.
- Exposure of patient and operating personnel to dangers of laser.

Indications
Non neoplastic disease
- Bilateral vocal cord paralysis.
- Glottic stenosis.
- Subglottic stenosis.
- Vascular laryngeal lesions.
- Removal of Teflon granuloma.
- Excision of supraglottic benign lesions, e.g. saccular cyst.

Neoplastic disease
- Recurrent respiratory papillomatosis.
- Glottic cancer (Tis, T1, selected T2).
- Supraglottic cancer (Tis, T1, T2).
- Debulking obstructing laryngeal cancers to avoid tracheostomy.

Procedure
Pre-operative
- Define 'laser case' on list.
- Allow extra 20min for theatre set-up.
- Laser alerting signs are posted.
- Protective eye wear available to all theatre personnel.
- Test-fire laser onto wooden tongue blade at 5W to check that the He–Ne visible aiming beam is well aligned with the CO_2 beam.
- Smoke extractor and fitter.
- The Laser Safe Endotracheal Tube cuff maybe filled with normal saline and methylene blue in order to give early warning of cuff damage.
- Jet (Venturi) ventilation may be used to laser the subglottis in adults.
- Anaesthesia should be run on as low oxygen concentration (preferably <30%) as safely tolerated.

- Patient protection:
  - Surround operative field and laryngoscope with wet towels.
  - Cover eyes with moist eyepads.
  - Cover cuff of laser safe metal endotracheal tube with moist neuropaties.

Operative

- Set up as per microlaryngoscopy.
- Use largest laryngoscope with plume evacuator built-in.
- Laser settings:
  - Super pulse continuous, 0.1 pulsed, 1.0 second repeat pulses.
  - Power (5–10W).
- Laser should be on standby whenever the procedure is intermittently discontinued.
- Foot pedal should only be manipulated by the operating surgeon.
- Adjust beam size with microspot manipulator:
  - Focused beam—precise cutting, poor haemostasis.
  - Slightly defocused beam—less precise cutting, better haemostasis.
  - Defocused beam—tissue vaporisation.
- Employ traction with counter-traction when cutting tissue with the laser, using microlaryngoscopy instruments.

Rigid oesophagoscopy

Indications
- Dysphagia.
- Removal of foreign bodies.
- Unknown primary.
- Dilation of strictures.
- Exclusion of 2nd primary tumour as part of a pan-endoscopy during assessment of a known ENT primary cancer.

Pre-operative
- Barium swallow if chronic dysphagia (useful to exclude pouch and prevent perforation or if dysmotility expected).
- Lateral and PA plain soft tissue X-rays to assess site of foreign body.
- Be aware of the anatomical and physiological narrowing of the oesophagus as a distance from the incisor teeth:
  - Cricopharyngeus 15cm.
  - Aortic arch 22.5cm.
  - Left main bronchus 27.5cm.
  - Diaphragm 40cm.

Method
- Supine position.
- Neutral head position.
- Follow down the right-hand side of the ETT beyond the epiglottis.
- Pass scope into right piriform sinus and then behind the ETT to identify the cricopharyngeal spincter.
- Gentle pressure will allow the sphincter to open in front of the examiner.
- Do not apply excessive force.
- The scope may not advance for three reasons:
  - Not enough muscle relaxant.
  - Large osteophytes causing obstruction.
  - Cuff of ETT causing compression.
- Once in oesophagus, keep lumen central.
- Withdraw sharp objects into lumen and then withdraw scope from the patient.
- Soft foreign bodies can be removed piecemeal.
- Certain foreign bodies (e.g. dentures) require shears to remove them.
- Biopsies should be taken with sharp punch forceps—in order to avoid mucosal tearing.
- NBM 6h post-op and then free clear fluids until the following day.

Management of oesophageal perforation

- Insert nasogastric tube.
- Start broad spectrum IV antibiotics.
- Post-op CXR.
- Watch closely for pyrexia, tachycardia, or hypotension.
- Monitor closely for surgical emphysema in the neck, chest pain radiating to back, dysphnoea.
- NBM, NG feed, gastrograffin swallow 10 days.
- Cardiothoracic consultation if perforation persists.

Laryngeal cancer 1

This is the commonest head and neck malignancy and as such is covered here in some detail.

Demographics
- Four per 100,000 in the UK.
- 1% of all malignancies.
- 1/3 die of their disease.
- ♂ : ♀, 4 : 1.
- Commonest age of presentation = 6th decade.
- Incidence of distant metastasis = 1–5%.
- Incidence of 2nd primary at presentation = 1–5%.
- Metachronous 2nd primary rate = 10%.
- N0 neck: 30% histologically +ve.
- 95% treatable.
- 5% of tumours are untreatable because of distant metastasis, irresectability (e.g. T4N3), refusal of treatment, or the patient is too unfit.

Risk factors
- Smoking: ×6 > relative risk.
- Alcohol: ×5 > relative risk.
- HPV infection subtypes 16 and 18.
- Synergistic risk for smokers who drink is estimated to be >30 times that of individuals who do not smoke or drink.
- Gastro-oesophageal reflux disease.
- Dark sprits.
- Social class V.
- Urban.
- Previous radiotherapy.

Prognosis
5-yr survival by stage:
- Stage I: >95%.
- Stage II: 85–90%.
- Stage III: 70–80%.
- Stage IV: 50–60%.
- All stages: 68%.

Site of presentation
- Supraglottis: 40%: early lymphatic spread.
- Glottis 50%: late lymphatic spread, better prognosis.
- Subglottis 10%: lymphatic spread to paratracheal nodes, worse prognosis.

Histologic types
- Squamous cell carcinoma represents >90%.
  - There is a spectrum from normal–hyperplasia–dysplasia–carcinoma *in situ*–invasive carcinoma.
  - Invasive can be well, moderately, or poorly differentiated.
  - Variants include verrucous carcinoma, spindle cell carcinoma, basaloid squamous cell carcinoma, and adenosquamous carcinoma.
- Salivary gland cancers, e.g. adenoid cystic and mucoepidermoid carcinoma.

- Sarcomas.
- Other, e.g. carcinoid, lymphoma, metastases from other primary sites, invasion from the thyroid.

Box 8.1 Cancers of the larynx are staged according to the TNM system of the American Joint Committee on Cancer (2002)

TX Primary tumour cannot be assessed.
T0 No evidence of primary tumour.
Tis Carcinoma *in situ*.

Supraglottis
T1 Tumour limited to one subsite of supraglottis with normal vocal cord mobility.
T2 Tumour invades mucosa of more than one adjacent subsite of supraglottis or glottis or region outside the supraglottis (e.g. mucosa of base of tongue, vallecula, medial wal of pyriform sinus) without fixation of the larynx.
T3 Tumour limited to larynx with vocal cord fixation and/or invades any of the following: postcricoid area, pre-epiglottic tissues, paraglottic space, and/or minor thyroid cartilage erosion (e.g. inner cortex).
T4a Tumour invades through the thyroid cartilage and/or invades tissues beyond the larynx (e.g. trachea, soft tissues of neck including deep extrinsic muscle of the tongue, strap muscles, thyroid, or esophagus).
T4b Tumour invades pre-vertebral space, encases carotid artery, or invades mediastinal structures.

Glottis
T1 Tumour limited to the vocal cord(s) (may involve anterior or posterior commissure) with normal mobility.
T1a Tumour limited to one vocal cord.
T1b Tumour involves both vocal cords.
T2 Tumour extends to supraglottis and/or subglottis, or with impaired vocal cord mobility.
T3 Tumour limited to larynx with vocal cord fixation.
T4a Tumour invades cricoid or thyroid cartilage and/or invades tissues beyond the larynx (e.g. trachea, soft tissues of neck including deep extrinsic muscles of the tongue, strap muscles, thyroid, or oesophagus).
T4b Tumour invades pre-vertebral space, encases carotid artery, or invades mediastinal structures.

Subglottis
T1 Tumour limited to the subglottis.
T2 Tumour extends to vocal cord(s) with normal or impaired mobility.
T3 Tumour limited to larynx with vocal cord fixation.
T4a Tumour invades cricoid or thyroid cartilage and/or invades tissues beyond the larynx (e.g. trachea, soft tissues of neck including deep extrinsic muscles of the tongue, strap muscles, thyroid, or oesophagus).
T4b Tumour invades pre-vertebral space, encases carotid artery, or involves mediastinal structures.

Laryngeal cancer 2: presentation and assessment

The patient's symptoms will depend upon which site(s) within the larynx is (are) affected. A tumour on the vocal cord will cause a hoarse voice and usually presents early. However, a tumour in the supraglottis may present with few symptoms until advanced.

Early symptoms and signs
- Hoarseness.
- Dysphagia.
- Throat pain.

Signs of advanced laryngeal cancer
- Otalgia.
- Airway compromise and stridor.
- Aspiration.
- Neck mass.
- Haemoptysis.

Investigations
- Although a clinical diagnosis can often be suspected after examination of the larynx, a biopsy under general anaesthetic via direct laryngoscopy is essential, since conditions such as laryngeal papillomas, granulomas, and polyps may mimic laryngeal cancer.
- The suspected lesion is mapped and photographed and staged (see Box 8.1). The lesion is palpated to assess depth of invasion and passive mobility of both cords is checked. Spread to the laryngeal ventricle and subglottis is assessed with an angled Hopkin's rod.
- All patients should have a panendoscopy to check for a second primary tumour.
- Early stage glottic cancer with an N0 neck requires no imaging.
- Computerized tomography (CT) or magnetic resonance imaging (MRI) is useful to look for invasion of the paraglottic and pre-epiglottic space, laryngeal cartilage erosion, and cervical metastasis in clinically advanced tumours.
- 25–45% of cancers are clinically upstaged on the basis of CT or MRI scanning. All patients must have at least a CXR. CT scan of the chest is routine practice in many centres.

When performing a diagnostic endoscopy for laryngeal cancer, consider the following, as they will influence the decision to treat:
- Mid cord only?
- Involves anterior commissure?
- 1 cord/both cords?
- Subglottic/supraglottic extension?
- Posterior commissure involved?
- Are the vocal cords fixed?
- Does the lesion involve the aryepiglottic fold?
- Is the epiglottis involved? If so, both surfaces?

- Is the pyriform fossa clear (medial wall, apex and lateral wall).
- Any neck lymphadenopathy? Bilateral? Levels?
- Check tonsils, tongue base, major bronchi, oesophagus.
- Is my biopsy representative?
- Fitness for major surgery?

Benefits of staging

- Planning therapy.
- Aid to prognosis.
- Comparison of results.
- Epidaemiology.

Limitations of T-staging

- Crude system.
- Tumour size not related to prognosis.
- Hard to assess clinical extent.
- Debatable anatomical boundaries.
- Inconsistencies.
- Omissions.

Limitations of N-staging

- No mention of levels.
- No immunological status.
- No mention of extracapsular spread.
- Bilateral involvement (N2c) implies better prognosis than large nodes >6cm (N3).

Laryngeal cancer 3: treatment

As with all head and neck malignancy one must always consider treatment not only of the primary but also of the regional lymph nodes. All newly diagnosed cases should be discussed in a multidisciplinary clinic.

The primary

- T1a/b: XRT or transoral CO_2 laser (equivocal disease-free survival but no RCT yet—XRT may give better functional results).
- T2: XRT, transoral CO_2 laser, or partial laryngeal surgery.
- T3: Controversial! Radiotherapy or partial/total laryngectomy.
- T4: Total laryngectomy.

The neck

- N0: No treatment unless T3/T4, in which case XRT or selective neck dissection (SND).
- N+: SND/modified radical neck dissection (MRND) ± post-operative XRT.

Surgical management of laryngeal carcinoma

- The decision as to which type of surgery is performed is largely dependant on the size and extent of the tumour.
- In general, smaller tumours (T1 and T2) are more easily treated with endoscopic laser surgery, and larger T3 and 4 tumours are offered radical excisional surgery.

Transoral laser surgery

- Small tumours of the larynx can be removed safely and effectively with the use of the operating microscope, microlaryngeal instruments, and the CO_2 laser. Tumours are sectioned and removed in 'blocks' until clear margins are obtained on frozen section.
- A neck dissection is performed 2 weeks later, if required.
- Very good results claimed in experienced hands.

Conservation laryngeal surgery

- Any laryngeal cancer procedure that maintains physiologic speech and swallow function without the need for a permanent tracheostomy.
- The goal is to preserve maximum laryngeal function without compromising the cure rate.
- One must be able to confidently predict the extent of the tumour, particularly subglottic extension.
- Involvement of the cricoarytenoid joint is a contraindication to any organ preservation surgery.
- The patient should be consented for total laryngectomy, since extent of submoscal tumour involvement cannot be predicted pre-operatively. Frozen section control of margins is essential.
- FEV1 of <50% of expected for the patient's age suggests a high risk of associated pulmonary associated complications following conservation surgery.

Vertical partial laryngectomy

Indications
- <1cm subglottic extension below true vocal cords.
- Mobile affected cord.
- Unilateral involvement.
- No cartilage invasion.
- No extra-laryngeal soft-tissue invasion.
- Patient's sex, age, occupation, lifestyle, ability to travel to treatment centres, and reliability of follow-up are all important factors.

Contraindications
- A fixed, true vocal cord.
- Involvement of the posterior commissure.
- Invasion of bilateral arytenoids.
- Bulky transglottic lesions.
- Thyroid cartilage invasion.

Procedure (Figs. 8.5a–c)
- Tracheostomy.
- Apron incision.
- Subplatysmal superior flap raised up to the level of the hyoid bone.
- Care must be taken to avoid injury to the superior laryngeal nerves.
- Divide strap muscles in the midline.
- The external perichondrium is divided in the midline and along the superior and inferior margins of the thyroid alae.
- Elevate the perichondrium to a point parallel to the superior and inferior cornu of the thyroid alae.
- The thyroid cartilage is divided in the midline or slightly to the less affected side with an oscillating saw.
- Cut the cricothyroid membrane vertically.
- Elevate the internal perichondrium off the deep surface of the thyroid alae.
- Excise the tumour with a cuff of normal tissue under direct vision.
- The inferior line of excision should extend along the superior margin of the cricoid cartilage.
- The surgical specimen should include the lower ½ of the false vocal cord and all of the true vocal cord (including the arytenoid as necessary).
- Reconstruction:
  - With an intact ipsilateral thyroid lamina, options include a skin graft, buccal mucosa, and false cord advancement.
  - When all or part of the ipsilateral thyroid lamina is removed, options include a composite septal cartilage/perichondrial free graft, and an inferiorly and laterally rotated epiglottis.
  - In either case, a bipedicled strap muscle flap is an excellent option.

(a)

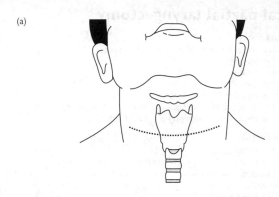

Fig. 8.5 a Skin incision.

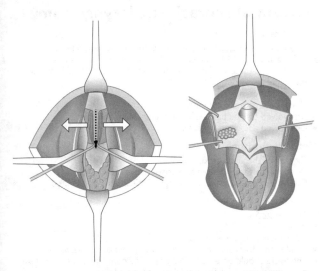

Fig. 8.5 b Diagrams showing a laryngofissure, splitting the thyroid cartilage in the midline to reveal a right-sided vocal cord cancer.

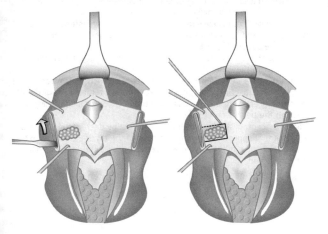

Fig. 8.5 c Elevation of the perichondrium off the deep surface of the thyroid alae and excision of tumour.

Horizontal supraglottic laryngectomy

Indications

- Laryngeal cancer situated above the plane of the ventricles.
- A T-stage of T1, T2 is, and certain T3 lesions, even though the pre-epiglottic space involved, since this can be removed by this operation.
- Mobile vocal cords.
- Uninvolved cartilage.
- Uninvolved anterior commisure.
- Uninvolved tongue base past the circumvillate papillae.
- Uninvolved apex of pyriform sinus.

Contraindications

- Fixation of the vocal cord.
- Extension to the arytenoid and post-cricoid area.
- Extension to the pharynx and tongue, unless early and limited.

Procedure

- Tracheostomy.
- Apron incision.
- Subplatysmal flaps are raised.
- Divide the infrahyoid straps close to the hyoid bone (Fig. 8.6a).
- The hyoid should be excised if there is any concern about the extent of the tumour or if the pre-epiglottic space is involved.
- Expose the greater cornu of the thyroid cartilage on the involved side.
- The incision is carried through the perichondrium along the upper border of the thyroid cartilage.
- The perichondrium is elevated from thyroid cartilage inferiorly to a point below the level of proposed cartilage incisions. This is higher in the female patient (Fig. 8.6b).
- Entry into the lumen should be performed either from the pyriform fossa or from the vallecula, under direct vision.
- After the upper incision has been completed, an incision is made on the lower margin, which passes through the lateral extent of the ventricle, preserving the mucosa over the vocal cords, and passing through the petiole anteriorly.
- Repair is accomplished by suturing the defect by deep, strong, absorbable material approximating the remnant of the thyroid cartilage to the base of the tongue if the hyoid was removed or around the hyoid if it was preserved.

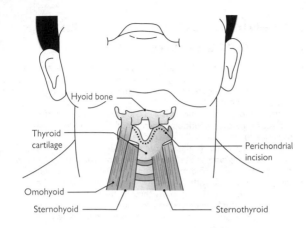

Fig. 8.6 a Perichondrium incision.

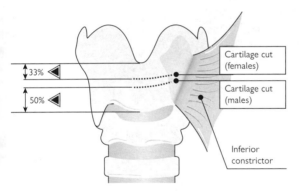

Fig. 8.6 b Extent of incision.

Supracricoid laryngectomy with cricohyoidepiglottopexy

- This is an expansion of the traditional supraglottic laryngectomy to preserve voice for individuals with cancers located at the anterior glottis, including the anterior commissure, or with more extensive pre-epiglottic space involvement.
- Surgically and oncologically, it is a difficult procedure to perform and its place in the therapeutic spectrum is not yet clearly established but may have a role in carefully selected cases.
- It consists of removal of the thyroid cartilage, both true and false cords, the paraglottic space, and one arytenoid with preservation of the epiglottis, the cricoid cartilage, one arytenoid, and the hyoid bone.
- The larynx is closed with three heavy absorbable stitches. These sutures encircle the cricoid, cross through the inferior edge of the epiglottis and the base of the tongue, and finally encircle the hyoid bone, thus bringing the cricoid into contact with the base of the tongue (cricohyoidoepiglottopexy).
- Half the patients remain dependent on their tracheostomy long-term.

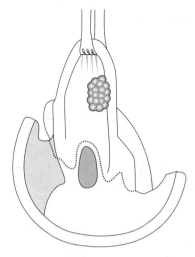

Fig. 8.6 c Internal laryngeal incision.

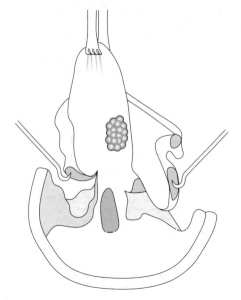

Fig. 8.6 d Supraglottic tumour excised with continuous traction.

Total laryngectomy

First described by Billroth more than 100 years ago, total laryngectomy remains the gold standard treatment to which alternatives must be compared. It has stood the test of time and remains the most commonly performed procedure for advanced laryngeal carcinoma. It is described in some detail below.

Preparation
- Re-scope and assess the patient to confirm diagnosis and staging.
- Place a sandbag between shoulders and head on a ring.
- Mark incisions.
- Infiltrate skin with LA.

Incisions
- Modified Gluck–Sorenson incision (Fig. 8.7a).
- Separate stomal incision if long neck.

Procedure
- Raise sub-platysmal flaps to level of hyoid above and suprasternal notch below.
- Divide investing layer of deep cervical fascia over sternocleidomastoid.
- Dissect medial to the great vessels in order to establish a 'paralaryngeal gutter' dividing the middle thyroid vein, if present.
- Divide omohyoid muscle and infrahyoid straps low in the neck.
- Identify inferior thyroid vessels. Divide these on ipsilateral side only.
- Divide suprahyoid straps close to the hyoid—beware XII at the greater cornu of the hyoid! (Fig. 8.7b).
- Identify superior thyroid vessels. Divide these on the ipsilateral side.
- Peel strap muscles off contra-lateral thyroid, divide isthmus, and reflect thyroid lobe off trachea (Fig. 8.7c).
- Divide constrictor muscles from the thyroid lamina (Fig. 8.7d).
- Reflect perichondrium on contralateral side and raise mucosa from inner surface of thyroid cartilage lamina in order to maximize mucosal preservation.
- Excise stomal skin when separate incision used.
- 2×2.0 silk stay sutures to anterior tracheal wall.
- Inform anaesthetist regarding tracheotomy.
- Divide trachea between 2nd and 3rd tracheal rings with adequate excision margins.
- Remove ETT and replace with laryngectomy tube through stoma.
- Contralateral suprahyoid pharyngotomy.
- Grasp the epiglottis with an Alis forceps (Fig. 8.7e).
- Divide pharyngeal mucosa aiming towards greater cornu of the thyroid cartilage. Preserve all non involved piriform sinus mucosa.
- Divide mucosa inferiorly below the level of the cricoarytenoid joints and continue inferiorly in the plane between the trachea and oesophagus to completely excise the larynx by dividing the posterior tracheal wall (Fig. 8.7f).
- Gloves and instruments are changed.

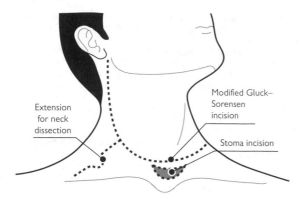

Fig. 8.7 a View of the neck from the right side showing the incisions for total laryngectomy with possibility of a right neck dissection. The stomal opening is shown below the inferior skin flap.

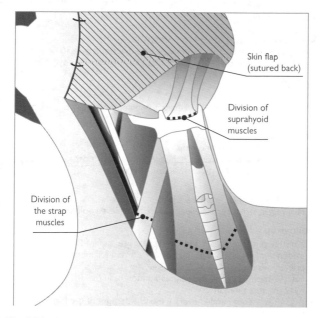

Fig. 8.7 b View of the neck from the right showing the initial steps in mobilising the larynx.

- Perform an upper-oesophageal myotomy by placing a finger in the oesophagus and cutting through the cricopharyngeal fibres until mucosa is seen.
- Some authors recommend a pharyngeal neurectomy at this stage.
- A primary puncture is performed by making a transverse incision 1cm below the cut edge of the trachea (Fig. 8.7g). Artery forceps are introduced via the oesophagus and the tips are introduced through the incision.
- Insert a size 14 Foley catheter through the primary puncture to facilitate post-operative feeding.
- Alternatively, insert an in-dwelling voice prosthesis.
- If placing a valve at the time of surgery, then a traditional nasogastric tube should be placed.
- Fashion stoma with 4/0 vicryl mattress sutures (Fig. 8.7h).
- 4/0 vicryl 3-layer meticulous longitudinal closure to pharynx. This avoids the 3-point junction when using a T-closure.
- 2 × 19Fr vacuum drains.
- 4/0 vicryl to platysma.
- Clips to skin.
- Stomal stent (Provox or Bivona) depending on surgeons preference.

Post-operatively
- Humidification.
- Remove the drains on days 4/5 or <20ml/24h.
- Organize a gastrograffin swallow or blue-dye test day 7–10 or later, if the patient has been previously treated with radiotherapy.

Complications
Operative
- Bleeding, air embolism (IJV damage), pneumothorax, hypogossal nerve damage.

Post-operative
- General—PE, UTI, septicaemia.
- Local—haematoma, wound dehiscence (especially post radiotherapy), pharyngocutaneous fistula, chyle leak, skin necrosis.

Late
- Stomal recurrence, stomal stenosis.
- Pharyngeal stricture, valve leak, failure to achieve good voice.

Follow-up
- Monthly outpatient visits for the 1st year are required to screen for evidence of recurrence at the primary site and for metanchronous primary lesions.
- Every 2 months in the 2nd year and 3 months in the 3rd year and every 6–12 months thereafter.
- A CXR is recommended every 6 months because of the high risk of lung cancer.
- Most recurrences occur with the first 2 years, and usually present with hoarseness, swallowing difficulties, cervical adenopathy, and pain.

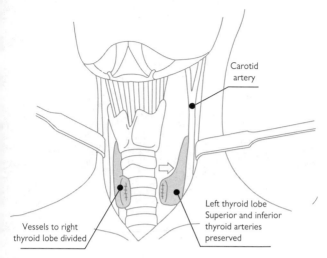

Fig. 8.7 c View of the neck from the front, showing the left thyroid lobe mobilised off the larynx, preserving its blood supply; the right lobe, on the side of the tumour, remains applied to the larynx.

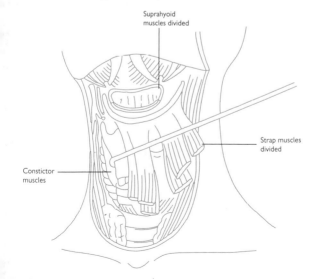

Fig. 8.7 d Identification of the posterior border of thyroid cartilage.

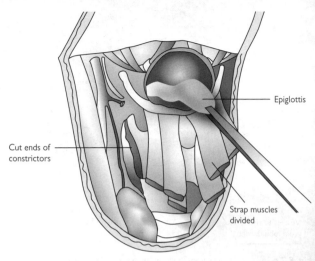

Epiglottis

Cut ends of
constrictors

Strap muscles
divided

Fig. 8.7 e Delivery of the epiglottis.

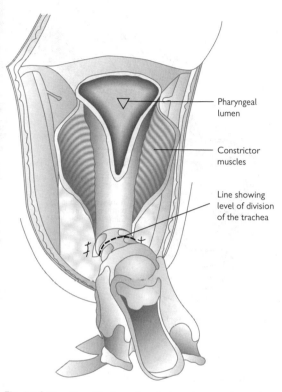

Pharyngeal
lumen

Constrictor
muscles

Line showing
level of division
of the trachea

Fig. 8.7 f Dissection of the larynx from the hypopharynx and cervical oesophagus.

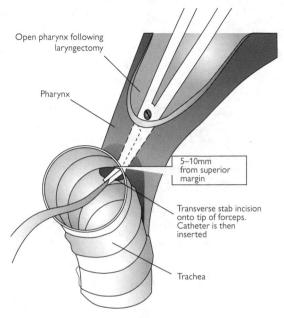

Open pharynx following
laryngectomy

Pharynx

5–10mm
from superior
margin

Transverse stab incision
onto tip of forceps.
Catheter is then
inserted

Trachea

Fig. 8.7 g Creation of tracheal-oesophageal fistula.

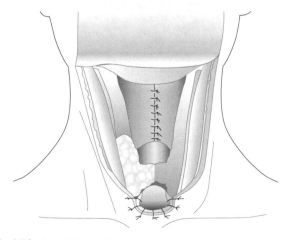

Fig. 8.7 h Method of suture for the tracheostome.

Voice restoration after laryngectomy

Oesophageal speech (Fig. 8.8a)

- Oesophageal speech offers near normal verbal communication in those who can achieve it.
- The basic principle is that air is swallowed into the stomach and then regurgitated into the pharynx.
- This causes vibration of the pharyngo-oesophageal segment (PE segment) similar to a belch.
- This can be modified with the lips and teeth into intelligible speech.
- However, often only small amounts of air can be swallowed resulting in speech comprised of short phrases at best.

Tracheo-oesophageal puncture (Fig. 8.8b)

- An artificial communication is created between the posterior wall of the trachea and the anterior wall of the pharynx/oesophagus.
- The tracheo-oesophageal fistula is usually performed at the time of the initial surgery (primary puncture) but can be performed at anytime thereafter (secondary puncture).
- A one-way valve is inserted into this tract, which allows the passage of air from the trachea to the oesophagus, vibrating the PE segment as above.
- In order to activate the valve, the patient must occlude their stoma and try to breathe out.
- This may be done with a finger or by using a second manually operated valve, which sits over the stoma as part of a heat and moisture exchanger (HME).
- The HME also filters the inhaled air and prevents excess water vapour being lost from the respiratory tract—in effect this replaces some of the functions of the nose.

Artificial larynx (servox) (Fig. 8.8c)

- Some patients cannot achieve either of the above forms of speech, and require an external vibrating source.
- The vibrating end of this device is held firmly onto the patient's neck, floor of their mouth or cheek, and this causes these tissues to vibrate.
- As a result, the air within the pharynx and oral cavity vibrates and sound is produced.
- The voice produced does sound rather unnatural but this is a simple and effective means of communication.

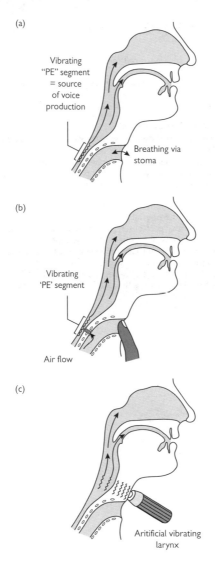

Fig. 8.8 a-c (a) Oesophageal speech, (b) Tracheo-oesophageal puncture, (c) Artificial larynx (servox).

Pharyngolaryngectomy

Indications
- Hypopharyngeal squamous cell carcinoma with anterior–inferior extension.
- Occasionally, laryngeal cancers that have spread posteriorly.
- Massive benign disease.
- Aspiration/stricture formation following trauma.

Early spread to lymph nodes
- 70% of hypopharyngeal cancers have palpable nodal disease at presentation.
- Of the clinically N0 necks, 60% will have microscopic nodal involvement.
- Often present with a very small 'silent' primary with large metastasis.
- Submucosal spread is common, often inferiorly.

Procedure
- The initial part of the operation is similar to a laryngectomy.
- Instead of preserving part of the pharynx it is separated off the pre-vertebral fascia by blunt dissection. The superior incision is level with hyoid and the inferior incision level with tracheal incision, with at least a 2cm margin from the tumour.
- Reconstruction is with a jejunal-free flap or tubed myo/fascio-cutaneous free flap using the thyroid, facial, or transverse cervical vessels for anastomosis.

Pharyngolaryngo-oesophagectomy

- The otolrayngologist's role in total pharyngolaryngo-oesophagectomy with stomach pull-up is little different to his/her role in pharyngolaryngectomy with jejunal conduit, except for a few points.
- The operation is more suitable for lower lesions, since the stretch of the stomach on the tenuous blood supply of the right gastro-epiploic artery places great strain on the superior anastomosis.
- A decision between a two-stage (abdomen and neck) and three-stage (abdomen, neck, and chest) must be made.
- The stomach requires a pyloroplasty for drainage, since the operation cuts vagal nerves.
- The hypopharynx must not be separated from the oesophagus until the stomach is delivered into the neck.
- A primary voice puncture is usually not successful due to the capaciousness of the stomach.
- Special problems of acid reflux into the mouth and 'dumping' may be a sequalae of this surgery.

Benign laryngeal lesions

Although not cancer, these lesions can inflict a significant morbidity and are particularly prominent in patients who use their voice professionally (e.g. singers, lecturers). Once a neoplastic cause has been excluded, patients should be managed in a voice clinic, in conjunction with a qualified speech and language therapist, with access to video laryngeal stroboscopy.

Clinical assessment

History
- Age.
- Occupational voice demands.
- Dysphonia (hoarseness):
  - Onset.
  - Duration.
  - Progress
  - Preceeding URTI.
  - Trauma.
  - Intubation.
- Previous surgery? thyroid.
- Smoking.
- Fluid intake—caffeine/alcohol.
- Nasal allergy/sinusitis.
- GORD.
- Hypothyroidism.

Examination
- Full ENT examination.
- Detailed examination of the larynx using viseostroboscopy.

Vocal cord granulomas (Fig. 8.9a)
- Arise posteriorly, adjacent to the vocal process and not on the vibrating segment of the vocal cord; thus dysphonia may not be a significant feature.
- Usually associated with a history of trauma to the larynx, commonly intubation.
- More common in men and associated with reflux.
- The granuloma arises due to chronic inflammation of the exposed arytenoid cartilage (perichondritis).
- Treatment involves laryngoscopy to confirm the diagnosis and exclude any malignancy, with limited removal trying to avoid further damage to cartilage.
- Treatment of reflux is essential.

Laryngeal cysts (Fig. 8.9b)
- Intracordal cysts are often found within the middle-third of the vocal cords.
- Cysts may be located in the supraglottis and may present with dysphagia without hoarseness.
- They are either mucous retention or epidermoid cysts.
- Speech therapy fails to correct the dysphonia.

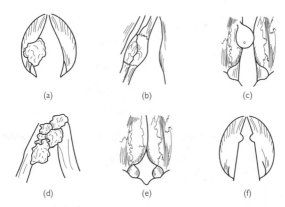

Fig. 8.9 The vocal cords are viewed as at microlaryngoscopy. a–f Benign laryngeal lesions. (a) vocal cord granuloma; (b) intracordal cyst; (c) pedunculated vocal cord polyp; (d) laryngeal papillomatosis; (e) reinkes oedema; (f) vocal cord nodules.

- Treatment is excision either by de-roofing and marsipulization (supraglottic) or enucleation (vocal cord).
- Care is taken not to damage the free edge of the vocal cord.

Vocal cord polyps (Fig. 8.9c)

- Usually unilateral, pedunculated lesions.
- Associated with smoking and voice abuse.
- Most common between middle- and anterior-thirds of the vocal folds.
- Histology shows deposits of hemosiderin and iron within the lamina propria.
- Primary treatment is surgical excision, exclusion of underlying malignancy, post-operative speech therapy, and avoidance of risk factors.

Papillomatosis (Fig. 8.9d) See 📖 p. 710.

Reinkes' oedema (Fig. 8.9e)

- Strong association with cigarette smoking and heavy voice abuse.
- Diffuse polypoid changes of vocal cords secondary to accumulation of fluid in the superficial layer of the lamina propria.
- Usually bilateral.
- Treatment involves stopping smoking and speech therapy. Refractory cases are treated by surgery in the form of a lateral cordotomy, extravasating the fluid, trimming then replacing mucosa.

Vocal cord 'singers' nodules (Fig. 8.9f)

- Affects children or professional voice users.
- History of voice abuse common.
- Bilateral whitish lesions at the junction of the anterior one-third and posterior two-thirds of the vocal cords.
- Primary treatment is speech therapy, then microlaryngeal surgery for refractory cases.

Vocal cord palsy

- Vocal cord paralysis signifies immobility of the 'true vocal cord' secondary to disruption of the relevant motor innervation of the larynx.
- The long course of the recurrent laryngeal nerve (RLN) makes it susceptible to damage in a variety of sites.
- The site of disruption of the nerve supply leads to a characteristic pattern in the position of the cords.
- This should be differentiated from fixation of the vocal cord secondary to direct pathological infiltration of the vocal fold, larynx, or laryngeal muscles, or fixation of the cricoarytenoid joint encountered in patients with rheumatoid arthritis or following traumatic intubation.
- Palsy or paralysis of the vocal cords will mean that the patient may have a weak, breathy voice, rather than the harsh, hoarse voice of laryngeal cancer. They will have a poor, ineffective cough, and aspiration is common.
- Any condition that affects the brainstem (CVA, trauma, or tumour) will affect the function of the vagus nerve and as such the recurrent laryngeal nerve.
- With these conditions, the voice problems may be less a cause for concern than the lack of protection of the airway, which can lead to life-threatening aspiration.
- Any systemic neurological or neuromuscular condition, such as multiple sclerosis or muscular dystrophy, may also affect the voice. It is rare for these conditions to present first to an ENT surgeon as voice problems.

Semon's law

- In recurrent laryngeal nerve lesions, the abductors paralyse before the adductors.

Causes

- 1/3 idiopathic.
- 1/3 surgery (thyroidectomy).
- 1/3 neoplasia (thyroid, malignant cervical nodes, carcinoma of the oesophgus, hypopharynx, or bronchus), aortic aneurysm, TB.

Investigation

Where there is no history of recent surgery:
- CT scan—skull base to diagphragm.
- ± USS thyroid.
- ± oesophagoscopy.

If the above are negative, then post-viral neuropathy is the most likely cause. An endoscopy, together with palpation of the cricoarytenoid joint, is necessary to exclude vocal cord fixation, if suspected.

Phonosurgery

Phonosurgery

This must be distinguished from conservation laryngeal surgery where the primary aim is to eradicate cancer and voice conservation or restoration is of secondary importance. The mainstay of phonosurgery is the treatment of patients with unilateral vocal cord palsy. The two main approaches are vocal cord injection and laryngeal surgery.

Vocal cord injection

Materials

- Teflon—a polymer of polytetrafluoroethylene (PTFE). Causes a localized granuloma but final space-occupying lesion is unpredictable ∴ good immediate results may deteriorate with time.
- Gelfoam—a hamostatic material. Only lasts for 3 months. Commonly used in conjunction with a re-innervation procedure to provide temporary improvement while neural regeneration occurs.
- Fat—autogenous material. Easily harvested, readily available, and does not give a foreign-body reaction.
- Collagen—natural constituent of the lamina propria of the vocal cord. Becomes incorporated and even replaced by new host tissue. Hypersensitivity reactions have been reported ∴ skin testing is performed pre-operatively.
- 'Bioplastique'—polymethylsiloxane gel widely used in Europe but not approved for the USA. Gives sustained improvement of phonation up to 7 years.

Operative techniques

- GA: direct laryngoscopy, no patient feedback via phonation during injection.
- LA: direct laryngoscopy.
- Indirect laryngoscopy can be performed in outpatients but, technically demanding.
- Transcutaneous route through the cricothyroid membrane. Outpatient procedure with the advantage that the head can be placed in a more anatomical position (Fig. 8.10).
  - Position patient sitting upright in an examination chair.
  - Topically anaesthetize the nose, oropharynx and larynx with 4% xylocaine spray.
  - 1% lignocaine is used to anaesthetize the skin anterior to the cricothyroid membrane.
  - Insert needle through the membrane just above the cricoid and, once into the lumen, inject 2–4ml of 4% xylocaine to anaesthetize the subglottic area.
  - A flexible nasendoscope with camera is passed via the nose to obtain a view of the larynx on the video screen.
  - A 90-degree smoothly curved 18-guage needle is pre-loaded with Teflon on a Luer-lock 5ml syringe.

- Introduce the needle through the cricothyroid membrane in the midline.
- Rotate needle to enter the inferior surface of the vocal fold at the level of the vocal process and place laterally, close to the medial surface of the thyroid cartilage.
- Teflon can then be injected until the fold lies in the desired position.
- Patient cooperation by phonation gives a clear indication of the amount of material required for good voice.

(a)

(b)

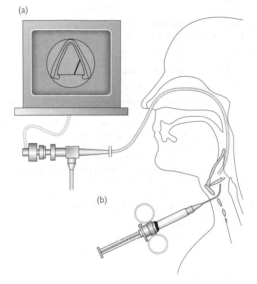

Fig. 8.10 Transcutaneous injection laryngoplasty.

Laryngeal framework surgery

- First described by Payr and re-introduced by Ishiki in 1974.
- Variety of materials used for implants:
  - Autologous cartilage.
  - Silastic.
  - Hydroxypatite.
  - Goretex.
  - Titanium.
- Advantages:
  - Permanent, but surgically reversible.
  - Excellent at closing anterior gap.
- Disadvantages:
  - More invasive.
  - Poor closure of posterior glottic gap.

Type 1 thyroplasty – procedure

- Horizontal incision is made over the mid-portion of the thyroid cartilage and the cartilage is exposed.
- A window is created in the thyroid ala approximately 8mm posterior to the midline providing a sufficient strut inferiorly to support the implant (Fig. 8.11a and b).
- The cartilage from the window is removed.
- The perichondrium is elevated from the medial aspect of the thyroid ala. (Fig. 8.11c).
- A depth-gauge is used to medialize the vocal cords in the anterior, middle, and posterior aspects of the window and measurements recorded (Fig. 8.11d).
- An implant is fashioned from a silastic block using the measurements.
- The point of maximal medialization is at the level of the vocal process.
- The implant is rotated into place and the patient asked to phonate and the voice assessed (Fig. 8.11e).

Other techniques

- Arytenoid adduction (Fig. 8.12).
  - First decribed by Ishiki with modifications by Zeitels and others.
  - Addresses posterior glottic gap by pulling arytenoid into adducted position.
  - Difficult to predict which patients will benefit pre-operatively.
  - Most advocate use in combination with anterior medialization.

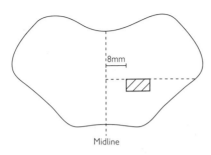

Fig. 8.11 a

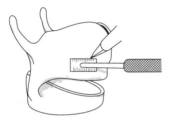

Fig. 8.11 b A guide is used to accurately mark the size and position of the window.

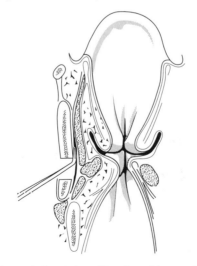

Fig. 8.11 c The perichodrium is elevated from the medial aspect of the thyroid ala.

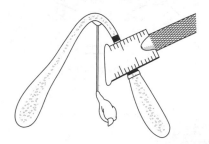

Fig. 8.11 d A depth-gauge is used to measure the size of the implant.

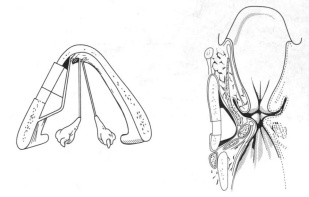

Fig. 8.11 e The implant is rotated into place.

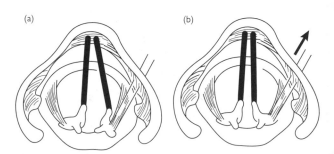

(a)   (b)

Fig. 8.12 a–b Arytenoid adduction.

Bilateral vocal cord paralysis

Bilateral abductor paralysis

- Patients exhibit lack of abduction during inspiration, but good phonation.
- Maintenance of airway is the primary goal.
- Management options.
  - Tracheostomy:
    - Gold standard.
    - Most adults will require this.
    - Speaking valves aid in phonation.
  - Laser cordectomy.
  - Laser cordotomy.
  - Woodman arytenoidectomy.
  - Phrenic to posterior cricoarytenoid anastamosis:
    - Allows abduction during inspiration.
    - Preserves voice when successful.
  - Electrical pacing:
    - Timed to inspiration with electrode placed on posterior cricoarytenoid.
    - Long-term efficacy not yet shown.

Bilateral adductor paralysis

- Patients have good airway with breathy voice.
- Goal is to prevent aspiration and improve phonation while preserving airway.
- Aforementioned medialization techniques can be applied.
- Patients may need tracheostomy if over-medialized.

Microlaryngeal surgery for benign lesions

General principles

- A thorough knowledge of the micro-architecture of the vocal folds and location of pathology is essential.
- The layered structure of the vocal fold and its different mechanical and physical properties allows the superficial layer to oscillate independently for phonation.
- This explains the mucosal wave seen on stroboscopy.
- Poor lymphatic drainage of Reinkes' space predisposes this layer to collect tissue fluid.
- Pre- and post-operative analysis is important to ensure preservation of the mucosal wave.
- Some lesions are difficult to diagnose with white light and therefore require stroboscopy.
- An academic approach should also utilize acoustic parameters for objective pre- and post-surgical analysis.
- A range of laryngoscopes and micro-instruments is required.
- Surgery should be superficial, staying out of the vocal ligament, with limited mucosal incisions only.
- There is currently no role for stripping of the mucosa of the vocal fold for benign disease.
- Laser is advantageous for vascular lesions that may bleed on removal, such as papillomastosis or granulomas.

Surgical techniques

Set up as for microlaryngoscopy (see 📖 p. 138).

Nodules

- The centre of the nodule is held with grasping forceps and pulled medially towards the opposite cord.
- Microscissors are used to cut the nodule close to its base, thus preserving normal mucosa.
- The opposite cord can be excised in a similar manner, taking care to not damage the anterior mucosa.

Polyps

Similar techniques to nodules ensuring preservation of mucosa.

Reinkes' oedema

- Lateral cordotomy incision on the superior surface of the vocal cord.
- The mucosa is elevated with a blunt dissector and the myxomatous contents either aspirated or removed with cupped forceps.
- The flap is then replaced and any excess mucosa is trimmed with microscissors.
- Fibrin glue or welding microspot laser may be used to replace the flap.

Intracordal cysts
Lateral cordotomy then blunt dissection releases the surgical planes, allowing the cyst to be released anteriorly and posteriorly.

Papillomas
- CO_2 laser is the treatment of choice.
- Setting of 4W on pulsed laser (0.1s) with a spot size of 0.3mm are used.
- Papillomata are grasped gently, as they may be friable, and the laser is used to excise the base.

Granulomas
- CO_2 laser (6W, 0.8mm spot size, 0.1s pulsed) is used to remove the lesion flush with perichondrium.
- The patient is placed on strict anti-reflux medication, together with intensive voice therapy.

The voice clinic

This is a multidisciplinary clinic involving an ENT surgeon with a special interest in voice and speech therapy. This approach allows accurate assessment of patients with voice disorders and tailored medical and surgical therapy.

Assessment

History

- Employment voice use.
- Singing.
  - Vocal fatigue.
  - Vocal cracking.
  - Pain on phonation.
- Alcohol and tobacco usage.
- Voice abuse.
- Allergic rhinitis.
- Reflux.
- Neurologic disorders.
- History of trauma or surgery.
- Systemic illness—e.g. rheumatoid.
- Duration.

Examination

- Complete head and neck examination.
- Flexible fibre-optic laryngoscopy.
- 90-degree Hopkins' rod telescope.
- Check for adequacy of airway, gross aspiration.
- Assess position of cords:
  - Median, paramedian, lateral.
  - Posterior glottic gap on phonation.

Evaluation

- Videolaryngoscopy—for documentation.
- Videostroboscopy—assesses the mucosal wave of the vocal fold and demonstrates subtle mucosal motion abnormalities (Fig. 8.13).
- Laryngeal electromyography (Fig. 8.14).
  - Assesses integrity of laryngeal nerves.
  - Differentiates denervation from mechanical obstruction of vocal cord movement.
  - Electrode placed in thyro-arytenoid and cricothyroid.
  - Localization of lesions in the superior laryngeal/recurrent laryngeal nerve network and identifies signs of re-innervation in a paralysed cord.

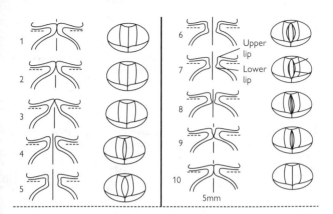

Fig. 8.13 The mucosal wave.

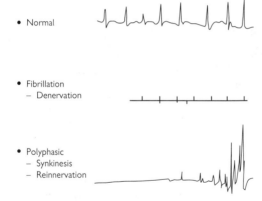

Fig. 8.14 Electromyography.

Stridor

Stridor is a high-pitched noise caused by a restricted airway. It is most common in children, due to the anatomical differences between the paediatric and the adult larynx (see p. 676). The timing of the stridor in respiration indicates the site of the obstruction or restriction:
- Laryngeal stridor = inspiratory.
- Tracheal stridor = expiratory—a wheeze.
- Subglottic stridor = biphasic.

A small reduction in the diameter of the airway leads to a dramatic increase in the airway resistance (Poiseuilles law: resistance = r4) and hence the work of breathing.

Causes of stridor

Congenital
- Laryngomalacia.
- Vocal cord web.
- Bilateral vocal cord palsy.
- Subglottic stenosis.

Acquired
- Trauma.
- Foreign body.
- Epiglottitis/supraglottitis.
- Croup.
- Carcinoma.
- Airway compression, e.g. thyroid.

Assessment

Stridor is an ominous sign. Even if the patient appears to be coping, be sure that they are closely observed and that facilities to secure the airway are readily at hand. Patients rapidly decompensate with devastating consequences.
- Take a rapid history.
- Measure O_2 saturation.
- Take temperature.
- Note respiratory rate.

In children, pyrexia, drooling, dysphagia, and a rapid progression of the illness, suggests epiglottitis. Take the patient to a place of safety, such as a resuscitation room or operating theatre, and call for a senior ENT surgeon and an experienced anaesthetist. A similar history in adults suggests supra-glottitis. This diagnosis can usually be confirmed by a careful nasolaryngoscopy (contraindicated in children).

The emergency airway

Patients presenting with upper-airway obstruction must be evaluated quickly, efficiently, and accurately. Remember to keep calm! The airway should be managed with an anaethestist, preferably the most senior in the hospital, and good communication is essential.

The following questions should be answered first

- Will admission and observation be sufficient for the time being or do you need to intervene to secure the airway? If the patient is safe to be observed, this should either be in ITU, theatre recovery or an experienced ENT ward where expertise to recognize a decompensating airway is available and where suitable action can be instigated quickly.
- If intervention is required, do you need to do something now, or do you have time to wait for senior help to arrive?

Assessment

Follow these three stages: look, listen, and observe.

Look

- What is the patient's colour—are they blue?
- Is there any intercostal recession or tracheal tug?
- What is the patient's respiratory rate?

Listen

- Can the patient talk in sentences, phrases, words, or not at all?
- Do they have stridor? Is it inspiratory, expiratory, or mixed?
- What history can the patient give?

Observation

- Is the patient's respiratory rate climbing?
- Is the patient pyrexial?
- What is the patient's O_2 saturation? Is it falling?

Interventions

Consider the following options.

Non surgical

- Give the patient oxygen via a face mask or nasal prongs.
- IV broad-spectrum antibiotics, such as Augmentin (check they are not allergic).
- Nebulized adrenaline (1ml of 1 : 1000 with 1ml saline).
- Heliox—this is a mixture of helium and oxygen that is less dense than air. It is easier to breathe and it buys you time, during which you can take steps to stabilize the airway.
- IV steroids.
- Endotracheal intubation should be the first line of intervention where possible. If it proves difficult or impossible, move on quickly.

- Fibre-optic guided endotracheal intubation performed via the nasal or oral route can be used in an awake, spontaneously breathing patient with a difficult airway. The ETT is advanced over the endoscope and into the trachea using the endoscope as a guide.
- The laryngeal mask is a hybrid of a face mask and endotracheal tube, which can easily be inserted into the hypopharynx making it a useful tool in many emergency airway situations. However, it is unsuitable when there is gross swelling or distortion of the supraglottis.
- Oropharyngeal and nasopharyngeal airways can be useful in certain circumstances, such as angio-oedema of the floor of mouth and tongue.

Surgical measures

The two basic surgical techniques to obtain an airway are: Cricothyroidotomy and tracheotomy.

Cricothyroidotomy

This is generally considered the procedure of choice because it is fast and simple to perform and requires very few instruments. The Biro is famous for having being used in this way, but a wide-bore cannula, 'mini-trac', or trans-tracheal ventilation needle are probably more appropriate! If these are not available, a 1cm horizontal incision, just above the cricoid cartilage, will allow access directly into the subglottis. This can be held open with artery forceps until an ETT or tracheostomy tube is inserted. If you are unsure of your landmarks, fill a syringe with a little saline and use a needle to probe for the airway, with suction applied. A steady stream of bubbles will appear when the airway is entered.

Emergency tracheostomy

A longitudinal incision is made in the midline of the neck and deepened to the trachea, dividing the thyroid. Brisk bleeding is to be expected. The blade is plunged into the airway and twisted sideways to hold the tracheal fenestration open. A cuffed tracheostomy or ET tube is inserted into the airway and the bleeding thyroid is dealt with afterwards.

Tracheostomy

Indications

There are three principal types of indictation for tracheostomy. The first is upper-airway obstruction and the second is to provide ventilatory support and bronchial toilet. The third is to protect the airway from aspiration. If the airway obstruction is acute and presents as an emergency, a surgical airway may have to be performed rapidly under local anaesthetic if the anaesthetist is unable to intubate the patient transorally.

Causes of upper-airway obstruction

Congenital
See Chapter 23.

Trauma
- Maxillary and mandibular fractures.
- Laryngeal injuries.
- Foreign bodies in the airway.
- Traumatic or prolonged endotracheal intubation.
- Inhalational injuries.

Neoplasia
- Laryngeal and pharyngeal tumours.
- Malignant thyroid tumours.

Infection
- Acute epiglottitis/supraglottitis.
- Deep-neck space infections.

Inflammation
- Angioneurotic oedema.
- Oedema as a result of inhalation of smoke, fumes or corrosive agents.

Neurological problems
- Pharyngeal or laryngeal as a result of motor-neurone disease.
- Bilateral recurrent laryngeal nerve palsies (thyroid surgery).
- Myasthenia gravis.

Surgery on the upper airway, particularly major resections within the oral cavity and pharynx.

Elective tracheostomy

Procedure
- Head rest and shoulder bag.
- Horizontal incision through skin, subcutaneous tissue, and deep cervical fascia midway between cricoid and sternal notch.
- Divide strap muscles in the midline.
- Divide thyroid isthmus in midline and hemitransfix with 4/0 vicryl.
- Warn the anaesthetist, and ensure a tracheostomy tube (3/4 of the diameter of the trachea) is ready and the cuff has been tested and that a sucker is at hand.
- A cricoid hook can be used to elevate the trachea into the wound.
- Tracheotomy removing the anterior half of 3rd or 4th tracheal ring.

- Alternatives includes a cruciate incision or Bjork flap.
- Ask anaesthetist to withdraw ETT.
- Insert tracheostomy tube once tip of ETT has been withdrawn proximal to the stoma and inflate cuff.
- Secure tube with 2/0 silk sutures and tracheostomy tape (ensuring head is flexed).

Complications

Early
- Infection.
- Haemorrhage.
- Subcutaneous emphysema, pneumothorax, or pneumomediastinum.
- Tracheal oesophageal fistula.
- Recurrent laryngeal nerve palsy.
- Tube dislodgement.
- Tube obstruction secondary to secretions or mucous plug.

Delayed
- Tracheal innominate artery fistula.
- Tracheal stenosis.
- Delayed tracheoesophageal fistula.
- Tracheocutaneous fistula.

Tracheostomy tubes

The choice of tubes may seem bewildering (Fig. 8.15). The basic principles are as follows.

Trache tubes with inner tubes

- The inner tube is slightly longer than the outer, and crusting tends to occur at the distal end and on the inner tube.
- The inner tube can easily be removed, cleaned, and replaced without removing the outer tube.
- Any patient who is likely to require a tracheostomy for more than 1 week is probably best fitted with a trache tube with an inner tube.

Cuffed and non-cuffed tubes

- The cuff, as in an endotracheal tube, is high-volume and low-pressure. This prevents damage to the tracheal wall.
- The cuff prevents fluid and saliva leaking around the tube and into the lungs.
- In addition, it makes an airtight seal between the tube and the trachea, allowing for positive pressure ventilation.
- Most tubes are cuffed, but when a tracheostomy is in place long-term, a non-cuffed tube may be used to prevent damage to the trachea.

Metal tubes

- Metal tubes are non-cuffed and are used only for patients with permanent tracheostomies.
- They have the advantage of being inert and 'speaking valves' can be inserted, and are cosmetically more acceptable to most patients.

Fenestrated tubes

- Most tubes are non fenestrated.
- The advantage of a fenestrated tube (one with a hole in its side wall) is that air can pass through the fenestration, through the vocal cords, enabling the patient to talk.
- The disadvantage is that saliva and liquids may penetrate through the fenestration, into the lower respiratory tree. For this reason most fenestrated outer tubes are supplied with both fenestrated and non-fenestrated inner tubes which can be interchanged appropriately.

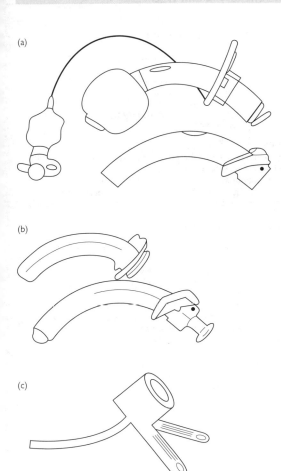

Fig. 8.15 Diagram of tracheostomy tubes: (a) cuffed fenestrated tube;
(b) non-cuffed, non-fenestrated tube; (c) paediatric tube.

Post-tracheostomy care

- In the first few days after a tracheostomy, special care needs to be taken.
- The patient should be nursed by staff familiar with tracheostomy care.
- The patient should be given a pad and pencil with which to communicate.
- Be aware that being rendered aphonic is likely to lead to frustration—be patient and understanding.

Precautions

- The tube should be secured with tapes and knotted at the side of the neck until a tract is well-established.
- The tapes should be tied with the neck slightly flexed.
- The cuff should not be over-inflated, in order to prevent ischemic damage to the tracheal wall. Use a pressure gauge to check the cuff's pressure.
- Release the pressure in the cuff after 24h, unless the patient is being ventilated.
- The patient must be given humidification for at least the first 48h to reduce tracheal crusting.
- Regular suctioning of the airway to clear secretions may be needed.
- A spare tracheostomy tube and an introducer should be kept by the patient's bed in case of accidental displacement of the tube.
- Tracheal dilators should also be close by for the same reason.
- The first tube change should take place after about 4–5 days, when a track is well formed. Good illumination and suction are necessary.
- Position the patient as close as possible to the operative position.
- Once the tube has been changed, a speaking valve may be applied to restore the patient's voice.
- Where a difficult tube change is anticipated, or where orotracheal intubation is not possible, changing the tracheostomy tube 'over' a Bougie or guide-wire avoids a false passage of the new tube.

Head and neck reconstruction

General principles

- Plan resection incisions to avoid the sacrifice of potential reconstructions.
- Conserve vital structures if oncologically safe since these can improve the reconstructive effort considerably, e.g. facial artery for anastomosis, lingual nerve for sensation.
- Recognize the uniqueness of structures.
- Restore like with like where possible.
- Respect the functional role of the area.
- Reconstruct in cosmetic units (see 📖 p. 654).
- Anticipate the consequences of healing.
- Cover vital structures with full-thickness, well-vascularized tissue.
- Restore bony architecture accurately.
- Understand the reconstructive ladder (see Fig. 22.1a 📖 p. 639).
- See 📖 p. 654 for local flaps.

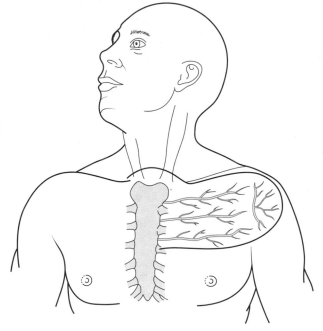

Fig. 9.1 Deltopectoral flap.

Pedicled flaps in head and neck reconstruction

Deltopectoral flap

- Medially based chest flap based on the axial branches of the first four internal mammary perforating vessels (Fig. 9.1).
- The flap can be transposed (tubed or untubed, lined or unlined, and delayed or undelayed) to almost any region in the head and neck.
- It can be used to resurface the chest, neck, and face, to reconstruct within the pharynx and oesophgaeal region, and to create a tracheal stoma.
- The flap is often outlined as a surgeon plans a pectoralis major flap to allow for defensive incisions to ensure that it could be used at a later stage, if necessary.

Pectoralis major flap

- The pectoralis major muscle is a flat, fan-shaped muscle originating from the medial half of the anterior surface of the clavicle, half the width of the sternum, all the adjacent costal cartilages to the sixth or seventh rib, and the aponeurosis of the external oblique muscle.
- The blood supply to this axial pattern flap is through the pectoral branch of the thoraco-acromial artery.
- Usually a narrow strip of muscle is elevated with the pedicle at the same time to protect the arterial pedicle.
- Main uses are resurfacing of the face and neck, reconstruction within the oral cavity, oropharynx or hypopharynx, and mandibular reconstruction.
- Rib can be harvested *en bloc* for mandibular bony reconstruction.

Procedure

- Draw a line between the acromial and xiphoid process, and then from the mid-point of the clavicle, a perpendicular line to join and meet the original line. The meeting point marks the line of the acromiothoracic artery (Fig. 9.2).
- The incision commences at the lower border of the flap to identify correctly the lower margin of the pectoralis major muscle (Fig. 9.3).
- Stitch the skin to the muscle as the paddle is elevated.
- Fig. 9.4 shows the flap being elevated in conjunction with a deltopectoral flap.
- The pectoralis flap is swung over the clavicle and under the neck skin into wherever the reconstruction is required, ensuring that the pedicle does not become twisted.
- The donor site can either be closed primarily by undermining the adjacent skin widely or by placing a skin graft over the defect.
- Insert a suction drain.
- Close wound in two layers with a deep layer of absorbable sutures and a cutaneous layer of non-absorbable sutures.

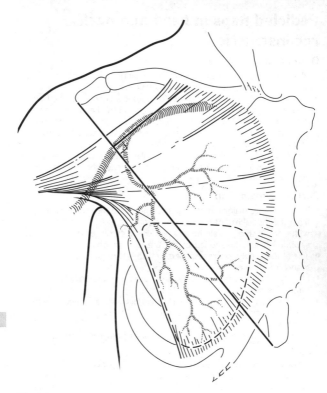

Fig. 9.2 Pectoralis major flap. Vascular pedicle runs along a line between the acromium and xiphisternum.

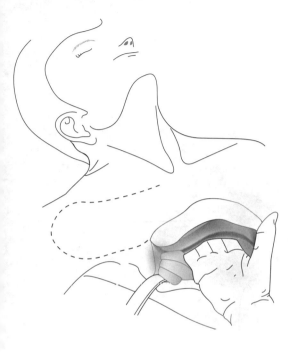

Fig. 9.3 Note the outlined Deltopectoral flap which can be raised 'defensively'.

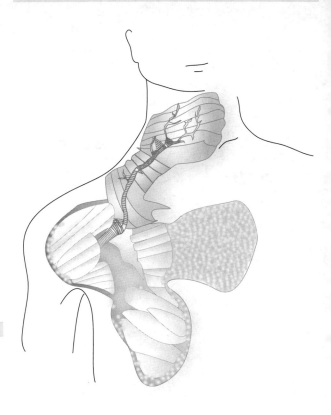

Fig. 9.4 Pectoralis major flap in conjunction with a deltopectoral flap.

Free tissue transfer in head and neck reconstruction

Indications
- Oromandibular defects.
- Anterior mandibular defects.
- Cranial base lesions.
- Orbito-maxillary defects.
- Circumferential hypopharyngeal or upper-oesophageal defects.
- Soft-tissue augmentation of the face and neck.
- Coverage of heavily irradiated and radionecrotic wounds.
- Facial reanimation procedures.

Relative contraindications
- Diabetes mellitus: macro and microvascular disease. Atherosclerotic disease is particularly problematic in the lower extremity vasculature, and the facial artery.
- Cardiac disease: long operative time, reduced perfusion.
- Smoking: hypercoagulation, decreased perfusion, impaired wound healing.
- Coagulopathies: warfarin, ethanol induced hepatic insufficiency.
- Collagen vascular disease: particularly active vasculitic processes.
- Obesity: dissection of pedicle, anastomisis, insetting and flap tailoring are compromised.

Absolute contraindication
- Hypercoagulable state, e.g. polycythaemia, sickle-cell disease.

Types of free flap
- Cutaneous/fasciocutaneous: scapular, radial forearm, lateral arm, lateral thigh.
- Musculocutaneous: latissimus dorsi, rectus abdominis.
- Osseous/osseouscutaneous: fibular, scapular.
- Osteomusculocutanous: deep circumflex iliac.
- Free visceral flaps: jejunum.

Advantages
- Immediate functional and aesthetic reconstruction.
- Simultaneous two-team approach.
- Large variety of donor sites.
- Unrestricted flap positioning and reach.
- Large amount of composite tissue.
- Potential for functional reconstruction (sensate/motor).
- Improved vascularity.
- Primary placement of osteointegrated implants.

Disadvantages
- Mircovascular expertise required.
- Prolonged operating time.
- Labour-intensive.
- Recipient vessels maybe unavailable or unusable.
- Muscle pedicle not always available for carotid protection.
- Functional disability at donor site.

Specific advantages and disadvantages of each flap

Free flap (vasculature)	Advantage	Disadvantage
Radial forearm fasciocutaneous flap. Radial artery and paired venae comitantes.	Intra-oral soft tissue reconstruction. Easy to harvest. Long vascular pedicle. Thin, pliable flap. Can be sensate when harvested with lateral antebranchial nerves. Radial bone or vascularised tendon may be included. Good sized vessels.	Donor site morbidity. Skin graft may be required to the donor site (can be avoided with V-Y advancement flap). If radial bone included, its length is limited, difficult to contour, and donor defect is unsightly. Predisposes to pathological fractures.
Lateral arm. Profunda brachii and venae comitantes.	Fasciocutaneous, composite with bone (humerus) or vascularised nerve graft. Donor site can be closed primarily. Limb ischaemia is never seen since blood supply is non-essential.	Donor site requires a pressure dressing which has been associated with radial nerve palsies.
Lateral thigh. Third perforator of the profunda femoris artery and venae comitantes	Long vascular pedicle. Large skin paddle. Two-team approach. Donor site closed primarily. Pliable skin, usually hairless. Can be senate (preservation of the lateral femoral cutaneous nerve).	Bulky in obese patients. Inconsistent vascular pedicle.
Rectus abdominis myocutaneous flap. Deep inferior epigastric artery and vein.	Versatile, bulky and pliable. Can provide entire length of muscle from xiphoid to the pubis. Largest skin paddle of all the free flaps. Good for reconstructing orbitomaxillary and glossectomy defects.	No bone. Depending on the patient's body habitus, it may be too thick. Harvesting either the muscle alone or a different thickness of subcutaneous tissue and applying a skin graft can avoid this.

	Long and wide calibre vessels facilitate microvascular anastomosis.	Possible ventral hernias.
	Easy to harvest.	
	Simultaneous two-team approach.	
Latissimus dorsi myocutaneous flap. Thoracodorsal artery and vein (branch of the subscapular artery).	Good for reconstruction of large defects on the face, neck, oral cavity and skull base. Long pedicle. Donor defect well-tolerated. Re-innervation of the muscle is possible if harvested with the thoracodorsal nerve, preventing muscle atrophy and maintaining bulk. Cosmetic advantage, especially females. Can be tubed.	Bulky flap may be a disadvantage in some patients. Patient positioning prevents dual team approach thus pro-longing operative time. Reduction in upper limb power. Occasional donor site dehiscence.
Fibular free flap. Peronneal vessels.	Reconstruction of segmental mandibular defects (angle to angle). Strong cortical bone. Allows osteo-integrated implants for dental rehabilitation. Course of vessels parallels that of bone allowing multiple osteotomies for contouring with preservation of blood supply. Thickness similar to body of mandible. Simultaneous dual-team approach. Limited donor site morbidity—limited to local sensory loss and weakness of dorsiflexion of great toe.	Septocutaneous blood supply is often variable (in 10% of the popula-tion the peronneal artery is the dominant supply to the foot). Short vascular pedicle. Limited cutaneous paddle and soft tissue bulk often requiring a second flap.
Deep circumflex iliac osseomyo cutaneous flap.	Good for oromandibular reconstruction. Large amount of bone up to 16cm. Contoured.	Advanced skill requirements.

(Contd.)

Free flap (vasculature)	Advantage	Disadvantage
Tripartite flap consisting of skin, internal oblique, and iliac crest. Deep circumflex artery and vein.	Muscle provides well vascularized tissue. When grafted with a SSG, can line buccal and lingual sulci and preserve mobility of tongue. Skin paddle can restore external defects and can act as an external monitor (good retention of anatomical relationship to bone maintains vascularity). Simultaneous dual-team approach reduces operative time. Allows placement of osteo-integrated implants.	Because skin paddle relies on musculocutaneous perforators for its vascularity, its ability to rotate is limited. Poor colour match. Significant post-operative hip pain and weakness. Possible late ventral hernias.
Jejunal free flap. Jejunal branches of the superior mesenteric artery.	Reconstruction of circumferential defects of the hypopharynx and cervical esophagus. Jejunum is of comparable size to oesophagus. Harvest and micro-vascular anastomosis are fairly easily accomplished. Eating by post-operative 7–10 days. Tracheo-oesophageal speech can be accomplished. Neck can be irradiated. No intestinal impairment. Chest not violated.	Laparotomy is required. Jejunum does not tolerate ischaemia well. Short pedicle. Total reliance on pedicle for blood supply, since serosa prevents neo-vascularisation from the recipient bed. Late graft failure. Difficult to monitor postoperatively.
Scapular and para-scapular free flaps. Cutaneous branch of the circumflex scapular artery.	Wide range of tissue types based on a single pedicle. Thin hairless skin. Large surface area. Thicker skin than RFFF. Inside and outside cover in oral reconstruction of mandibular defects. Separation of soft tissue and bone allows freedom in the 3D setting.	Cannot re-innervate skin. Patient must be turned ∴ simultaneous two-team approach not possible. Brachial plexus injury. Shoulder weakness.

Assessing flap failure

In combined head and neck cases the otolaryngologist may be asked to review the patient post-operatively who has had a reconstruction with a pedicled flap where there is concern over tissue-viability. Flap failure can be either due to arterial hypoperfusion or venous stasis.

Arterial hypo-perfusion

- Initially the flap will become paler and shrink.
- The flap then stops bleeding around the edges, there is reduced bleeding on pin-prick, and the capillary refill becomes longer.
- Eventually the flap becomes mottled and dusky due to under-perfusion with oxygenated blood.

Venous stasis

- Initially the flap becomes engorged with arterial blood.
- There is increased bleeding on pin-prick and oozing from around the edges.
- Eventually the flap becomes blue/purple and oedematous with engorged blood.

NB: See also 📖 p. 79.

The oesophagus and swallowing

Gastro-oesophageal reflux disease (GORD)

Demographics
- Most common upper-gastrointestinal (GI) disorder in the Western World.
- Experienced by 20–40% of adults.
- Prevalence likely to be higher than reported.
- Increases with age.
- Sex ratio $\male = \female$.
- More common during pregnancy.

Pathogenesis
- Abnormal retrograde flow of gastric contents into the oesophagus resulting in symptoms, mucosal damage, or both.
- Most commonly due to a defective lower oesophageal sphincter (LES).
- In 40–60% of patients, abnormalities of oesophageal peristalsis are also present. These patients also have more atypical symptoms, such as a cough or hoarseness.
- Hiatus hernias also contribute to reflux by altering the relationship between the LES and oesophageal crus.

Symptoms and signs
- Typical (oesophageal):
  - Heartburn.
  - Regurgitation.
  - Dysphagia.
- Atypical (extra-esophageal):
  - Cough.
  - Wheeze.
  - Chest pain.
  - Hoarseness.
  - Dental erosions.
  - Laryngitis and sore throat.
  - Vocal cord glanuloma.
  - Globus.
  - Otitis media.

Investigations
- Barium swallow is useful for detecting hiatus hernia and strictures.
- Endoscopy is useful for detecting complications of GORD.
- Oesophageal manometry provides information on the LES.
- Ambulatory pH monitoring is the most reliable test (sensitivity and specificity of 92%).

Treatment

Non-surgical

- Life-style modifications—frequent, small meals; avoid fatty foods, spicy foods and chocolate; last meal of the day at least 2h before going to bed; elevate head of bed; stop smoking; lose weight.
- Antacids.
- H2 antagonists.
- Proton-pump inhibitors.

Surgical

- Laparoscopic fundoplication—90% success rate in patients with typical symptoms.

Neurological causes of swallowing problems

The swallowing mechanism is a complex process involving both sensory and motor functions. It is initiated voluntarily but progresses as a dynamic reflex. A neurological condition that affects a patient's motor or sensory function may ∴ also cause problems with swallowing.

Neurological causes of swallowing problems

- CVA (stroke).
- Bulbar palsy.
- Motor neurone disease.
- Multiple sclerosis.
- Tumours of the brain stem.
- Cranial nerve lesions, e.g. vagal neuroma.
- Systemic neurological conditions, e.g. myasthenia gravis.

Investigations

- Assessment will involve taking a detailed swallowing history and asking the patient about any coughing or choking attacks, indicating aspiration.
- A general neurological examination and a specific cranial nerve examination should be done.
- A CXR may show lower-lobe collapse or consolidation if aspiration is present.
- A video swallow gives detailed information about the function of the oesophagus (such as delay, pooling, unco-ordination, spasm, etc).
- Functional endoscopic evaluation of swallowing (FEES) gives real-time information on laryngeal penetration and aspiration.

Treatment

Wherever possible the patient's underlying condition should be treated, but there will be times when treatment aims to control the symptoms. This could involve:

- Swallowing therapy as directed by a speech and language therapist.
- Dietary modification, such as thickened fluids.
- Cricopharyngeal myotomy.
- Vocal cord medialization procedures.
- Tracheostomy.
- Percutaneous endoscopic gastrostomy (PEG).
- Tracheal diversion or total laryngectomy (see p. 158).

Post-cricoid web

- This is a rare condition and its cause is unknown.
- An anterior web forms in the lumen at the junction of the pharynx and oesophagus, posterior to the cricoid cartilage.
- Patterson Brown–Kelly (UK) and Plumber–Vinson (USA) both describe this condition—their names are frequently used in association with the syndrome.
- A post-cricoid web is linked with iron-deficiency anaemia, and it has the potential to become malignant ∴ an endoscopy and a biopsy is recommended.
- It may also cause dysphagia and can be seen on a barium swallow.
- The web may be dilated and/or divided with the help of an endoscope.

Achalasia

- This is a rare condition where there is absence of oesophageal peristalsis and hypertonia in the lower oesophageal sphincter muscle that fails to relax completely on swallowing.
- ♂ = ♀.
- Any age.
- 1 in 100 000.
- Aetiology is unclear, but a degeneration of the myenteric plexus of Auerbach has been documented, with loss of post-ganglionic inhibitory neurones resulting in increased LES resting pressure and insufficient relaxation.

Signs and symptoms
- Progressive dysphagia.
- Regurgitation.
- Weight loss.
- Aspiration when supine.
- Heartburn.
- Chest pain.

Investigations
- A barium swallow may show a narrowing at the level of the gastro-oesophageal sphincter.
- A dilated, sigmoid oesophagus may be present in patients with long-standing achalasia.
- An endoscopy is needed to exclude an oesophageal tumour as this can produce similar radiological appearance and symptoms.
- Absence of peristalsis is seen on manometry.
- Ambulatory pH monitoring is performed to rule out abnormal gastro-oesophageal reflux.

Treatment
Non-surgical
- Calcium-channel blockers.
- Intra-sphincteric injection of botulinum toxin.
- Pneumatic dilatation.

Surgical
- Laparoscopic Heller myotomy (involves a controlled division of the muscle fibres of the lower oesophagus and proximal stomach follwed by a partial fundoplication.
- Bypass procedures.

Pharygneal pouch (Zenker diverticulum)

- Originates from the posterior wall of the oesophagus in a triangular weakness limited inferiorly by the cricopharyngeus muscle and superiorly by the inferior constrictors (i.e. Killian's triangle).
- As the diverticulum enlarges it tends to deviate towards the left.
- Thought to be due to either a hyperactive upper-oesophageal sphincter or lack of pharyngeal co-ordination.
- There is progressive herniation of mucosa and submucosa through Killian's triangle resulting in the diverticulum lying between the pharyngo-oesophagus and the prevertebral fascia.

Incidence

- 1 case per 100 000 per annum in the UK.
- ♂ : ♀, 2 : 1.
- Most commom between 6th and 9th decades.
- Mainly affects Caucasians.

Symptoms and signs

- Dysphagia.
- Regurgitaion of undigested food (with risk of aspiration).
- Gurgling sounds in the neck.
- Halitosis.
- Pulmonary complications from aspiration.

Investigations

- A barium swallow will clearly demonstrate the position and size of the diverticulum.
- A video swallow gives information about the function of the pharyngeal muscles as well as the presence or absence of gastric reflux.
- Either study should include an examination of the oesophagus and stomach to exclude a synchronous carcinoma.

Treatment

- It is important to consider the overall health of the patient as well as assessing the effect the pouch is having on the individual's quality of life.
- Traditional external-approach surgery has now been mostly superceded by the use of trans-oral approaches.
- However, ENT surgeons should be familiar with both approaches since complications from trans-oral approaches may require external exploration.

Surgery for pharyngeal pouch

Open approach

Pre-operatively
- Treat any malnutrition, chest infection, dehydration, or GORD.
- Clear fluids 24h prior to surgery.

Procedure
- Pharyngoscopy to aspirate any contents and to exclude any malignancy.
- Pack the pouch with ribbon gauze.
- 32Fr bougie is inserted into the oesophagus.
- The neck is extended on a head ring and shoulder bag.
- Left-transverse cervical incision at the level of the cricoid cartilage through platysma.
- Raise subplatysmal flaps.
- Divide the investing layer of deep cervical fascia along the anterior border of sternomastoid.
- Identify and divide omohyoid and middle-thyroid vein.
- Rotate the ipsilateral lobe of the thyroid forward to expose the posterolateral surface of the pharynx and the oesophagus within the operative field.
- Enter the retropharyngeal space anterior to the vertebral bodies at a level superior to the inferior cornu of the thyroid cartilage, thus avoiding injury to the recurrent laryngeal nerve.
- Identify the sac in the midline and deliver into field identifying the neck of the sac by sweeping away tissue until only musosa is seen protruding through the muscular defect of the pharynx.
- Cricopharyngeal myotomy is performed prior to excision of the sac to prevent recurrence.
- The sac is then excised (diverticulectomy) and sent for histology. The defect is closed with a continuous inverting Connell suture placed in the horizontal plane and reinforced with a second layer of interrupted sutures. Other second-line procedures, such as sac inversion and suspension (diverticulopexy), have been described.
- Haemostasis.
- Suction drain.
- Close wound in layers.
- Patient should be fed via a nasogastric tube for 5 days and then a water-soluble contrast study performed to exclude a leak.

Complications
- Recurrent laryngeal nerve palsy.
- Cervical emphysema.
- Mediastinitis.
- Pharyngo-cutaneous fistula.
- Pharyngeal stenosis.

Endoscopic approach (Dolman's procedure)
- The diverticuloscope is introduced to expose the hypopharyngeal bar.
- The scope has blades which can be manoeuvred to give optimum exposure.
- Clear food from the pouch using a soft-tip sucker.
- Inspect the lining of the pouch with a Hopkins' telescope and biopsy any suspicious lesions.
- The bar is divided with either diathermy, laser, or staples.
- Assuming there is no chest pain, surgical emphysema, or tachycardia, the patient can commence on free fluids initially and then soft diet the following day.

Advantages
These include:
- Shorter procedure and anaesthetic (these patients are usually elderly and have several co-morbidities).
- Less invasive.
- Quicker resumption of oral intake and shorter stay in hospital.

Oesophageal tumours

Benign oesophageal tumours are rare and arise from the local tissue elements, e.g. leiomyoma, adenoma, lipoma.

Barrett's oesophagus

- Metaplasia of the oesophageal mucosa caused by the replacement of the physiological squamous epithelium with columnar epithelium due to GERD.
- More common in caucasians over 50.
- May progress to high-grade dysplasia and eventually adenocarcinoma.
- Endoscopy reveals a salmon-pink epithelium.
- Treatment consists of proton-pump inhibitors or a fundoplication and regular follow-up with endoscopy and biopsy.

Malignant oesophagal tumours

Risk factors

- Smoking.
- High alcohol intake.
- Achalasia.
- Plummer–Vinson syndrome (squamous).
- Caustic injuries (squamous).
- GERD (adeno).

Demographics

- 80% of malignant tumours occur in males over 60 years old.
- Squamous cell carcinoma of the thoracic oesophagus used to be the most common but now adenocarcinoma of the lower-third of the oesophagus accounts for over 50%.

Signs and symptoms

- Weight loss.
- Pain in the throat and/or epigastrium.
- Progressive dysphagia initially for solids.

Investigations

- Barium swallow may show a stricture or mucosal abnormality suggesting a malignant tumour.
- Endoscopy and biopsy will confirm the diagnosis.
- CT scan of the chest and abdomen assesses the extra-mucosal extent and metastatic spread of the tumor (PET can also be used).
- Endoscopic ultrasound is the most sensitive test to determine the penetration of the tumour, the presence of enlarged perioesophageal lymph nodes, and invasion of structures adjacent to the oesophagus.

Treatment

All tumours must be discussed at the upper-gastrointestinal multidisciplinary team meeting.

Curative

• Trans-hiatal oesophagectomy (abdominal and cervical incisions).
• Trans-thoracic oesophagectomy (abdominal and thoracic incision).
• These may be offered with pre-operative chemotherapy (neoadjuvant), and post-operative chemo- and/or radiotherapy (adjuvant), but no increase in survival has been shown in randomized controlled studies, to date.

Palliative

Because most patients already have lymph-node metastases at the time of surgery, the 5-year survival rate remains poor at 25–30%. Options include:

• Radiotherapy.
• Laser-debulking of the mass (Nd:YAG).
• Endoscopic stenting with expandable, coated, metallic stents.
• PEG tube for long-term feeding.

The thyroid and parathyroid glands

Anatomy and embryology

Thyroid problems are frequent topics in both undergraduate and post-graduate exams. Many ENT surgeons perform thyroidectomy and it is a common problem seen in neck lump clinics. It is ∴ well worth investing some time in understanding the thyroid.

Embryology of the thyroid

The thyroid begins its development at the foramen caecum at the base of the tongue. The foramen caecum lies at the junction of the anterior two-thirds and the posterior third of the tongue in the midline. The thyroid descends through the tissues of the neck and comes to rest overlying the trachea.

Anatomy of the thyroid

The thyroid gland is surrounded by pre-tracheal fascia and is bound tightly to the trachea. The thickening of fascia at this point is known as Berry's ligament and results in movement of the thyroid superiorly during swallowing. The gland is also enveloped by a fine capsule from which septa pass into the gland. Dissection between this capsule and the pre-tracheal fascia comprises the 'capsular dissection'. The istmus is at the level of the 3rd and 4th tracheal rings and the superior pole overlies the cricoid cartilage and cricothyroid muscle. The recurrent laryngeal nerves (branches of the vagus) lie very close to the posterior aspect of the thyroid lobes having ascended from the mediastinum in the tracheo-oesophageal grooves. On the right side the nerve may lie outside the groove and approach from a more oblique angle. The nerve is intimately related to the inferior thyroid artery, which runs from lateral to medial when the gland is retracted. The nerve passes behind Berry's ligament to enter the larynx behind the cricothyroid joint. In approximately 1% of cases, the right nerve is non-recurrent and is closely related to the inferior pole of the thyroid as it passes from lateral to medial, directly from the vagus. The external laryngeal nerve arises from the superior laryngeal nerve at the thyrohyoid membrane and passes down beneath the lateral border of the sternothyroid muscle and on the middle constrictor to run along the lateral surface of the cricothyroid muscle, which it supplies (Fig. 11.1).

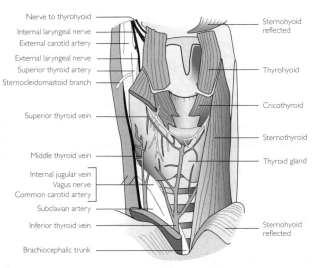

Nerve to thyrohyoid
Internal laryngeal nerve
External carotid artery
External laryngeal nerve
Superior thyroid artery
Sternocleidomastoid branch

Superior thyroid vein

Middle thyroid vein

Internal jugular vein
Vagus nerve
Common carotid artery
Subclavian artery

Inferior thyroid vein

Brachiocephalic trunk

Sternohyoid reflected

Thyrohyoid

Cricothyroid

Sternothyroid

Thyroid gland

Sternohyoid reflected

Fig. 11.1

Benign thyroid disease

Hashimoto's thyroiditis

- Autoimmune condition.
- Often associated hyperthyroidism.
- Many patients develop a large compressive or persistently painful goitre.
- Thyroxine replacements may be necessary.
- Increased risk of developing a thyroid lymphoma.
- Surgery is rarely indicated.

Reidel's thyroiditis (invasive fibrous thyroiditis)

- Uncommon.
- Woody, hard goitre.
- Infiltrates adjacent structures.
- Steroids, tamoxifen, or methotrexate can be useful in the early stages.
- Surgery is the last resort.

Non-toxic goitre

- Benign multi-nodular goitre.
- Commonest thyroid problem.
- Caused by episodic periods of thyroid hypo-function and subsequent thyroid-stimulating hormone (TSH) hyper-secretion that leads to hyperplasia of the gland. This is followed by involution of the gland.
- Prolonged periods of hyperplasia and involution are thought to be responsible for the nodular enlargement of the gland found in a multi-nodular goitre.
- A finding of a single nodular enlargement of the thyroid raises the question of malignancy and is managed as described in Fig. 11.2.
- Thyroidectomy may be necessary for one or all of the following signs:
  - Pressure symptoms in the neck.
  - Dysphagia.
  - Airway compression.
  - Cosmetic deformity.
- In cases of airway obstruction or dysphagia, a CT is required to assess the degree of tracheal compression and retrosternal extension. Usually the goitre can be removed through the cervical approach, but occasionally a sternotomy maybe required.

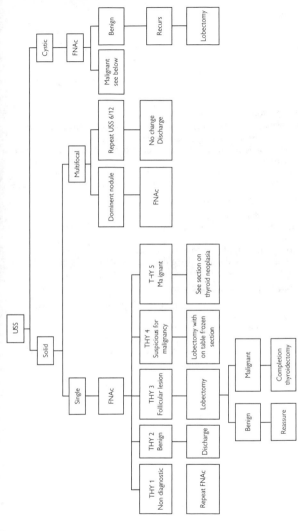

Fig. 11.2 Management of a solitary thyroid lump.

Graves' disease

- Toxic goitre.
- Autoimmune condition where antibodies are produced that mimic the effect of TSH.
- A hyperthyroid state develops and there is often a smooth goitre.
- Eye signs may be most impressive (the actor Marti Feldman had this condition).

Treatment

- Hormonal manipulation with carbimazole and propylthyouracil for 6–18 months followed by a period of withdrawal.
- Radioactive iodine or surgery is the definitive long-term therapy of choice.
- A patient who is lactating, pregnant, or who wants to become pregnant within 6 months of treatment, should not receive radio-iodine.

Indications for total thyroidectomy

- Severe opthalmopathy.
- Patients who do not want to spend a period away from their child.
- Large retrosternal goitres.
- Large toxic goitre for cosmetic reasons.
- Nodular Graves' disease where there is a suspicion of a malignant tumour.

Perioperative management

- Hyperthyroid patients must be made euthyroid pre-operatively to prevent a thyroid storm.
- An endocrinologist is often involved.
- Iodine (lugol's solution) 7–10 days pre-operatively decreases vascularity of the gland and beta-blockade stabilizes the patient intra-operatively.
- The patient requires life-long thyroxine supplements post-operatively.

Thyroid eye disease

- Organ-specific autoimmune condition characterized by inflammation of the orbital fat and eye muscles.
- Commonly associated with Graves' disease.
- Two phases:
  - Acute—marked oedema.
  - Chronic—fibrosis of orbital contents.
- Graves' orbitopathy results from the infiltration of orbital fat, extra-ocular muscles, and the lacrimal gland by lymphocytes and fibroblasts during the acute phase.
- Orbital fibroblasts are phenotypically unique and in patients with Graves' disease are stimulated to secrete glycosaminoglycans (GAGs) at a rate 100-fold higher than normal extra-orbital fibroblasts.
- Activated orbital fibroblasts participate in the inflammatory event through CD-40 ligation and, in turn, lymphocyte activation.
- As a result, the orbital soft-tissue volume undergoes expansion.
- Orbital soft-tissue fibrosis persists in the stable phase of the disease.
- The signs and symptoms of the orbitopathy are related to the both fibrosis and compression of the intra-orbital contents.

Symptoms and signs

- Heavy, 'gritty' feeling around the eyes.
- Proptosis.
- Diplopia (20–60%).
- Dry eyes (exposure keratitis).
- Reduced visual acuity (10–50%).

Management

- These cases should be managed jointly between a Rhinologist and Ocular-plastic surgeon.
- Ensure the patient is euthyroid.
- Steroids if the orbital oedema develops rapidly.
- Radiotherapy can be used with the risk of cataract formation.
- Orbital decompression is the usual treatment of choice.

Endoscopic orbital decompression

Orbital decompression

- Involves removal of between 1 and 4 of the bony walls of the orbit to allow orbital contents to prolapse into the adjacent spaces.
- Historically, the indications for surgical decompression of the orbit have been to relieve exophthalmos accompanied by corneal exposure and disfigurement, and to reduce the increased orbital pressure produced by swelling of extra-ocular muscles, which can lead to compressive optic neuropathy and visual loss.
- With recent advances in techniques it is now more common to perform cosmetic decompressions.

Relevant anatomy

- The middle turbinate insertion at the skull base represents the medial limit of dissection.
- The fovea ethmoidalis represents the superior limit.
- Lamina papyracea represents the lateral limit.
- The lamina extends from the nasolacrimal system anteriorly to the annulus of Zinn posteriorly.

Aim

To remove the medial wall and part of the floor of the orbit in order to allow the orbital contents to prolapse into the nasal cavity.

Procedure

- Step 1: endoscopic speno–ethmoidectomy; exposure of the whole medial wall from orbital floor to skull base, from agger nassi cell to the sphenoid sinus.
- Step 2: maxillary antrostomy is enlarged to include all the medial wall of the maxillary sinus superior to the inferior turbinate and posterior to the nasolacrimal duct. The infra-orbital nerve is visualized and forms the lateral boundary of the orbital-floor excision. The floor is removed with a Blakesley forceps.
- Step 3: the medial orbital wall is skeletonized (Stamburger drill and a diamond burr) then dissected free off the orbital periosteum using a Frear elevator and an angled curette, while preserving the bone at the frontal recess and optic canal.
- Step 4: periosteal incisions in the lamina papyracea periosteum are perfromed longitudinally in a posterior to anterior direction, to allow herniation of periorbital fat. The orbital-floor periosteal incision begins in the most lateral aspect of the floor and proceeds medially. Incisions are made with a Beaver sickle knife. The fat can be further indrawn by teasing through each incision with a Strumpel–Voss forceps.
- Step 5: the degree of decompression is assessed by gentle manual pressure on the globe.

Other surgical approaches

Three or four wall decompression

May be performed in severe cases but complications such as strabismus, orbital hypothesia/pain, sinusitis, or orbital cellulitis, changes in visual quality and loss of vision occur at a higher frequency.

Balanced two-wall decompression

Endoscopic approach to the medial wall in combination with a lateral decompression (anterior or deep lateral) may reduce the incidence of the above complications. Preservation of the strut of bone between the ethmoids and the floor of the orbit reduces the incidence of post-operative diplopia.

Thyroid neoplasia

- Primary thyroid tumours may arise from either the follicular cells or the calcitonin-secreting cells of neuroendocrine origin found in the normal gland. Papillary and follicular adenocarcinomas are referred to as well-differentiated thyroid tumours.
- The management of thyroid tumours should be undertaken in the context of multidisciplinary teams in specialized units following evidence-based guidelines.
- Core members should include an endocrinologist, surgeon, clinical oncologist and nuclear medicine physician.
- Other key members of the team include a pathologist, radiologist, biochemist, and specialist nurse.

Classification

- Well differentiated:
  - Papillary adenocarcinoma.
  - Mixed-follicular variant of papillary carcinoma.
  - Follicular adenocarcinoma.
- Poorly differentiated:
  - Anaplastic adenocarcinoma.
- Calcitonin-secreting cells of neuroendocrine origin:
  - Medullary carcinoma.
- Lymphoma.
- Metastasis.

Well-differentiated thyroid cancer 1

Papillary
- 65%.
- Age 30–40y.
- ♀ : ♂, 3 : 1.
- Bilateral disease in 30–87%.
- Lymphatic metastases.
- Histology: calcified psammoma bodies, nuclear grooving, 'Orphan Annie' nuclei.

Mixed-follicular variant of papillary carcinoma
- Microfollicular histological pattern.
- Demographics and clinical behaviour similar to papillary.

Follicular
- 30%
- ♀ > ♂.
- 5th decade.
- Seen in endemic goitres associated with iodine deficiency.
- Haematogenous spread.
- Variants: minimally invasive encapsulated, invasive, Hurthle cell carcinoma.

Predisposing factors
- Radiation.
- Age.
- Sex.
- Gardner syndrome.
- Iodine deficiency.
- Endemic goitre.
- Family history (rare for well-differentiated tumours).
- RET proto-oncogene (for medullary only).

Presentation
- Solitary nodule or dominant nodule in a multi-nodular thyroid in a euthyroid patient.
- 10–30% of solitary nodes are malignant.
- Sudden rapid growth.
- Hard, fixed, irregular thyroid swelling.
- Pain.
- Hoarsness.
- Haemoptysis.
- Dyspahagia.
- Stridor.
- Horner's syndrome.
- Cervical lymphadenopathy.

Assessment

- Clinical examination.
- Thyroid-function tests and auto-antibody status.
- FNA (86% sensitive, 89% specific).
- USS.
- Vocal-cord movement.
- Distinguishing between hyperplastic nodule, adenoma, and follicular carcinoma requires histological assessment since it is not possible to identify capsular and vascular invasion by FNAc alone.
- CT/MRI for tumours where the limits cannot be determined or for patients with haemoptysis.

Poor prognostic factors

- Age: <10 years or >40 years.
- Male gender.
- Grade: poorly differentiated.
- Extent: size, extracapsular spread, cervical lymph node metastases, and distant metastases.
- Completeness of resection.

Prognostic scoring systems

- MAICS (metastasis, age, invasion, complete surgical excision, size; see Table 11.1a).
- AMES (age, metastasis, extent, size; see Table 11.1b).

Staging

See Box 11.1.

Table 11.1 Prognostic scoring systems

(a) MAICS

Prognostic Variables	Score			
Presence of distant **M**etastasis	Yes = 3, No = 0			
Age at the time of diagnosis	<39 years = 3.1 >40 = 0.08 × age			
Invasion beyond the thyroid gland	Yes = 1, No = 0			
In **C**omplete surgical resection	Yes = 1, No = 0			
Size of the tumour	0.3 × size (in cm)			
20-year survival rate according to MAICS score				
MAICS Score	<6.00	6.00–6.99	7.00–7.99	>8.00
20-year survival	99%	89%	56%	24%

Table 11.1 (Contd.)

(b) AMES

Low Risk = 1.8% Mortality Rate	High Risk = 46% Mortality Rate
Men <41 years old and women <51 years old	All patients with distant metastases
All men >41 years old and women >51 years old with:	All men >41 years old and women >51 years old with
Intrathyroidal papillary carcinoma with minor capsular involvement	Extra-thyroidal papillary carcinoma
OR	OR
Follicular carcinoma with minor capsular involvement	Follicular carcinoma with major capsular involvement
AND	AND/OR
Primary tumour <5cm in diameter	Primary cancer >5cm in diameter
AND	
No distant metastases	

Box 11.1 TNM staging of well-differentiated thyroid cancer

TX Primary tumour cannot be assessed.

T0 No evidence of primary tumour.

T1 Tumour 2cm or < in greatest dimension limited to the thyroid.

T2 Tumour >2cm but not >4cm in greatest dimension limited to the thyroid.

T3 Tumour >4cm limited to the thyroid or any tumour with minimal extrathyroid extension (e.g. extension to sternothyroid muscle or perithyroid soft tissues).

T4a Tumour of any size extending beyond the thyroid capsule to invade subcutaneous soft tissues, larynx, trachea, oesophagus, or recurrent laryngeal nerve.

T4b Tumour invades pre-vertebral fascia or encases carotid artery or mediastinal vessels.

† Anaplastic carcinomas:

T4a Intrathyroidal anaplastic carcinoma—surgically resectable.

T4b Extrathyroidal anaplastic carcinoma—surgically unresectable.

All categories may be subdivided: (a) solitary tumour, (b) multifocal tumour (the largest determines the classification).

† All anaplastic carcinomas are considered T4 tumours.

Well differentiated thyroid cancer 2: surgical treatment

Guidelines from the British Thyroid Association consensus document (2002)

- A microadenoma (<1cm) which is node-negative is treated with a lobectomy including istmus followed by TSH suppression.
- Tumours >1cm, multifocal disease, extra-thyroidal spread, familial disease, clinically involved nodes, distant metastases, or previous neck irradiation are treated with total thyroidectomy, subsequent radio-iodine ablation, long-term TSH-suppression with thyroxine (T4) and thyroglobulin levels.
- Small tumours with unfavourable histology e.g. Hurthle cell carcinoma may also be managed with total thyroidectomy.
- Central compartment of the neck (level 6) is routinely cleared for tumours >1cm.
- A selective neck dissection levels II–IV is performed when nodal involvement is present.

Surgical treatment of locally advanced disease

- Complete macroscopic clearance, if possible.
- 'Shave' excision may be appropriate.
- Tracheal resection and anastomosis of resected segment, if <6cm.
- Tracheal stents can be used for palliation of acute airway obstruction secondary to poorly differentiated tumours as a palliative procedure.

Post-surgical treatment

- Check calcium (see Table 11.2).
- Start triiodothyronine (T3) 20mcg tds.
- Stop T3 2 weeks prior to radio-iodine ablation.
- Thyroglobulin every 3 months for the first 2 years to check for disease recurrence. Levels <50cg/L signify no evidence of tumour recurrence.
- Follow-up should be life-long.
- Recurrent disease is treated with further surgery and radio-iodine treatment.

Recombinant human TSH

- Avoids symptomatic hypothyroidism following withdrawal of thyroid hormone supplementation.
- Expensive and less sensitive than thyroid hormone withdrawal alone.
- Currently limited to patients in whom thyroxine withdrawal is undesirable.

Table 11.2 Guidelines for the management of hypocalcaemia following total or completion thyroidectomy

Reference range (adjusted):	2.1–2.6mmol/L.

Symptoms of hypocalcaemia:

Weakness/lethargy.

Perioral tingling.

Fingertip tingling.

Carpopedal spasm.

When to measure:

Pre-operatively, 1st evening and morning post-operatively, or any time in the first 36h if hypocalcaemic symptoms occur.

1. Serum calcium normal:	no further action.

2. Mild hypocalcaemia >2.0mmol/L and asympomatic:

No specific treatment.

Calcium check at 6 weeks.

3. Moderate hypocalcaemia 1.81–2.0mmol/L or 2.01–2.10mmol/L with symptoms:

Sandocal 1000 up to 3 tablets b.d. then re-check calcium at 24h.

If >2.0mmol/L, then discharge on 5 weeks of Sandocal then stop. Check calcium at 6 weeks.

If still low, switch to alpha-calcidol 0.5mcg b.d. and Sandolcal 1000 b.d. Discharge patient once calcium >2.0 on two occasions 24h apart. Check calcium at 6 weeks.

4. Severe hypocalcaemia <1.8mmol/L and/or symptoms:

Medical emergency. For an adult, give 10ml bolus of 10% calcium gluconate IV slowly over 4min.

Start alpha-calcidol 0.5mcg b.d. and Sandolcal 1000 b.d. and repeat calcium in 6–8h time.

Radio-iodine ablation therapy

- Destroys microscopic disease.
- Reduces loco-regional recurrence.
- Requires a minimum level >30mU/L of circulating TSH for thyroid remnant to take up iodine.
- Typical dose 3.7GBq.
- Usually performed at 6 weeks following surgery.
- Patient required to be in isolation with specialized shielding facilities for 4–5 days.
- A diagnostic scan is performed 3–5 days following treatment and at 4–6 months following ablation.
- T4 is used for long-term suppression. The dose is adjusted by 25mcg until the serum TSH level is <0.01mU/L.
- Routine follow-up includes measurement of serum thyroglobulin and TFTs every 3–6 months.

Medullary C-cell carcinoma

- Originates from the parafollicular cells (C cells) of the thyroid.
- 5–10% of malignant thyroid conditions.
- Sex ratio ♂ = ♀.
- Regional lymph node involvement 50%.
- 85% occur sporadically.
- 15% familial—three forms:
  - Multiple endocrine neoplasia type 2a.
  - Multiple endocrine neoplasia type 2b.
  - Non-multiple endocrine neoplasia familial.
- Diagnosis is made by FNAc with typically raised serum calcitonin.
- Mutation of the RET proto-oncogene is seen in most cases of familial medularry carcinoma and family members should be screened for this point-mutation.
- Patients with the mutation for MEN2a should undergo prophylactic thyroidectomy before the age of 6; those with the more aggressive MEN2b mutation should undergo thyroidectomy before the age of 2.

Treatment

- Exclude a concomitant pheochromocytoma.
- Total thyroidectomy with a central neck clearance is the only effective treatment.
- A modified radical neck dissection is performed for cervical metastases.
- Mean survival is 50%.

Anaplastic thyroid cancer

- Rare.
- Peak incidence 7th decade.
- Must be distinguished from lymphoma of the thyroid (similar clinical presentation).
- Usually associated with pre-existing thyroid disease supporting the theory that these tumours arise as a result of de-differentiation from more differentiated thyroid cancer.
- Usually presents with a rapidly growing mass with tightness or pressure on the neck.
- Thyroid gland usually diffusely involved and fixed to surrounding structures.

Investigation

- FNAc, incisional or core biopsy, MRI/CT.
- In a patient presenting with stridor, a frozen section may be useful in deciding whether or not the tumour is anaplastic or lymphoma.
- A lymphoma will respond to high-dose steroids, an anaplastic carcinoma will not.

Treatment

- Usually palliative.
- Initial objectives are to ensure airway protection and a route for nutritional support.
- Treatment modalities include: appropriate surgery, chemotherapy, and external-beam radiotherapy.
- Performance status, comorbidities, and patient wishes must be taken into account when making treatment plans.

Thyroid lobectomy

A good way to think about this operation is to consider the structures you will encounter, working from superficial to deep. These are:
- Skin.
- Platysma.
- Strap muscles.
- Middle/inferior thyroid veins.
- Inferior parathyroid.
- RLN.
- Superior parathyroid.

Identification of the RLN is of uppermost importance and can be aided by use of operating loops and nerve-monitoring devices.

Preparation
- GA.
- Reverse Trendelenburg.
- Head ring, shoulder bag to extend the neck.

Incision
- Prep and drap to expose neck from mandible to clavicles.
- Incision two-fingers' breaths above the clavicles extending to the sternocleidomastoid (Fig. 11.3a).

Procedure
- Elevate subplatysmal flaps to the level of the thyroid notch superiorly and surprastrenal notch inferiorly.
- Separate sternohyoid then sternothyroid in the mid line (Fig. 11.3b).
- Identify the trachea inferiorly and cricoid superiorly.
- Dissect the strap muscles off the underlying thyroid lobe to expose the superior and inferior poles.
- The assistant retracts the straps throughout the procedure.
- The straps may need to be divided to provide access.
- The sternothyroid can be divided at the larynx.
- Using a Lahey swab mobilize the inferior pole (Fig. 11.3c).
- Ligate and divide the inferior thyroid veins and middle thyroid vein.
- The assistant retracts the gland medially and using a Lahey swab the fascia on the undersurface of the gland is broken down to find the inferior parathyroid gland which is preserved.
- Identify the recurrent laryngeal nerve using a Lahey swab to sweep the fascia in the direction of the nerve (Fig. 11.3d).
- Mobilize superior pole.
- Identify, ligate, and divide the superior thyroid artery and vein close to the gland dissecting medial to the vessels to avoid damage to the external laryngeal nerve (Fig. 11.3e).
- Identify and preserve the superior parathyroid gland at the level of the cricothyroid junction posterior to the RLN.
- Reflect the parathyroids posteriorly from the thyroid gland, always visualizing the recurrent nerve. A mosquito forceps passed along the course of the nerve facilitates dissection (Fig. 11.3f).

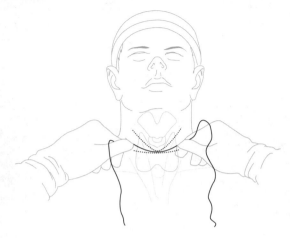

Fig. 11.3 a Some surgeons use a suture pulled tight onto the neck to mark the line of the incision.

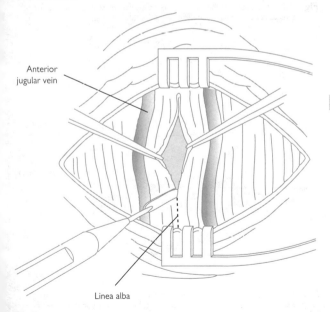

Anterior
jugular vein

Linea alba

Fig. 11.3 b Separation of strap muscles with monopolar diathermy.

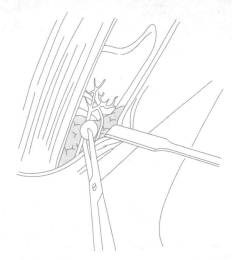

Fig. 11.3 c Dissection of the inferior pole to display the trachea and Inferior thyriod veins. A Lahey Swab is an ideal dissection tool for this.

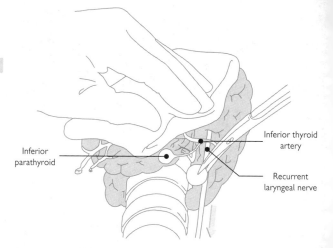

Inferior parathyroid

Inferior thyroid artery

Recurrent laryngeal nerve

Fig. 11.3 d Identification of the inferior parathyroid gland (forceps) and the recurrent laryngeal nerve. A Lahey Swab is swept in the direction of the nerve.

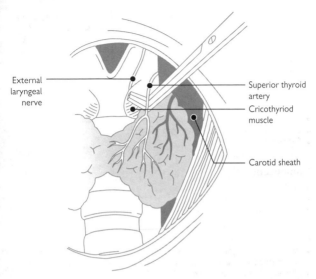

Fig. 11.3 e Dissection of the superior pole. The superior thyroid artery and vein are cleared of fascia and a plane is developed between them and the cricothyroid muscle and external laryngeal nerve.

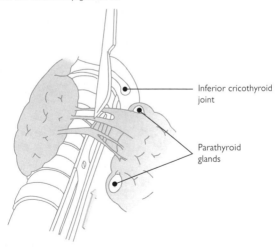

Fig. 11.3 f Division of Berry's ligament. A mosquito forceps is passed along the nerve and opened, allowing safe incision of the ligament.

- Divide the ligament of Berry under direct vision. Be aware that a small leaflet may extend posterior to the RLN making dissection difficult until this leaflet is divided.
- Once the nerve is seen passing behind the cricothyroid joint, the lobe can be dissected free from the trachea across the midline to the istmus.
- Any parathyroid tissue taken with the specimen can be diced and re-implanted in the sternocleidomastoid muscle.
- Haemostasis.
- Saline flood with valsalva helps identify bleeding vessels.
- Loosely re-approximate the strap muscles.
- 3/0 vicryl subcutaneous.
- 4/0 nylon or clips to skin.

Complications
Operative
- Recurrent laryngeal palsy.
- External laryngeal nerve palsy.

Post-operative
Early
- Airway obstruction secondary to haematoma, bilateral recurrent laryngeal palsy, tracheomalacia, or laryngospasm from hypocalcaemia.
- Hypocalcaemia (see Table 11.2).

Late
- Unrecognized hypothyroidism.
- Recurrence.

The parathyroid glands

Anatomy and physiology

- Oval, 6mm in size, weigh up to 60mg.
- Usually four glands (range 2–6).
- Characteristic caramel colour.
- Superior parathyroids arise from the 4th branchial arch, usually located adjacent to the deep aspect of the thyroid gland, posterior to the recurrent laryngeal nerve and inferior thyroid artery, at the level of the cricothyroid joint.
- The inferior parathyroid glands arise from the 3rd branchial arch and descend with the thymus gland and consequently their location is more variable. In the majority they lie within 1cm of the lower pole of the thyroid gland but may be in the thymus gland outside the surgical field.
- Parathyroid hormone acts directly on bone and the kidneys to increase plasma calcium influx and stimulates absorption of calcium from the gut by stimulating 1,25—dihydroxyvitamin D synthesis.

Primary HPT

- Only cause of elevated PTH in the presence of hypercalcaemia.
- Incidence is 25–28/100,000.
- Majority related to a single parathyroid adenoma.

Secondary HPT

- Due to renal disease, vitamin-D deficiency or malabsorption.

Management

- Multidisciplinary thyroid/parathyroid clinic with an endocrinologist, otolaryngologist and oncologist.

Medical

- Bisphosphonates.
- Cinacalcet (oral calcimimetic).
- Oestrogen in post-menopausal women.

Indications for surgery

- Serum calcium >3.0mmol/L.
- Previous episode of life-threatening hypercalcaemia.
- Radiological evidence of nephrocalcinosis or renal stones.

Relative indications

- Serum calcium levels 1mg/dL above upper limit of normal.
- 24-h urinary calcium excretion >400mg.
- A 30% reduction in creatinine clearance compared with age-matched controls.
- Bone mineral density >2.5 standard deviations below peak at any site.
- Age less than 50.

Pre-operative localization

- A combination of sestamibi with ultrasound has been shown to have 96% sensitivity and 100% specificity.
- Sestamibi is a small protein that is labelled with technetium-99 and preferentially taken up by the parathyroid.
- Scintigraphy is used to locate the parathyroids.

Surgical techniques

- If the imaging identifies a solitary adenoma, the patient is offered a minimally invasive parathyroidectomy. Some units will perform intra-operative parathyroid hormone assay to confirm excision of the adenoma.
- If the imaging is negative, the patient is offered bilateral cervical exploration.

For a single adenoma

- Unilateral mini-cervicotomy.
- Methylene blue dye can be administered intravenously pre-operatively.
- The adenoma appears as a smooth, vascular, dark-brown nodule, often bilobed with a rim of fat. Its position is as described above.

Parathyroid carcinoma is treated by *en bloc* tumour resection with ipsilateral thyroid lobectomy.

The neck

Anatomy and nodal levels

Muscles of the neck (Fig. 12.1a)

The deep cervical fascia (Fig. 12.1b)

This comprises of three layers:
- Superficial (investing) layer: arises from the spinous processes and ligamentum nuchae and surrounds the entire neck. It divides to enclose the trapezius muscle, but forms a single layer as it crosses the floor of the posterior triangle. It then splits again around the inferior belly of the omohyoid and sternocleidomastoid.
- Middle (visceral) layer: found in the anterior neck surrounding all the visceral structures.
- Deep layer (pre-vertebral): covers the vertebral muscles and extends laterally on the anterior and medial scalene and levator scapulae muscles, forming the fascial floor of the posterior triangle. The carotid sheath is formed by the fusion of all three layers.

Lymph-node levels

The boundaries of the cervical lymph-node groups are shown in Box 12.1. These levels are referred to clinically when examining a patient with a neck node and intra-operatively when performing a neck dissection; they are vital for histopathology. There are ∴ clinical and operative landmarks that delineate the boundaries.

Lymphatic drainage

The lymphatic system is divided into the deep and superficial systems. The deep system lies alongside the carotid sheath, deep to the investing layer of deep cervical fascia. Understanding the lymphatic drainage patterns from sites in the head and neck is crucial to understanding where a potential primary tumour may be situated and which nodal groups are most at risk. Predictable patterns of spread are recognized. The first group of nodes that a cancer involves is called the first echelon-nodal level. For example the first echelon nodes for tonsil cancer are level III, for nasopharyngeal cancer level V.

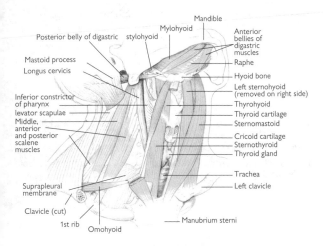

Fig. 12.1 a Muscles of the neck. Reproduced from Oxford Textbook of Functional Anatomy Volume Three (second edition), (2005), by Pamela McKinnnon and John Morris (Oxford; Oxford University Press).

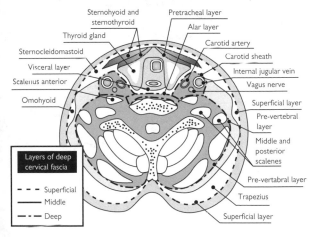

Fig. 12.1 b Layers of deep cervical fascia.

Box 12.1 Boundaries of cervical lymph node groups (Memorial Sloan Kettering Group)

Level I   Submental and submandibular triangles, area bounded by anterior belly digastric, hyoid, posterior belly digastric and the body of the mandible.

Level II   Upper 1/3 IJV, carotid bifurcation to skull base.

Level III   Middle 1/3 IJV, carotid bifurcation to omohyoid.

Level IV   Lower 1/3 IJV, omohyoid to clavicle.

Level V   Posterior triangle, between posterior border of SCM and an anterior border trapezius including supraclavicular nodes.

Level VI   Anterior compartment.

Level VII   Paratracheal nodes.

▶ Clinically the bifurcation of carotid is at the level of the hyoid bone at C4 and the omohyoid is at the level of the cricoid.

Neck masses

Neck masses are relatively common. The majority in children are benign, while in adults most are malignant. When establishing the cause for a neck mass it is worthwhile having a surgical sieve at hand to avoid missing pathology.

Congenital
- Branchial cyst.
- Thyroglossal cyst.
- Laryngocele.
- Plunging ranula.
- Lymphangiomas.
- Haemangioma.
- Teratoma.
- Dermoid cyst.
- Thymic cyst.
- Sternocleidomastoid tumours of infancy.

Infective
- Viral lymphadenopathy, e.g. glandular fever.
- HIV associated.
- Bacterial:
  - Suppurative.
  - Toxoplasmosis.
  - Brucellosis.
- Granulomatous:
  - Cat scratch.
  - Actinomycosis.
  - Atypical mycobacteria.
  - Tuberculosis.
  - Sarcoidosis.
- Fungal.

Inflammatory disorders
- Sinus histiocytosis.
- Kawasaki disease.
- Castleman's syndrome.

Neoplastic
- Metastatic SCC.
- Thyroid masses.
- Lymphoma.
- Salivary neoplasms.
- Paraganglioms.
- Lipoma.

Vascular
- Carotid artery aneurysm.
- Carotid body tumor.

Neck masses 1: congenital

Lymphangioma

- Cystic hygromas are thought to arise from sprouting endothelial fibrillar membranes from the walls of embryological cysts that normally extend centrifugally to form the peripheral lymphatic system. These membranes penetrate the surrounding tissue, canulise it, and produce more cysts, infiltrating planes of least resistance between large muscles or vessels.
- Simple lymphangioma: thin-walled, capillary-sized lymphatic channels (40%).
- Cavernous lymphangioma: dilated lymphatic spaces (35%).
- Cystic hygroma: cysts of various sizes (25%).
- ♂ : ♀, 1 : 1.
- 35% oral, 25% cervical, 15% axillary.
- 60% present at birth, 75% by 1 year, 90% by 2 years.
- Sudden increase in size due to haemorrhage may be fatal.
- Treatment is either excision or injection with sclerosing agent OK432.

Dermoids

- Always midline when in the neck.
- ♂ : ♀, 1 : 1.
- Epidermoid cyst:
  - Most common.
  - No adnexal structures.
  - Lines by squamous epithelium.
  - Contains cheesy keratinous material.
- True dermoid cyst:
  - Lined by squamous epithelium.
  - Contains skin appendages:hair follicles, sebaceous and sweat glands.
  - Congenital along lines of fusion.
  - Acquired through implantation of epidermis in a puncture wound.
- Teratoid cyst:
  - Rarest variant.
  - Lined by either squamous or respiratory epithelium.
  - Contains elements of ectoderm, endoderm and mesoderm: nails, teeth, glands.
- Treatment is complete local excision.

Thyroglossal duct cysts

- Embryological remnant of the duct in which cysts develop.
- The duct runs from the thyroid gland, behind, through, or in front of the hyoid bone and ends deeply at the foramen caecum of the tongue.
- ♂ : ♀, 1 : 1.
- Mean age 5 years.
- 90% midline.
- Most common midline neck cyst.
- Three times more common than branchial cysts.
- Mostly painless, mobile on swallowing or protruding the tongue.
- 75% prehyoid.

- 25% at the thyroid cartilage, the cricoid cartilage or above the hyoid.
- 5% have tenderness and enlargement due to infection.
- 15% have fistulae at presentation.
- Investigations includes TFTs and neck ultrasound to ensure that there is a normal thyroid.
- Treatment is excision including the middle-3rd of the hyoid and tract (Sistrunk's procedure).
- 7–8% recur.

Branchial cysts

- Theories of origin:
  - Remains of pharyngeal pouches or branchial clefts, or a fusion of these two elements.
  - Remains of the cervical sinus of His, which is formed by the second arch growing down to meet the 5th.
  - Inclusion theory suggests that the cysts are epithelial inclusions in lymph nodes; explains why branchial cysts have lymphoid contents and no internal opening.
- Arch of origin:
  - 5–25% 1st.
  - 40–90% 2nd.
  - 2–8% 3rd and 4th.
- Branchial cysts are lined by stratified squamous epithelium, 80% have lymphoid tissue in the wall and they contain straw coloured fluid in which cholesterol crystals are found.
- ♂ : ♀, 3 : 2.
- Peak age 3rd decade.
- 70% clinically cystic, 30% feel solid.
- 1st-arch anomalies are of two types: dorsal and ventral.
- The dorsal type runs medial to the conchal cartilage, extending psoteriorly to the retroauricular scalp. The ventral type presents as a sinus, cleft or fistula, inferior to the cartilaginous ear canal.
- The lesions are variably related to the facial nerve.
- Treatment is total excision with recurrence up to 20% in some series.

Branchial fistulae

- 2nd-arch fistulae result in a skin-line tract from the skin along the junction of the middle to lower two-thirds of the sternocleidomastoid to the anterior aspect of the tonsillar fossa. The tract travels below the stylohyoid and posterior belly of digastric, above the hypoglossal nerve and between the internal and external carotid arteries.
- Presents in young infants as a discharging sinus, which may or may not have an internal fistulous communication.
- Those from the first arch open at the junction of the bony and cartilaginous meatus.

- Fistulae from the 3rd and 4th arches have opening at the level of the piriform sinuse or below. These fistulae route caudal to the glossopharyngeal nerve, over the superior laryngeal nerve, posteromedial to the internal caroid artery piercing the thyrohyoid membrane to enter the pharynx.
- Treatment is excision using several stepladder incisions removing the mouth of the pit in an ellipse.

Neck masses 2: infective/inflammatory

Tuberculous cervical adenitis

- Lymph-node tuberculosis remains a very common manifestation of TB outside the Western World, especially in Asia.
- Presents as a painless enlargement of the node, which caseates and liquefies producing a fluctuant mass.
- Sinus formation is common (50% in Asia), skin involvement, or cold abscesses.
- Diagnosis is by positive skin test, demonstration of acid-fast bacilli in the lymph-node biopsy and growth of *M. tuberculosis* from the biopsy.
- Treatment is with antituberculous chemotherapy followed by excision of any residual disease.

Toxoplasmosis

- World-wide infection caused by *Toxoplasmosis gondii*, a protozoan transmitted by the ingestion of cysts excreted in the faeces of infected cats, or from eating undercooked beef or lamb.
- Symptoms include isolated lymphadenopathy, generalized aches and pains, fever, cough, malaise, macular papular rash.
- Peripheral blood film shows atypical mononuclear cells.
- Diagnosis is confirmed by serum antibodies, lymph-node biopsy, cerebrospinal fluid analysis.

Actinomycosis

- An anaerobic organism that is commensal in the normal healthy oral cavity.
- The organism may become pathogenic when the mucous membrane is injured.
- Clinical features include:
  - Severe dental caries.
  - Firm indurated mass with indefinate edges, usually lateral to the mandible.
  - Untreated, invades adjacent tissue and becomes bony hard.
  - Multiple sinuses which discharge pus and watery fluid containing sulphur granules.
- May be difficult to culture ∴ have a high index of suspicion and treat 'clinically'.
- Treatment is IV benzylpenicillin for several weeks.

Cat-scratch disease

- Acutely tender lymphadenopathy.
- 30% pyrexial.
- 90% give a history of contact with cats.
- Primary papule or vesicle develops at the site of a scratch after 1–2 weeks.
- Papule subsides after a few weeks but may be helpful in the diagnosis.
- Slowly progressive chronic regional lymphadenopathy ensues 1–2 weeks later.

Brucellosis
- Primarily a disease of domesticated animals.
- Human spread occurs by direct contact of infected tissue with conjuctiva or broken skin, ingestion of contaminated meat or dairy products, and by inhalation of infectious aerosols.
- Very varied symptoms in humans.
- 20% have cervical and inguinal lymphadenopathy.
- Undulating fever with sweats, chills and malaise.
- Definitive diagnosis is made by recovering the organism from blood, fluid or tissue specimens.

Infectious mononucleosis (Glandular fever)
See 📖 p. 104.

Investigation of a neck lump

- In an adult, a mass in the neck should be considered neoplastic until proven otherwise. Open biopsy should be deferred until an exhaustive diagnostic work-up, including clinical examination, radiological studies, panendoscopy, FNAc has been completed in an effort to detect the primary lesion.
- If the neck lump is due to metastatic SCC, a thorough history detects most lesions and in asymptomatic patients the examination will detect 65% of lesions.
- FNAc will usually define the problem and identify cell type and tissue of origin.

Indication for open biopsy

- Failure of diagnostic work up to establish diagnosis.
- Cytology suggestive of lymphoma.
- Enlarging neck node in a child.
- Possibility of TB or atypical mycobacterium infection.

Pre-operative management

History

- Hoarseness.
- Dysphagia.
- Pain.
- Otalgia.
- Nasal obstruction.
- Bleeding.
- Night sweats.
- Malaise.
- Weight loss.
- Smoking.
- Alcohol.
- Contact with TB, HIV.

Examination

- Full ENT examination.
- Particular attention to the post-nasal space, oral cavity, posterior 3rd of tongue, tonsil, larynx, pharynx, and thyroid.
- Position, size, and character of node.
- Hard and fixed nodes implies SCC.
- Soft and rubbery nodes implies lymphoma.
- Pulsatile mass implies a carotid body tumour.
- Mobile node in only one direction implies a vagal schwannoma.
- Supraclavicular nodes usually suggest metastatic spread from outside the head and neck region—think chest/breast/GIT.

Investigations

- FNAc (except in young children)—send for microbiology and cytology.
- FBC, ESR, CRP.
- Consider: Paul-Bunnell, Toxoplasma, HIV test.
- Mantoux skin test if there is a suspicion of TB.

- CXR.
- CT neck ± chest.
- MRI.
- Barium swallow.
- USS thyroid.

Endoscopy

- A panendoscopy is indicated if the initial management has failed to reveal a primary site or to make a diagnosis.
- Ideally this should be done by the surgeon who will be responsible for the further management of the patient.
- If this does not reveal any obvious primary, then biopsies should be taken from the PNS, tongue base, piriform fossae and both tonsils should be excised.

FNA—procedure

- Lie the patient down.
- Clean the skin with alcohol.
- Fix the lump between finger and thumb.
- Use a fine needle (blue or orange) attached to a 10ml syringe.
- Pass the needle into the lump.
- Apply suction.
- Move the needle back and forth through the lump using small vibration-type movements—this can prevent contamination by sampling other tissues.
- Make some rotary movements in order to remove a small core of tissue.
- Release the suction, then remove the needle.
- Detach the needle from the syringe and fill it with air.
- Replace the needle and expel the contents onto a microscope slide.
- Remove the needle and repeat, as necessary.
- Check the inside of the barrel of the needle for any tissue which may have become lodged there.
- Take a second slide and place it on top of the first, sandwiching the sample between the two.
- Briskly slide the two apart, spreading the sample thinly and evenly.
- Fix and label the slides.

Lymph-node biopsy: operative technique

Preparation
- GA or LA with sedation, if patient unfit.
- Supine with head elevation.
- A sandbag under ipsilateral shoulder can be helpful.
- Mark incision then turn head away to contralateral side.
- Careful planning of incision is needed if a future neck dissection is planned. This should lie over the node and in a relaxed skin line.
- Infiltrate marcaine 0.25% with 1 : 200 000 adrenaline.
- Prep and drape.

Incision
- Skin.
- Subcutaneous tissue.
- Platysma.

Procedure
- Elevate subplatysmal skin flaps.
- Identify marginal mandibular nerve or accessory, as appropriate.
- For access to the jugular chain of lymph nodes, divide the investing layer of deep cervical fascia along the anterior border of sternocleidomastoid and retract muscle laterally.
- Identify carotid artery, internal jugular vein and any other significant structures such as cranial nerves, e.g. X, XI, XII.
- Identify node by palpation, and exclude any other pathology such as a carotid body tumour.
- Dissect around node to allow an excisional biopsy, where possible.
- If the node is part of a matted mass or adherent to important structures, then an incisional biopsy should be performed.
- Little advantage in excisional versus incisional biopsy if lymphoma is suspected but careful handling to prevent damage to the pathology specimen is needed.
- Haemostasis.

Closure
- Vacuum drain if large cavity.
- Close would in layers.
- 4/0 vicryl to platysma, 5/0 nylon to skin.

Complications
- Intra-operative:
  - Haemorrhage.
  - Carotid sinus reflex.
  - Air embolism.
  - Pneumothorax.
  - Nerve damage.
- Post-operative:
  - Haematoma.
  - Wound infection.

Neck dissection

Four types:[1]
- Radical neck dissection.
- Modified radical neck dissection.
- Selective neck dissection.
- Extended radical neck dissection.

Radical neck dissection

A radical neck dissection involves removal of lymph node levels I–V, SCM, IJV and IX. The main indication is the N-positive neck (however a single node <2cm may be treated with XRT with equal success) or where the treatment of the primary is surgical. Access to the neck may also be required in order to facilitate free tissue transfer.

The radical neck dissection can be modified depending on which non-lympahatic structures, either the SCM, IJV, or IX, are preserved:
- Type I modified RND—preservation of one structure.
- Type II modified radical neck dissection—preservation of two structures.
- Type III (also known as a functional neck dissection)—preservation of all three structures.

An extended radical neck dissection is removal of all the structures in a radical neck dissection plus either a further lymph-node group, e.g. level VI, level VII, or retropharyngeal lymph nodes, or a further non-lymphatic structure, e.g. the posterior belly of digastric or the external carotid artery.

Selective neck dissection

A selective neck dissection describes preservation of one or more lymph node groups and all three non-lymphatic structures, and removal of those nodal groups thought to be at highest risk. There are four different named types based on potential distribution of nodal metastases.
- Supraomohyoid neck dissection (levels I, II, and III) performed for oral cavity tumours.
- Lateral neck dissection (levels II, III, and IV) performed for laryngeal and hypopharyngeal tumours.
- Posterolateral neck dissection (levels II, III, IV, and V) for skin tumours, e.g. melanoma.
- Anterior compartment neck dissection (level VI) for thyroid cancer and some laryngeal cancers.

---

1 American Academy Committee for Head and Neck Surgery and Oncology (1991).

Box 12.2 N-staging for all head and neck sites except the nasopharynx and thyroid[2]

Nx Regional lymph nodes cannot be assessed.

N0 No regional lymph node metastasis.

N1 Metastasis in a single ipsilateral lymph node, 3cm or < in greatest dimension.

N2 Metastasis in a single ipsilateral lymph node, >3cm but not >6cm in greatest dimension; or in multiple ipsilateral lymph nodes, none >6cm in greatest dimension; or in bilateral or contralateral lymph nodes, none >6cm in greatest dimension.

N2a Metastasis in a single ipsilateral lymph node >3cm but not >6cm in greatest dimension.

N2b Metastasis in multiple ipsilateral lymph nodes, none >6cm in greatest dimension.

N2c Metastasis in bilateral or contralateral lymph nodes, none >6cm in greatest dimension.

N3 Metastasis in a lymph >6cm in greatest dimension.

---

2 American Joint Committee on Cancer (AJCC) (2002).

Radical neck dissection: operative technique

Preparation
- GA.
- Reverse trendelemburg.
- Head-ring, shoulder sandbag.
- Turn head to contralateral side.
- Prep and drape.

Incision
- 1 : 100 000 adrenaline infiltration.
- Mastoid to mental incision.
- Lower portion two-fingerwidths below mandible.
- T arm 90 degrees to above, behind carotid bifurcation, overlying the sternocleidomastoid extending to the mid-clavicular point (see Fig. 12.2a).

Procedure
- Subplatysmal flaps raised to body of mandible superiorly, anterior border of trapezius posteriorly, clavicle inferiorly and to the midline.
- Identify and preserve the marginal mandibular nerve (MMN).
- Alternatively identify and ligate the common facial vein and incise the submandibular gland capsule and reflect surpeiorly, thus protecting the MMN. This should not be performed if a facial node is involved with tumour.
- Divide SCM 1cm above insertion.
- Divide omohyoid at the tendon.
- Identify IJV, X, CCA inferiorly.
- Double-tie IJV with 2/0 silk, transfix with 3/0 vicryl, and divide.
- Clamp and ligate any fibrofatty tissue lateral to the IJV stump since this may contain large lymphatic ducts.
- Identify pre-vertebral fascia overlying posterior triangle.
- Look for and divide the tranverse cervical vessels.
- Continue dissection posteriorly 2cm above clavicle until trapezius is reached.
- Divide fascia superiorly along anterior trapezius preserving IX, where possible.
- Roll specimen forward on pre-vertebral fascia preserving phrenic and exposing the levator scapulae and splenius capitus superiorly).
- The roots of the cervical plexus are identified and divided (Fig. 12.2b).
- Expose CCA and X by sharp dissection.
- Divide SCM just below the insertion to the mastoid tip.
- Identify XII above the posterior belly of digastric in Lesser's triangle or between the IJV and the bifurcation of the CCA.

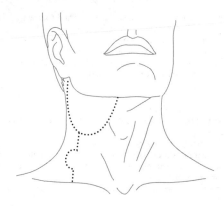

Fig. 12.2 a Incision.

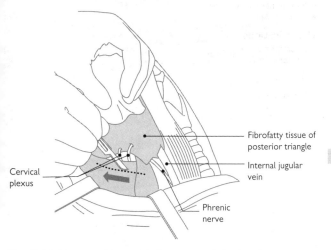

Fig. 12.2 b The roots of the cervical plexus are identified and divided.

- Alternaltively identify descendans hypoglossi and follow this superiorly.
- Identify upper IJV, and divide as per the lower end.
- Dissect IJV with the neck specimen off the carotid artery.
- Now approach the dissection from the medial aspect.
- Identify the contralateral anterior belly of digastric and dissect tissue off the geniohyoid towards the specimen.
- Divide tissue between the inferior border of the mandible and the SMG.
- Identify and ligate facial artery.
- Identify post-border of mylohyoid, retract this anteriorly to reveal lingual nerve.
- Divide submandibular ganglion and duct.
- Ligate facial artery as it crosses under the posterior belly of digastric.
- The level I dissection can now be connected with the rest of the specimen from level II–V.
- The stump of the omohyoid is dissected up to and off the hyoid.
- Water wash.
- Meticulous haemostasis.
- Two size 19 drains.
- Subcutaneous 3/0 vicryl.
- Clips to skin.

Complications
- Haematoma.
- Chylous fistula.
- Infection.
- Carotid artery rupture.
- Nerve damage.
- Facial oedema.
- Failure to control disease.

Deep neck-space infections

The incidence of these potentially life-threatening infections has significantly reduced with the availability of antimicrobial agents, but the diagnosis can still remain confusing and the treatment challenging. Knowledge of the fascial planes of the neck is the key to understanding how these infections start and may spread.

Indications for surgery
- Deep neck-space abscess.
- Protection of an embarrassed airway.
- Prevention of aspiration into the respiratory tract.

Clinical features suggestive of deep neck-space abscess
- Fluctuating pyrexia.
- Pain.
- Dysphagia.
- Odynophagia.
- Neck swelling.
- Trismus.
- Torticollis.
- Airway compromise with retropharyngeal and parapharyngeal abcesses and with Ludwig's angina.

Management
- Dependent drainage of the compartment involved.
- Appropriate high-dose systemic antibiotics.

Retropharyngeal space abscess
Symptoms and signs
- Dysphagia.
- Severe URTI.
- Stiff neck.
- Torticollis.
- Vertebral dislocation.
- Cervical lymphadenopathy.
- Airway compromise.
- Midline swelling of the posterior pharyngeal wall.
- ❶ Infections can rupture into the airway inducing laryngeal spasm and aspiration, as well as spread through the alar fascia into the danger space (pre-vertebral space) and thus into the posterior mediastinum.

Operative approach to a retropharyngeal space abcess
Peroral
This may be the most appropriate approach in a child in extremis. The procedure should ideally be managed with a paediatric anaesthetist or the most experienced anaethetist in the hospital.
- Head down.
- Plenty of suction and light.
- Mouth gag.
- Vertical incision in posterior pharyngeal wall.
- Aspirate contents—MC&S.
- Be prepared to perform a tracheostomy!

External approach
- Skin incision along anterior border of sternocleidomastoid between sternum and hyoid.
- With blunt finger dissection, the SCM and carotid sheath are retracted laterally and the thyroid, superior thyroid vessels and superior laryngeal nerve are reflected medially exposing the abscess at the level of the hypopharynx. The omohyoid, middle thyroid vein and inferior thyroid vessels may need to be divided for access.
- Insert corrugated drain.
- Close skin incision loosely with interrupted sutures.
- High-dose IV antibiotics until clinically improved.
- Watch for signs of mediastinitis over the next week.

Parapharyngeal space abscess

The parapharyngeal space is cone-shaped, with its base located at the skull base and its apex at the hyoid bone. It is divided by the styloid process into two:

- The anterior compartment is related to the tonsillar fossa medially and the medial pterygoid muscle laterally;
- The posterior compartment contains the carotid sheath and the last four cranial nerves.

Signs and symptoms

- Anterior compartment:
  - Marked trismus.
  - Medial displacement of lateral pharyngeal wall and tonsil.
  - Induration at the angle of the mandible.
- Posterior compartment:
  - Medial displacement of the posterior pillar of the tonsil and posterior pharyngeal wall.
  - External induration.
  - Thrombosis of IJV.
  - Rarely haemorrhage from the ICA.

Both are associated with significant sepsis.

Operative approach

- The important landmark is the greater cornu of the hyoid bone.
- Transverse skin incision at this level.
- Identify tip of greater cornu.
- ECA will lie just lateral to this.
- Slide a finger along the posterior belly of digastric and stylohyoid muscles to reach the styloid process in the parapharyngeal space.
- Alternatively identify the carotid sheath in the neck and trace this superiorly to enter the space.
- Send pus for MC&S.
- Insert corrugated drain.
- Close skin loosely with interrupted sutures.

Ludwig's angina

This is a rare infection of the submandibular space. It usually occurs as a result of dental infection. It is more common in adults than in children.

Signs and symptoms

These include pyrexia, drooling, trismus and airway compromise due to backward displacement of the tongue. There may be firm thickening of the tissues of the floor of mouth—best appreciated on bi-manual palpation.

Treatment

High doses of IV broad-spectrum antibiotics (Augmentin). Secure the airway (try a naso-pharyngeal airway first since this will often suffice, but were necessary consider a tracheostomy). Surgical incision is often unsatisfying since little pus may drain away.

Parapharyngeal space tumours

- Arise in the parapharyngeal space.
- 0.5% of head and neck tumours.
- 80% benign, 20% malignant.
- 50% salivary gland in origin, mainly deep lobe of parotid.
- 30% neurogenic in origin (vagal).

Clinical presentation

- Benign tumours usually present late displacing the palatine tonsil anteromedially.
- Malignant tumours present by invasion of surrounding structures.

Imaging

MRI and CT is essential in evaluation of these lesions, and where indicated selective angiograpghy.

Contents of the PPS	
Pre-styloid	Post-styloid
Pterygoid muscles	ICA
Ramus of mandible	IJV
Deep lobe parotid	IX, X, XI, XII
Mandibular branch V	Lymph nodes
Lymph nodes	

Surgical approach

There are three basic surgical approaches to the parapharyngeal space that will depend on the type and extent of the tumour:

- Transcervical approach.
- Transcervical approach with parotidectomy.
- Transcervical approach with midline mandibulotomy.

Allied health professionals

Who are allied health professionals?

This term covers a number of different professional groups including.
- Audiologists.
- Hearing therapists.
- Speech and language therapists (SALT).
- Head and neck specialist nurses.
- Dietician.
- Aural care nurse.

They all have different roles and these are explained in the following pages.

Modern ENT practice has become multidisciplinary and the involvement of these professionals, alongside members of the medical team, has enhanced patient care significantly.

There are many other personnel who are equally important to patient care, such as physiotherapists and occupational therapists. These are not discussed in this handbook.

It is important to use these professional services properly. Get to know the names of the staff in your department, and find out their particular skills and interests. Try to sit in on their clinics to obtain first-hand knowledge of their areas of expertise.

Communicate with these other professionals and give them the respect that their expertise deserves.

The audiologist

The majority of an audiologist's work is with older people and young children. These age groups comprise the majority of hearing problems. The audiologist has a wide-ranging role, encompassing many aspects of patient care.

The main duties of an audiologist are:
• To assess hearing problems.
• To rehabilitate hearing loss with aids.
• To assess balance disorders.
• To rehabilitate balance disorders.
• To give counselling for hearing problems.

Many audiologists specialize within the field of audiology. Particular specialities include:
• Paediatric audiology.
• Cochlear-implant rehabilitation.

The role of the audiologist is extended to allow for liaison with peripatetic services in the community. A child of school age will require support in school if their hearing loss has an educational impact. The audiologist can provide an effective route of communication between the school and the ENT department.

You will need to understand audiological tests and investigations, as they are an important aspect of ENT care. Audiologists are able to offer advice on appropriate tests and their interpretation.

Every practicing otolaryngologist should be able to perform an audiogram and a tympanogram. This is important for clinical practice, in particular, for out of hours assessment when no audiological staff are available. Watching an experienced audiologist perform an audiogram is a good way to become familiar with the technique.

The hearing therapist

This profession has evolved from duties previously undertaken in the audiology department. Many hearing therapists are fully trained audiologists.

The duties of a hearing therapist can include.

- Tinnitus counselling.
- Auditory training.
- Counselling for people with hearing impairment.
- Supportive counselling for families.
- Providing lip-reading advice.

The hearing therapist can spend a considerable amount of time with each patient. This allows for an in-depth discussion of a person's difficulties. This can help to improve the quality of life of affected individuals.

Vestibular rehabilitation

Many patients have vestibular dysfunction arising from the causes discussed in Chapter 13. Central compensation for these problems is often complete and unaided. However, a large number of patients have problems in fully compensating for this type of problem. Their symptoms are often compounded by psychological problems caused by the fear of experiencing a vertigo attack. Targeted exercise programmes combined with counselling by a hearing therapist can overcome these difficulties.

Speech and language therapists (SALT)

Speech and language therapists have an important role to play in some ENT conditions. Many patients who are under the care of the ENT department will need specialist input from the SALT team. A major component of their work is dealing with swallowing disorders.

The main duties of a speech and language therapist are:
- Managing communication disorders. This includes:
  - Assessing the communication capacity of a patient.
  - Helping to determine the prognosis for regaining speech.
  - Determining the patient's need for communication and the aids required.
  - Providing appropriate advice.
- Managing dysphagia. This includes:
  - Assessing the type of swallowing problem.
  - Assessing the risk of aspiration.
  - Assessing possible interventions.

As well as their general duties, the SALT team form part of the multidisciplinary team managing patients with head and neck cancer and voice disorders.

Voice rehabilitation after laryngectomy

Patients undergoing laryngectomy often fear that they will be unable to communicate after surgery. SALTs may help by introducing patients, who have already undergone surgery, to the range of options for rehabilitation. The options for communication after surgery can include:
- Pen and paper.
- Magnetic writing tablets such as Etch-a-sketch.
- Oesophageal speech.
- Electric larynx.
- Tracheo-oesophageal valves.

The head and neck specialist nurse

This nurse specialist is often the glue that holds the head and neck cancer multidisciplinary team together. The role of the head and neck specialist nurse spans the whole of patient care from diagnosis to pre-operative planning to follow-up.

These nurses are uniquely placed to manage patient care; their job flexibility allows them to be active in the community and to extend their care into the home environment. Patients will often view the head and neck nurse as their first point of contact. They are involved early on at the diagnosis stage, up to the patient's final discharge from the clinic.

The main duties of the head and neck specialist nurse are:
- Counselling the patient and their family.
- Explaining and giving information on every aspect of care.
- Liaising with other members of the multidisciplinary team.
- Assessing the suitability of care options, e.g. how the patient might cope with radical surgery.
- Mobilizing support from the family and community services.

Background of head and neck specialist nurses

These are usually very experienced senior grade nurses from head and neck specialties. They will have had previous responsibility, usually at ward sister/charge-nurse level. They will have a degree-level qualification and experience in head and neck or oncological care.

They will also have good counselling skills and the personality to cope with this demanding job.

Extended roles

A head and neck specialist nurse may also have additional roles:
- Nurse trainer.
- Research co-ordinator.
- Protocol design.
- Independent follow-up clinics.

Dietician

From a nutritional point of view, head and neck cancer patients present a wide variety of challenges. The dietician is an extremely important member of the multidisciplinary team.

The main duties of a dietician are:
- To assess the nutritional status of patients.
- To identify specific nutritional concerns.
- To plan dietary interventions.
- To monitor the patient's response to an intervention.

Specific problems and areas of work dealt with by a dietician
- Pre-operative malnutrition:
  - Due to dysphagia from primary tumour.
  - Cachexia of malignancy.
  - Associated alcohol abuse.
- Planning pre-operative feeding regime.
- Planning pre-operative route of nutrition such as PEG/NG tube.
- Post-operative nutrition:
  - Avoiding re-feeding syndrome.
  - Managing nutrition in the absence of swallowing.
  - Non-functioning alimentary tract.
  - Intolerance to enteral nutrition.
  - Electrolyte disturbance.
- Discharge planning.
- On-going care including liaising with community nurses and the patient's family.
- Dietary review in outpatients.

Box 13.1 Houseman's tip

Dieticians often have essential knowledge of electrolyte replacement and supplementation. This expert knowledge can help in planning nutritional requirements for the optimum care of patients. They will also give advice about the frequency and type of investigations needed to monitor these parameters.

Aural care nurse

Aural care nurses provide an important service in the management of ear disorders and have taken on many aspects of otological care. They are trained to recognize problems in the ear canal and the tympanic membrane. They are also skilled in using the operating microscope. Shared care of patients is important and these nurses should be supervised by, or in close contact with, an otologist.

Areas of expertise of an aural care nurse include:
• Wax removal.
• Pre- and post-operative care of patients undergoing ear surgery.
• Continued aural care for chronic ear disorders.
• Diagnosis and management of otitis externa.
• Treatment of mastoid cavity problems.

The aural care nurse's efficient management of these conditions—which represent a large amount of clinical otological practice—has led to increased capacity in the outpatient department.

Aural care nurses are graded 1–3 depending on their level of experience. Grade 3 aural care nurses are able to undertake the full range of aural care from a simple de-wax to the maintenance and cleaning of complex ears with distorted anatomy.

Areas of potential for extending the role of aural care nurses are:
• Direct referral from GP or A&E.
• Nurse prescribing.
• Research and development.
• Guideline and protocol development.

Time spent working and learning from an aural care nurse can help you develop the skills necessary to perform ear surgery. Experience in using instruments with the operating microscope significantly enhances hand and eye co-ordination.

Audiology

Tuning-fork tests

Tuning-fork tests are a basic hearing screening tool to use in conjunction with other methods of hearing assessment; they may or may not support other audiological findings.

There are five tuning-fork test frequencies used clinically to test the hearing (as the C0 fork at 128Hz frequency is used for vibration testing rather than hearing testing): the C1-256Hz to the C5-4096Hz. The most useful fork is C2-512Hz because of the intermediate length of decay to allow enough time for a test to be carried out, and at the same time minimizing the vibratory (rather than auditory) stimulus when the fork is pressed against skin/bone, as happens with the lower frequencies forks.

Several tests can be performed with a tuning fork, the first two are the most commonly used.

Rinne test (Fig. 14.1)

- Compares the air and bone conduction of the patient.
- The tuning fork is made to resonate and its base placed in the mastoid process of the ear to be tested and the patient asked if he/she can hear it (rather than feel it). A gentle but firm pressure is applied with the other examiner's hand to the opposite side of the patient's head to guarantee good contact of the fork's base against the mastoid prominence.
- Then the tines of the fork are placed in line with the external auditory canal (approximately at 2.5–4cm of distance).
- The patient is asked if he/she can hear the sound louder in front or behind the ear, or the same in both.

Results

- **Positive Rinne** (normal hearing or sensori-neural hearing loss): louder at the front or equally loud front and back. It means that air conduction is equal or better than bone conduction (AC≥BC).
- **Negative Rinne** (conductive hearing loss): louder at the back. It means that bone conduction is better than air conduction (BC>AC).
- **A Rinne test** will detect a conductive defect in 50% of patients with an air–bone gap of 20dB, and in 90% of patients with an air–bone gap of 40dB.
- **A false-negative Rinne** test may appear when there is a severe unilateral sensori-neural hearing loss. BC is heard louder than AC, as the sound is transmitted through the skull to the contralateral cochlea of the better hearing ear. Masking the opposite ear with a Bàràny box will likely prevent this situation.

A Bàràny box produces a broadband noise of 90dB A if the instrument is held at a right-angle to the ear and 100dB A when held directly against the ear. There is a potential cross-masking of the test ear as the sound will also travel around the skull to the other ear.

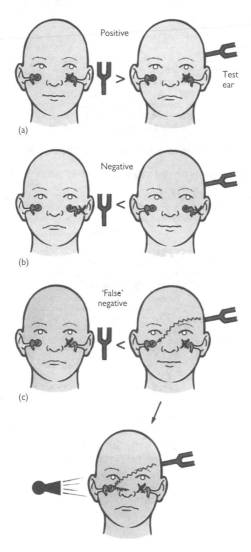

Fig. 14.1 Diagram of Rinne's tests. Reproduced with permission from the Oxford Handbook of ENT and Head and Neck Surgery, Oxford University Press.

Weber test (Fig. 14.2)
- Uses the bone conduction only and tests the lateralization of the sound.
- A resonating tuning fork is placed in the midline of the patient's skull (vertex) or forehead and the patient asked if he/she can hear it in the midline or towards one of the ears. Again, pressure may be applied to achieve good contact of the fork's base against the skull. If the patient cannot hear it at all, try placing the fork against the mandible or upper incisors (protecting the teeth with a surgical glove or similar).
- Normal patients or those with equal hearing loss will hear the fork's sound centrally.
- Unilateral conductive hearing-loss patients will lateralize the sound to the poorer ear.
- Unilateral sensori-neural hearing-loss patients will lateralize the sound to the better ear.
- However, in some cases of unilateral hearing-loss or bilateral mixed hearing-loss the Weber test may not lateralize. It is important to conjugate Rinne and Weber tests results for a more accurate diagnosis.

Stenger test
- A test for 'non-organic hearing loss'.
- Uses air conduction only and is based on the principle that when two sounds of the same frequency are presented simultaneously at the same distance to both ears, only the better hearing ear will perceive the sound.
- Two identical tuning fork tests (512Hz) are activated and presented behind the patient (to prevent any visual clues) in line with the ears and at approximately 15cm.
- Both the genuine and non-genuine patient will report hearing the sound in the better hearing ear.
- Then the tuning fork of the worse (or so alleged) hearing ear is approximated to 5cm of the ear.
- The patient with non-organic hearing loss (NOHL) will deny hearing any sound. The tuning fork held near the worse ear (at 5cm) will mask the sound of the tuning fork near the better ear (at 15cm).
- The genuine patient will only hear the tuning fork near the better ear (at 15cm).
- There are other tuning fork tests (Bing, Gellé, Schwabach), however these have largely been replaced by pure-tone audiometry and are mainly of historical interest only.

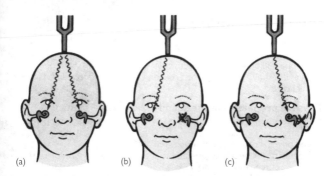

Fig. 14.2 Diagram of Weber's tests. Taken from the Oxford Handbook of ENT and Head and Neck Surgery. Reproduced with permission by Oxford University Press.

Pure-tone audiometry

(see Table 14.1 on 📖 p. 308 for summary table)

Pure-tone audiometry is a subjective test that aims to establish pure-tone hearing threshold, i.e. the quietest sound that can be perceived at different frequencies.

Physical properties of the sound—the decibel scale

Sound travels in waves. In air it travels at 340m/s (at standard temperature and atmospheric pressure).

The physical properties of sound are:
- Frequency (or pitch), determined by the frequency of vibration of the sound source; and
- Intensity, which is the sensation of sound loudness (dependant on the energy applied by the sound source).

The bel is a logarithmic unit that indicates the ratio between two different intensities (the measured one and a reference one). In practice a smaller unit, the decibel (dB) is used:

$$n\text{dB} = 10 \log_{10} I_1/I_2$$

where I_1 and I_2 are the measured and reference intensities, respectively.

The decibel scale is therefore a logarithmic scale. A change of intensity of 2-fold equals to a 3dB change, a 10-fold increase equals to a 10dB change, and a 100-fold increase to a 20dB increase.

Interestingly by coincidence, 1dB is the least perceptible difference of loudness detected by the human ear at speech frequencies.

There are several decibel scales that can be used to measure hearing thresholds.

Decibel hearing-level (HL) scale

This is the most commonly used. A decibel scale of human hearing was created, and the 0dB value designated for each frequency was the median value of the minimal audible intensity (threshold) of pure tones in a group of healthy (normally hearing) individuals, in accordance with the International Standards Organization (ISO).

The amount of energy at 0dB HL for each frequency is not the same. The representation of a normal hearing individual in dB HL scale will be a flat audiogram. In clinical work:
- The threshold of hearing is defined as 0dB HL.
- A whisper from 1m distance has an intensity of 30dB.
- Normal conversation, 60dB.
- A shout, 90dB.
- Discomfort is felt at 120dB.

Decibel sound pressure level (SPL) scale

In this dB SPL scale there is an equal amount of energy at each frequency, but it was considered that the use of this scale in an audiogram would make abnormalities difficult to identify in the normal U-shape nature of this audiogram.

Decibel A scale

The reference intensity (I_2) is adjusted to reflect ambient low frequencies and is closer to normal hearing sensitivity. It is used in industrial noise measurements.

Decibel sensation level (SL) scale

The reference intensity (I_2) is an individual's threshold. If a person has a threshold of 20dB HL at 1000Hz, the 40dB SL for that person will be 60dB HL.

Standard manual audiometric testing 1

The audiometer is an electronic instrument that delivers pure tones at frequencies between 125 and 8000Hz (hertz) at selected intensities.

Equipment

It consists of:

- a stimulus selector (pure tones, or warbled, narrow-band, white or speech noise);
- an output selector (right, left, or both headphones, or insert earphone, or speakers, or bone oscillator);
- a frequency dial (125–8000Hz); output attenuator (in 5dB steps from – 10dB to +110dB); and
- an interrupter switch/bar (to present or interrupt the stimulus).

The equipment should meet the performance requirements and be calibrated daily, weekly, and every 3 months to 1 year (pure tone within 3% of intended frequency and ± 1dB of accuracy) in accordance to British Standard and ISO criteria.

Environment

The test is carried out preferably in a sound-proof room, or with an ambient noise not exceeding 35dBA; if it is higher than this, it is recommended not to proceed with audiometry.

The subject should be clearly visible to the tester (within the same room, or from outside the room through a window or CCTV system), and in turn the subject should not be able to see or hear the tester adjust the audiometer controls.

Preparation of test subjects

- Before starting the test, otoscopic examination should be done and removal of occluding wax carried out, if necessary.
- The subject should be asked about any recent noise exposure, any tinnitus, and which one is the better hearing ear.
- Start the test with that ear, and also make an informal assessment of the extent of the hearing loss.
- Remove any hearing-aids and glasses, and any other accessories that may interfere with the correct placement of the test transducers (headphones, or if not possible insert earphones).
- Prolonged test time (over 20min) will fatigue the subject and can affect the result. In this situation, a short break may be beneficial.

Instructions

Give clear information about the task:

'I am going to test your hearing by measuring the quietest sounds that you can hear. As soon as you hear a sound, press the button. Keep it pressed for as long as you hear the sound, no matter which ear you hear it in. Release the button as soon as you think you no longer hear the sound. Whatever the sound and no matter how faint the sound is, press the button as soon as you think you hear it, and release it as soon as you think it stops.'

Standard manual audiometric testing 2: procedures

Air conduction pure-tone audiometry without masking

- Start with the better-hearing ear at a frequency of 1kHz.
- Next test 2, 4, 8, 0.5, and 0.25kHz in that order. Then retest at 1kHz. Testing other frequencies (3 and 6kHz) may also be needed.
- Test the opposite ear in the same order.
- When presenting a tone, the duration of it should be between 1 and 3s.
- Be careful not to create a pattern.
- The first tone presented to the subject should be clearly audible (i.e. at 40dB). If there is no response increase the level of the tone in 20dB steps until a response occurs.
- Following a satisfactory response, reduce the level of the tone in 10dB steps until no further response occurs.
- Increase the level of the tone in 5dB steps until a response occurs.
- Continue this procedure, as required, until the individual has 50% or more of the responses correct.

Bone conduction pure-tone audiometry without masking

- Without masking it is not possible to determine which ear is responding to BC testing.
- The bone vibrator is placed over the mastoid prominence of the worse hearing ear; alternatively, it can be placed on the forehead (but requires a series of correction values).
- The test is similar to that used in AC but is only performed in the 500–4000Hz frequencies range.
- Vibrotactile responses may appear at 55dB at 500Hz and 70dB at 1000Hz, and care should be taken not to misinterpret this as hearing response.

Masking in pure tone audiometry

It is not always certain that the intended tested ear is the one actually detecting the sound. Masking is necessary when there is a risk of cross-hearing due to inter-aural (transcranial) transmission of sound to the contra-lateral cochlea. This can vary from 40 to 80dB in AC and from 5 to 15dB in BC, depending on individuals and type of earphone used.

Masking is carried out by placing a masking (narrow band) noise into the non-tested ear of the appropriate intensity to prevent it from detecting the test signal (10dB above threshold).

Rules of masking

There are three rules of masking:

Rule 1: air conduction audiometry i.e. AC (test) – AC (non-test) ≥40dB. Where the difference between the not-masked air conduction of the test and non-test ear is ≥40dB. Mask the better (on air conduction) ear.

Rule 2: bone conduction audiometry. i.e. AC – BC ≥10dB.

Where the difference between the not-masked air and bone conduction (air–bone gap) is ≥10dB. Mask the better (on air conduction) ear.

Rule 3: air conduction audiometry. i.e. AC (test) – BC (non-test) ≥40dB.

Where the difference between the not-masked air conduction of the test ear and the not-masked bone conduction of the non-test ear is ≥40dB. Mask the better (on bone conduction) ear.

Uncomfortable loudness levels

This is the lower intensity level that is judge to be uncomfortably loud to the subject. This information is helpful for a hearing-aid fitting.

Recruitment

The loudness recruitment phenomenon occurs in hearing-impaired ears, especially those with sensori-neural hearing loss (i.e. presbyacusis) and is defined as a greater increase in the perception of sound loudness in relation to an increase in sound intensity than in normal ears. The dynamic range of the affected ear to perceive different sound intensities is reduced.

Recruitment is thought to occur because in sensori-neural hearing-loss there is a greater reduction in the number of outer hair cells than of inner hair cells.

When a loud sound is presented to the cochlea, the activation of cochlear nerve fibres will be dependant on the number of inner hair-cells, and these ones, being less affected than the outer ones, will create a greater sensation of loudness.

Audiogram format, examples, and results

In Fig. 14.3 are representative audiograms of normal hearing (Fig. 14.3a), conductive hearing loss (Fig. 14.3b), and sensori-neural hearing loss (14.3c). The British Society of Audiology recommends the description or interpretation of hearing thresholds on an audiogram as:

- 'Normal' hearing thresholds are considered to be 20dB or better.
- 'Mild' hearing loss between 20 and 40dB.
- 'Moderate' loss from 41 to 70dB.
- 'Severe' loss from 71 to 95dB.
- 'Profound' loss worse than 95dB.

In the surgical world, audiometry is one of the main outcome measures to report in studies and to audit surgeon's results. In these cases, pure-tone average is calculated for the 500, 1000, 2000, and (more frequently now) 3000Hz frequencies AC thresholds, and for the 500, 1000, and 2000Hz frequencies BC thresholds. Then AC, BC, and the air–bone gap average can be calculated and compared pre- and post-intervention.

To see the recommended format and symbols for audiogram forms, go to: http://www.thebsa.org.uk/docs/RecPro/PTA.pdf

Békésy audiometry

This technique, rarely used now but of historical importance, uses a specialized audiometer, which presents a continuous or pulsed tone, sweeping from low to high frequencies. The subject adjusts the intensity of the tone by pressing a button when the tone is heard that lowers the intensity of the signal. When the signal cannot be perceived the button is released, which increases the intensity of the signal. A zig-zag printout is obtained for the entire frequency range.

This test can be self-administered and is ideal for screening, and also gives additional auditory information such as abnormal adaptation (also known as tone decay), recruitment, and non-organic hearing loss.

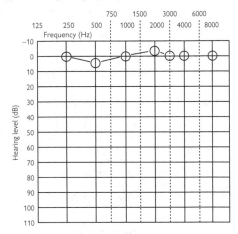

Fig. 14.3 a Normal hearing (right ear). Reproduced from *Diseases of the Ear* (Harold Ludman and Tony Wright), with permission of Edward Arnold (Publishers) Ltd ©1997 Arnold.

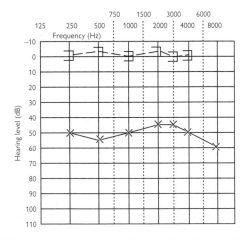

Fig. 14.3 b Left conductive hearing loss. Reproduced from *Diseases of the Ear* (Harold Ludman and Tony Wright), with permission of Edward Arnold (Publishers) Ltd ©1997 Arnold.

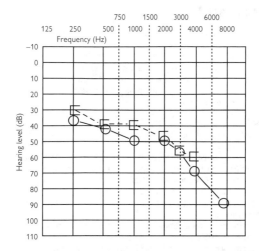

Fig. 14.3 c Right sensoneural loss. Reproduced from *Diseases of the Ear* (Harold Ludman and Tony Wright), with permission of Edward Arnold (Publishers) Ltd ©1997 Arnold.

Speech audiometry

Speech audiometry is a method to assess auditory discrimination. It offers a more realistic representation of an individual's hearing as opposed to pure-tone audiometry (PTA). In PTA the hearing is tested for the ability to hear a pure tone (thus establishing hearing thresholds), whereas speech sounds are a complex amalgamation of a large number of tones and other noises, ∴ speech audiometry has a better role in assessing the impact of the hearing impairment.

Method

- The test can be delivered to only one ear through headphones or free-field to both ears.
- A standardized list of phonetically-balanced words, such as Boothroyd, Fry, and Medical Research Council are used. Alternatively a sentence list may be preferred in for children e.g. –Bamford–Kowal–Bench (BKB).
- The individual is asked to repeat the words.
- A score is created with the percentage of words or phonemes correctly identified.
- The optimum discrimination score (ODS) is the highest score achieved (maximum is 100%).
- The speech-reception threshold (SRT) is the sound level at which the individual obtains 50% of the score.
- The half-peak level (HPL) is the sound level at which the individual obtains half his/her ODS.
- Half-peak level elevation (HPLE) is the comparison (difference) of the HPL of the tested individual with the HPL of normal individuals.
- The speech audiogram curve (Fig. 14.4) distinguishes conductive from sensori-neural hearing-loss.
- In conductive hearing-loss the ODS is excellent with increased sound level. This curve is very similar to one of normal hearing but displaced towards the right.
- In sensori-neural hearing-loss, the ODS is smaller and speech discrimination deteriorates with increased sound levels—'roll-over'.

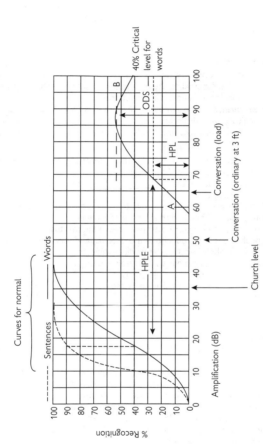

Fig. 14.4 Speech audiogram. Reproduced from *Diseases of the Ear* (Harold Ludman and Tony Wright), with permission of Edward Arnold (Publishers) Ltd ©1997 Arnold.

Acoustic impedance

Impedance has as principle the opposition to the flow of energy in a sound wave. There are two tests used in clinical practice:
- Tympanometry.
- Acoustic reflexes.

Tympanometry

It is an important objective test of middle-ear function. The sound transmission from the external to the middle ear is optimal when the pressure in the ear canal is the same as the middle ear.

The compliance of the tympanic membrane is measured as a function of mechanically varied air pressure in the external auditory canal and hence the middle-ear pressure is indirectly measured.

Method
- A probe is placed in the external auditory meatus creating an air-tight seal. The probe consists of three devices:
  - A sound producer, that delivers a continuous pure tone sound wave (probe tone).
  - A sound receiver, that transmits the waves back from the meatus into a microphone and then converted in electrical activity.
  - A pump that changes the air pressure in the meatus.
- The probe tone is introduced in the external auditory canal, of which some will be absorbed and some will be reflected.
- The air pressure in the ear canal is slowly raised to $+200mmH_2O$, and then gradually reduced to $-200mmH_2O$.
- The compliance can be measured by measuring the amount of sound energy reflected with the microphone. The compliance will be maximal (peak of the plotted curve) when there is no difference of pressure across the tympanic membrane.

Tympanogram graphs
There are several types of tympanogram graphs (Jerger classification, Fig. 14.5):
- **Type A**: normal. Peak is at $0mmH_2O$, range from -100 to $+200$. The peak can be shallow, and this could represent restricted tympanic membrane movement (as in otosclerosis or other ossicular fixation, and tympanosclerosis), or high, representing hyper-compliance (ossicular disarticulation, flaccid tympanic membrane).
- **Type B**: flat or very low, rounded peak. Has a 96% positive predictive value for middle-ear effusion. It can also represent a tympanic membrane perforation; ∴ the shape of the curve must be read jointly with the compliance (canal) volume, which will be normal in the effusion and high in the perforation.
- **Type C**: shows low pressure in the middle ear and represent Eustachian-tube dysfunction:
  - C_1: peak in the negative pressure region, range from -100 to $-200mmH_2O$.
  - C_2: as above but range from -200 to $-400mmH_2O$.

- **C_3**: range from −400 to −600mmH$_2$O. (Most tympanogram machines do not reach below the −400mmH$_2$O, ∴ it could be represented as a type B curve).

Ear-canal volume

In any type of curve, normal compliance volume is approximately 2ml in adults, slightly less in children. When larger canal volumes are obtained, they can represent either a tympanic membrane perforation or a very large pars tensa retraction, where the volume measured equals the ear canal and the middle-ear volumes.

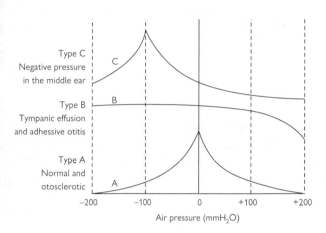

Fig. 14.5 Tympanogram graphs. Reproduced from *Diseases of the Ear* (Harold Ludman and Tony Wright), with permission of Edward Arnold (Publishers) Ltd ©1997 Arnold.

Acoustic reflexes

Acoustic-reflexes testing is an objective measure of the contraction of the stapedius muscle (bilateral), providing the facial nerve and brainstem function normally.

The acoustic-reflex pathway consists of:
- the ipsilateral auditory nerve;
- ipsilateral cochlear nucleus;
- bilateral superior olive complexes; and
- bilateral facial nucleus and nerves.

Measuring the threshold, latency, decay, and amplitude of the reflex gives diagnostic information to localize pathology (cochlear, retrocochlear, or in the brainstem).

The most used measurement is the acoustic or stapedial reflex threshold; i.e. the minimum sound intensity required to produce the stapedius muscle contraction, which is between 70 and 100dB above the normal hearing threshold.

Method

The same equipment as for tympanometry is used, with the addition of a mono-aural headset that delivers sound to the contralateral ear, when contralateral reflex is tested.

Reflexes can be stimulated using pure tones, or wide- or narrow-band noises. Usually one or two pure tones at 500, 1000, 2000, and 4000Hz are used.

At approximately 80dB HL there will be a deflection in the compliance plot that indicates there is a reflex present. If there is no deflection, the sound level is increased until a reflex is obtained or until the maximum output of the machine is reached (120dB).

Clinical applications of stapedial reflex

Facial paralysis
- A present reflex implies that the lesion of the facial nerve is distal to the branch that innervates the stapedius muscle.
- Also to monitor facial nerve function during recovery of the paralysis.

Otosclerosis
- Absent reflex due to stapedial fixation.

Retrocochlear lesion
- Abnormal reflex decay (or adaptation) was used for the diagnosis of acoustic neuroma pre-MRI.

Oto-acoustic emissions

Oto-acoustic emissions (OAEs) are sounds originated in the cochlea that can be recorded by a sensitive microphone fitted in the ear canal. These sounds are created by the movements (electromotility) of the outer hair cells in the cochlea as they respond to auditory stimulation. This mechanism, known as the 'cochlear amplifier', contributes significantly to the sensitivity and discrimination (fine tuning) of hearing by amplifying the sound-traveling wave in the basal membrane of the cochlea (see 📖 p. 458).

The OAEs can be as loud as 30dB SPL, and are generated only when the organ of Corti and the middle ear are in near normal condition. OAEs are affected by conductive and sensori-neural hearing losses.

Method

A tight-fitting ear canal probe containing:
- a loudspeaker;
- a sensitive microphone; and
- a signal-separating processor that can discriminate the sound of the OAE from the stimulus sound and other noise.

The testing does not require patient cooperation, but ear-canal patency is essential, and background room-noise levels should be below 40dB.

The acoustic stimulus inserted through the speaker can vary from no stimulus, to click stimuli (wide-band noise), or tones (narrow-band noise). The choice of stimulus determines what portion of the cochlea is stimulated (frequency specific response).

Each individual has his/her own characteristic repeatable OAE. Repeatability or reproducibility is used to verify the response.

Types of OAEs

Can be broadly classified into two groups:
- **Spontaneous OAEs (SOAEs)**: occur without any stimulus in about half of the population. They have little clinical use.
- **Evoked OAEs (EOAEs)**: occur during or after a stimulus, and can be classify into:
  - **Transient evoked OAEs (TEOAEs)**: occur between 4 and 20ms after a click stimulus of around 84dB SPL. The response contains multiple frequencies between 700 and 4000Hz, and only if hearing thresholds are 20dB HL or better.
  - **Stimulus frequency OAEs (SFOAEs)**: occur by the stimulation of a continuous pure tone. The response is at the same frequency. They are of little clinical use.
  - **Distortion product OAEs (DPOAEs)**: occur as a response to two simultaneous pure tones (typically 55 and 65dB SPL) at two different frequencies. By using different frequencies combinations a larger portion of the basilar membrane can be stimulated and its response analysed. The response occurs in the 1000–8000Hz frequency range. DPOAEs are, however, unreliable to estimate an individual's hearing threshold.

Clinical applications

- TEOAEs and DPOAEs are complementary, as the former is best detecting threshold elevation below 3000Hz, and the latter above it. The former gives an overview of cochlear activity, the latter specific information to one set of pure tones.
- TEOAEs main use is in neonatal screening, while DPOAEs are better suited for advanced clinical and research investigation mainly on adult patients.
- OAEs are also useful to monitor changes in cochlear status over time as in during surgery for acoustic neuroma, sudden hearing loss, Ménière's disease, loud noise, and ototoxicity exposure, and suspected non-organic hearing loss.

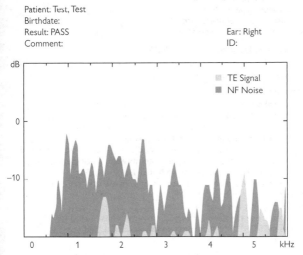

Patient. Test, Test
Birthdate:
Result: PASS   Ear: Right
Comment: ID:

Right: 24-Apr-07: Stab:100% : TE Screen, 70% at 3/4 freq. for pass: 07D23T00.TE

Frq (kHz)	Repro (%)	TE (dB)	NF (dB)	TE-NF (dB)	Result
1.0	97	4.5	−9.6	14.1	–
1.5	96	1.0	−10.0	11.0	Pass
2.0	83	5.3	−4.5	9.8	Pass
3.0	88	4.5	−6.1	10.6	Pass
4.0	73	2.7	−4.8	7.5	Pass
1.2–3.5	87	8.8	−1.6	10.4	–

Fig. 14.6 Transient evoked OAE (TEOAE).

Electric-response audiometry

Electric-response audiometry (ERA) records the bioelectrical potentials ('brainwaves') that arise in the auditory pathway in response to sound stimulation (auditory evoked potentials). These bioelectric potentials have very small amplitude, and they are difficult to separate from other neural activity. To achieve this, the summation of different responses to multiple sound stimuli is used to enhance the auditory electrical response and cancel other electrical background activity.

ERA testing does not require patient's active cooperation, but the complex tracings obtained must be interpreted by the tester, ∴ becoming subjective the test.

There are three types of ERA:
- Electrocochleography.
- Auditory brainstem response.
- Cortical electrical audiometry.

Electrocochleography (ECochG)

Measures the electrical output of the cochlea and the auditory nerve in response to an auditory stimulus.

Technique
- Subject lies comfortably in a sound-proof room.
- A ground electrode is placed on the forehead, and a reference electrode on the mastoid prominence of the tested ear.
- The active electrode can be extra-tympanic, placed close to the tympanic membrane in the external auditory canal, or trans-tympanic, via a needle (through the tympanic membrane) in contact with the promontory of the cochlea close to the round window niche.
- The test sound signal can be a series of wide-band clicks or tone bursts, which can be produced using headphones.
- Masking is not necessary in ECochG.
- The response obtained is measured over a 10ms period (usually between 1.5 to 4ms depending on the intensity), and consists of (Fig. 14.7):
  - The cochlear microphonic (CM) is an electrical wave-form that resembles the vibratory pattern of the basilar membrane and indicates that the cochlear hair cells are intact. Its precise mechanism of origin is not well-understood.
  - The summating potential (SP) also originated in the hair cells, and is an alteration of the electrical potential baseline in response to an auditory stimulus. It has a positive and a negative part. SP can be used in the diagnosis of Ménière's disease.
  - The action potential (AP) is the electrical response of the auditory nerve, and it is useful for determining thresholds.

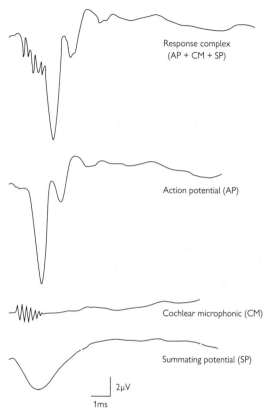

Fig. 14.7 Electrochleographic response complex. Reproduced from *Diseases of the Ear* (Harold Ludman and Tony Wright), with permission of Edward Arnold (Publishers) Ltd ©1997 Arnold

Clinical applications
- Threshold determination, to within 5–10dB at 3–4kHz. It is the most accurate objective test to determine thresholds at these frequencies.
- Ménière's disease diagnosis. There is an increased SP/AP ratio (>30%).
- Acoustic neuroma diagnosis. Broad AP with normal CM.

Auditory brainstem response (ABR)
Also known as brainstem evoked response (BSER), measures the electrical response in the auditory nerve and brainstem.

Technique
- Subject lies comfortably in a sound-proof room.
- The active electrode is placed on the forehead.
- A reference electrode is placed on the mastoid prominence of the tested ear, and the ground electrode on the contralateral side.
- The test sound signal is identical to EChocG, but with different settings and filters.
- Masking may be necessary.

The waveform created in ABR (Fig. 14.8) testing has five waves or levels of the auditory pathway where the responses originate:
I. Auditory nerve.
II. Cochlear nucleus.
III. Superior olivary complex.
IV. Lateral lemniscus.
V. Inferior colliculus.

The results are recorded in the 10–15ms after the stimulus, and analysed looking particularly at the latency of waves I–V, normal values being: 4.2 ± 0.2ms, and the inter-aural I–V latency 0 ± 0.2ms.

Clinical applications
- Acoustic neuroma diagnosis (pre-MRI time). Latency I–V > 4.2 ± 0.2ms, and the interaural I–V latency 0.2–0.4ms.
- Threshold determination. Especially in children (used with Oto-acoustic emissions in neonatal screening). Can detect threshold, but not frequency specific.
- Intra-operative testing. During acoustic neuroma surgery.

Cortical electrical audiometry (CERA)

Measures the electrical response (to a sound stimulus) in the cortex, and subsequently the entire auditory mechanism is tested.

Technique
- Subject sits comfortably in a sound-proof room, awake and avoiding mental or physical activity.
- A ground electrode is placed on the forehead, and a reference electrode on either mastoid prominence.
- The active electrode is placed on the vertex.
- The preferred test signal is tone bursts.
- The potentials are recorded between 30 and 100ms after the stimulus.

Clinical applications
- Threshold determination. The best of the three methods described in this section to determine thresholds across all frequencies.
- Assessing central problems.

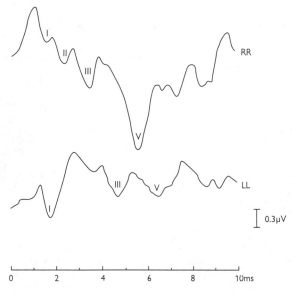

Fig. 14.8 Normal ABR (above) compare to abnormal ABR (below). Reproduced from *Diseases of the Ear* (Harold Ludman and Tony Wright), with permission of Edward Arnold (Publishers) Ltd ©1997 Arnold.

Table 14.1 Summary of hearing tests, their characteristics and applications

Type	Frequency specific	Screening	Objective	Subjective	Applications
PTA	yes	x	x	yes	• Hearing thresholds and type of loss
Speech audiogram	x	x	x	yes	• Hearing thresholds and type of loss • Acoustic neuroma[*]
Acoustic reflex	yes	x	yes	x	• Facial nerve palsy • Otosclerosis • Acoustic neuroma[*]
OAEs	yes	yes	yes	x	• Hearing thresholds • Intra-operative monitoring • Research
ABR	x	yes	x	yes	• Hearing thresholds • Intra-operative monitoring • Acoustic neuroma[*]

[*] Superseded by MRI.

Vestibular function testing 1

The vestibular organs, together with the eyes and the propioceptors in the muscles and joints of the body, are the sensory part of the system with connections to the brainstem, cerebellum, and brain, responsible for maintaining balance.

The aim of vestibular function testing is to assess whether the vestibular organs are responsible for the patient's symptoms, the side of the lesion, and whether the lesion is peripheral (labyrinth or vestibular nerve) or central (brainstem, cerebellum, brain). There are two main tests used for this purpose:

- Electronystagmography.
- Caloric testing.

Electronystagmography (ENG)

This is an electronic test to record eye movements by using the difference of potential between the cornea and the retina (the retina being negative respect to the cornea).

Technique

- An active electrode is placed close to the lateral canthus of each eye, and above and below the eye (to monitor horizontal and vertical movements).
- A ground electrode is placed on the forehead.
- Movement of the eyes will cause a difference of potential, between the two active electrodes, which is proportional to amplitude of the movement and can be recorded.
- Alternative to the electrode system is a pair of modified Frenzel glasses, incorporating a camera to video-record eye movement with the appropriate accompanying computer software.
- Eye movement to the right will produce (by convention) an upwards trace on the recording, and the opposite if movement to the left.
- A laser light is placed at 8.5m from the subject and, after calibration, the light is moved at different speeds and patterns to evaluate the slow-phase velocity, the frequency, and duration of the eye movements.
- The eyes are tested open, closed, and with mental exercises to remove any cortical suppression of the nystagmus.

ENG can be used to evaluate eye movements controlled by the visual system interacting with the vestibular and central nervous system (vestibulo-occular reflex, VOR). These movements are:

- saccades;
- smooth pursuit; and
- optokinetic nystagmus.

Their function is to maintain gaze stability to allow smooth tracking of a moving object (i.e. watching the ball at a tennis match), and their analysis helps to establish if the pathology is peripheral or central.

Saccades

These are very fast eye-movements (350–600 degrees/s), which bring the image of an object to the fovea as quickly as possible. They can occur normally if the target (i.e. laser light) is moved more than 30 degrees to either side of the midline. The presence of saccades depends on the brainstem function, but can also be affected by central nervous system pathology.

Abnormal saccades can be overshooting (hypermetric) or undershooting (hypometric). The former implies cerebellar pathology; the latter, brainstem or basal ganglia. Absence of saccades implies central nervous system pathology.

Smooth pursuit

This is responsible for maintaining gaze on a moving target, by keeping the image on the fovea. Eye and target velocities should be the same. If the eyes are unable to follow the target (too fast target or CNS disease), saccades will appear. The smooth pursuit depends on the brainstem, cerebellum and cortex. Impaired bilateral smooth pursuit occurs by the use of drugs (psychotropics, sedatives, antiemetics, anticonvulsants) and alcohol.

Optokinetic nystagmus (OKN)

This is responsible for tracking moving objects, by keeping the image on the retina (not the fovea as above). Stimulation of this system leads to a slow, tracking eye-movement (slow phase) followed by a saccade to the opposite direction (fast phase). It occurs in normal individuals when, e.g. looking at the landscape from a moving vehicle. The direction of the nystagmus is, by convention, the one of fast phase. The OKN depends on an intact brainstem and cortex.

Unilateral pathology produces abnormality of the OKN when the object is moving towards the affected side. In this case there will be abnormality also of the smooth pursuit, as this one overlaps with the slow phase of the OKN. Whereas the fast phase of OKN overlaps with the saccadic movement.

Caloric testing

First described by Bàràny in 1906, this tests the integrity of the vestibular system. The caloric test consists of altering the temperature of the endolymph, which induces convection currents and movement of the fluid in the lateral semicircular canals, leading to stimulation of the sensory cells and consequent nystagmus that can be measured.

The semicircular canals are paired structures that detect angular acceleration, this occurs when the endolymph fluid moves towards or away from the ampullae (ampullopetal or ampullofugal), which are the dilated ends of the canals. The movement of the fluid causes stimulation of the sensory cells (type I and II) in the crista ampullaris in the interior of the ampulla (see 📖 p. 456).

Ampullopetal flow, i.e. towards the ampulla, is excitatory in the lateral semicircular canal, but inhibitory in the superior and posterior canals. Ampullofugal flow (away from the ampulla) has the opposite effect.

Head and eye movement always take place in the plane of the canal stimulated and the direction of the endolymph flow (Edwald's law, 1892), or in other words the direction of the eye movement follows the direction of the movement of endolymph and the fast phase of the nystagmus will be in the opposite direction.

Technique
- The subject lies supine comfortably with their head elevated at 30 degrees of the horizontal (which brings the lateral semicircular canal into the vertical plane, being the ampulla at the superior end).
- The ear canals must be free of wax or debris, and the tympanic membrane must be intact (if water is used for the test). In the presence of tympanic perforation, or mastoid cavity, air may be used instead of water.
- Cold water (or air at 30°C) is run into one ear for about 40s. This cools the endolymph and induces movement of the fluid away from the ampulla, thus accompanying movement of the eyes in the same direction (Ewald's law) and subsequent nystagmus (fast-phase corrective movement of the eyes) to the opposite direction, away from the stimulated ear.
- The same procedure is repeated 5min later in the opposite ear with cold water, and then again in both ears with warm water (or air) at 44°C of temperature, in this case the specific gravity of the endolymph decreases and the fluid moves towards the ampulla, with the eyes following this direction and the nystagmus in the opposite direction, that is towards the stimulated ear.
- The mnemonic used to remember the direction of the nystagmus is COWS (Cold Opposite, Warm Same).
- The duration of the nystagmus is measured from the start of the irrigation to the end of the nystagmus response (lasting usually around 90s), while using Frenzel's glasses (that completely black out vision) to remove any central control. This duration is compared for both ears, separately and between themselves.
- If no response is obtained with the standard temperatures, an 'ice caloric' can be used with very cold temperature (10°C). Failure to obtain a response in this test indicates severe depression of the vestibular function of the affected ear.

Clinical applications
Caloric testing is the cornerstone of vestibular testing, and it is useful in all patients with vertigo. It only tests the lateral semicircular canal. The most common abnormalities found are canal paresis and directional preponderance.

Canal paresis (CP)
Unilateral canal paresis means that the response of one ear to cold and hot stimulation is reduced or absent *compared to the opposite side*. This usually represents a lesion in the periperal vestibular system (i.e. inner ear), with exceptions in multiple sclerosis and lateral brainstem infarction, where the lesion is at the level of the vestibular nerve root entry to the brainstem.

The degree of canal paresis can be calculated as a percentage using the following formula:

$$CP\ (\%) = (L30° + L44°) - (R30° + R44°)/L30° + L44° + R30° + R44°.$$

CP values above 25% are considered significant.

Directional preponderance (DP)

Indicates the nystagmus evoked in one direction is stronger that the one evoked in the opposite direction. DP suggests pathology either peripheral or central. In peripheral lesions usually is directed away from the diseased ear.

DP can be calculated with the formula:

$$DP(\%) = (L30° + R44°) - (R30° + L44°)/L30° + R44° + R30° + L44°.$$

Bilateral symmetrically decreased duration of nystagmus (<90s) suggests bilateral peripheral vestibular function. Increased response (>90s) can occur in cerebellar lesions (caused by the absence of cerebellar inhibitory effect on the vestibular nuclei).

Hearing-aids

Who benefits from a hearing-aid?

- Any individual with a hearing impairment (either conductive or sensori-neural in nature) confirmed by audiometry.
- The usual threshold that causes a hearing disability is 30–35dB HL in the better ear. However, the average hearing loss in individuals seeking a hearing-aid is 45dB HL in the better ear.
- Those with a hearing loss of 25–45dB HL will wear a hearing-aid 40% of the time.
- Those with >65dB HL loss will wear aids 90% of the time.

Classification of hearing-aids

Depending on the nature of the signal they use
These can be:
- Non-electrical: auricles, trumpets and speaking tubes.
- Electrical: the most commonly used. They have several components:
  - Microphone.
  - Amplifier.
  - Sound transmitter/output receiver (earphone, bone conductor).
  - Power source.

According to the type of signal processing systems
Analogue
- In which the acoustic signal is converted into electrical at the microphone. The amplitude of this electric signal can be adjusted to emphasize selected frequencies.
- To avoid discomfort caused by loud noises, the analogue hearing-aids can use two methods:
  - peak clipping ('cut off' the top of the peaks of the amplitude of the signal energy), or
  - automatic gain control (compressing the signal with a set maximum peak value), which causes less distortion.
- The analogue hearing-aids have external controls for volume, and a switch with three positions: Off (O), Telecoil (T, for television or telephone induction coil), and Microphone (M).

Digital
- The acoustic signal is also converted into its electrical analogue at the microphone, but then after passing through a frequency filter, the signal is converted into its digital equivalent (using a binary code) at the analogue to digital stage (A/D).
- Then the digital signal passes through a central processor unit (CPU) or microprocessor, where it is modified using programmable algorithms to control loudness, select amplification frequencies, or enhance signal over background noise.
- Finally this signal is converted back to analogue in the digital to analogue stage (D/A).

Generally is better to have binaural hearing-aids (as central summation of input from two ears can improve loudness by 6dB HL). If only one ear is aided, it should be the one with greater speech discrimination and loudness tolerance, irrespective of being the better or worse hearing ear (preferably in the moderate hearing-loss area of a pure tone audiogram). In asymmetric hearing, if the hearing thresholds are worse than 70dB HL in the worse ear, then the better ear should be fitted.

The hearing-aid must work in a relatively narrow dynamic range, i.e. the range of sound between being able to hear it and becoming uncomfortable. In a normal individual this range is 90–100dB HL, but in individuals with hearing loss this is reduced, by the elevated threshold, but also by recruitment.

Digital hearing-aids are more flexible, as they can manipulate more parameters of the received signal, and they have more audiometric configurations than their analogues counterparts. They have no loudness control, as this is automatically regulated by the aid.

According to the position of the aid

Behind the ear hearing-aids (BEHA)

- The most commonly used.
- The body of the aid sits in the post-auricular area and is connected through a hollow plastic tube to an ear mould, which allows the transmission of the sound to the ear.
- Moulds are usually made of hard acrylic, but when a tight-fitting is required (as in severe/profound hearing losss), they can be made of soft acrylic. Silicone can be used for individuals that develop an allergy to acrylic material. Loose moulds are more comfortable to wear but can cause feedback. An alternative to prevent this is to make a small ventilation channel in the ear mould.
- In unilateral unaidable ears a CROS (contralateral routing of signal) aid will pick up the signal in the worse hearing ear and pass it to the better ear (wireless or wired transmission—usually mounted on a pair of glassess) to a non-occluding ear mould.

In the ear/canal hearing-aid (ITE/ITC)

- They are less obvious, but more expensive than the BEHA.
- They are more likely to present feedback problems as the speaker and microphone are very close one to the other.
- They also may not be powerful enough in severe hearing-loss cases.

Body-worn hearing-aids (BW)

- The body of the aid is worn on the patient's chest, supported with a strap around the neck.
- They can be very powerful (for profound hearing loss). Feedback is rarely a problem as the distance from speaker to microphone is larger than in other aids.
- They are also useful in individuals with poor manual dexterity.
- Against them are:
  - larger size, restricting movement;
  - the possibility of picking up other noises, such as the rubbing of clothes;
  - cosmetic appearance.

Bone conduction hearing-aids
- Similar to body-worn aids but the output receiver feeds to a bone conductor.
- They are useful when air conduction is not possible: canal atresia or chronic otorrhoea or otitis externa.

Osseo-integrated—bone anchored hearing-aid (BAHA)
- This is a BC aid in which the output receiver is connected to a titanium osseo-integrated implant on the skull (see 📖 p. 420).
- BAHA offers a higher gain than conventional BC aids.
- It is not beneficial if there is a sensori-neural hearing-loss worse than 45dB HL or if speech discrimination score is worse than 60%.

Middle ear implantable hearing-aid
- This works on the principle of increasing the ossicular chain vibration by attaching a coil (output receiver) to the patient's incus.
- This coil is stimulated by a signal processor under the skin, connected via a magnet to the external body of the aid.

Spectacle aids
- These are useful when BEHA is difficult to fit, in patients that wear lenses to correct visual defects.
- They can be used also as a BC and as CROS aid.

Environmental aids
- These are general instruments used to enhance the sound quality and also to provide visual clues to improve the disability caused by hearing loss.
- They can be telephone and television amplifiers, induction coils, video-phone, text telephone, television headphones, and subtitles, doorbells, and alarms with visual and vibratory signals, and so on.

Hearing therapy

A hearing therapist's role is to provide a comprehensive rehabilitation service for adults who have hearing difficulties and/or associated disorders. This role requires a holistic approach, looking at the whole needs of the person, including the impact of hearing loss at work, home and in their social life.

Aims of a hearing therapist

- To create a consistent and continuous rehabilitation service for hearing-impaired individuals and hearing-aid users by fostering collaboration between statutory and voluntary organizations.
- To recognize and minimize the psychological consequences of hearing difficulties in adults by counselling, use of hearing-aids and assistive devices. The aim of the intervention is to reduce the disability effect of deafness.
- To increase independence, autonomy and quality of life.

Who can be help by a hearing therapist?

Patients who:

- are not suitable for a hearing-aid because they have too great or too small a hearing loss for an aid;
- do not wear their hearing-aid for physical (poor manual dexterity), psychological (reluctance), or acoustic reasons;
- would benefit from environmental aids at home or work, such as telephone aids, television adaptors, and other devices (e.g. doorbells, alarms);
- have communication skills that could be improved by lip-reading, auditory training, and/or hearing tactics;
- have been recently fitted with a cochlear implant for counselling and specialist auditory training;
- suffer from sudden hearing loss and those likely to suffer severe balance and/or hearing loss post-operatively;
- suffer from tinnitus, obscure auditory dysfunction (OAD)—thought to be a central-processing disorder in the presence of an otherwise normal hearing on pure-tone audiogram—and balance disorders requiring vestibular rehabilitation.

Aural rehabilitation

Aural rehabilitation consists of:

- Explaining the reasons behind hearing difficulties.
- Giving support and help, working towards acceptance of the hearing loss. Being able to discuss people's hopes and fears, and to improve confidence.
- Discussing how everyday life has been affected and working towards strategies to reduce difficulties that may rise at home, work, or socially.

- Maximizing residual hearing, use of hearing-aids, and environmental devices.
- Using lip-reading and other communication tactics.
- Improving other people's understanding of hearing loss. Meeting other people with similar problems.
- Advising in the management of tinnitus, OAD, and vertigo, usually by offering tailor-made programmes in auditory training, relaxation, and balance rehabilitation.

Tinnitus retraining therapy

In recent years increasing attention has been given to the method known as tinnitus retraining therapy (TRT). This is a therapeutic process that uses a combination of low-level, broad-band noise and counselling to achieve 'habituation'.

Aims

The aim of the treatment is to redirect the brain's 'attentional focus' away from the tinnitus signal, based on the principle that the persistence of tinnitus and the distress caused by it is due to problems at the central auditory processing level, involving signal detection and pattern recognition, which leads to 'normal' electrical noise being recognized and interpreted as a threat.

Method

TRT seems to be effective producing habituation, i.e. to remove the distressing emotions associated with tinnitus, and also to reduce the perception of persistent tinnitus. This process is carried out over a variable number of sessions through a 1–2y period.

- The first step is a full otological examination. This is followed by an explanation of the meaning of tinnitus to the patient, which is often thought as a noise within the head for which there is no cure and which will probably continue forever at the present level, or even get worse (a negative and frightening thought for most people).
- Then the patient needs help to understand the hearing mechanism in order to understand the origin of the tinnitus, any precipitating factor, and what makes it better or worse (including Jastreboff's neurophysiological model of tinnitus).
- This initial counselling session may be successful or may need modification to suit each individual's needs.
- Relaxation therapy can be very useful in recognition and control of tension.
- The next step is to break this 'vicious circle' of negative responses caused by the perception of tinnitus as a threat, by introducing a constant low-level noise (lower than the tinnitus itself) by means of a white-noise generator (subtly different from tinnitus 'maskers').
- This noise generator is constantly worn by the patient in the form of an instrument (hearing-aid, noise generator) or may even come from an environmental source such as a radio or cassette/CD player.
- The instrument is used to introduce a constant level of background noise for as many hours as possible during the day or at night time in which the patient is awake. It is particularly important to have such background noise during the quietest times awake: these are often when going to bed, on waking up in the morning, and if awake during the night.
- The principle of white-noise generators is that, by repeated exposure to low-level noise, the auditory system adapts and finds intrusive noise (tinnitus) less troublesome.

Results
- Significant reduction in tinnitus can take between 6 and 36 months.
- Success rate for tinnitus retraining therapy reaches 70% of cases in which tinnitus is less intrusive and in a further 20% of cases where tinnitus is virtually abolished.

Vestibular rehabilitation

Vestibular dysfunction and cerebral compensation

Balance disorders can result from peripheral (visual, proprioceptive, or vestibular system) or central nervous system pathology.

Chronic vertigo and unsteadiness associated with peripheral vestibular dysfunction will normally improve over a period of 6–12 weeks, as a result of what is known as 'cerebral compensation'. This cerebral compensation can occur in two ways:

- Habituation or adjustment of the central nervous system to the changes in signals from the peripheral vestibular system.
- Sensory substitution, in which the central nervous system relies more on other balance organs (vision and proprioception) than the affected vestibular system.

However, this compensation may not be complete and the patient may continue having symptoms intermittently or persistently of varying severity, particularly when placed in a challenging environment (i.e. uneven floor or poor lighting).

Compensation may be hindered by ongoing or intermittent insults to the peripheral vestibular system, such as in Ménière's disease. Drugs with an effect on the central nervous system (i.e. vestibular sedatives) may delay compensation as well.

Vestibular rehabilitation

Vestibular rehabilitation is a structured programme to enhance central compensation in order to improve the symptoms of patients mainly with unilateral peripheral vestibular dysfunction, but also in cases of bilateral peripheral and central vestibular pathology. This programme consists of:

- Initial assessment.
  - General physical condition, musculoskeletal, proprioception, and visual systems.
  - The validated vestibular rehabilitation benefit questionnaire (VRBQ) addresses all main areas of dizziness symptoms and its impact on everyday activities.
- Physical exercise programme, including:
  - General fitness programme.
  - Cooksey–Cawthorne exercises. These exercises are performed with the eyes open and closed, and at a speed or level of difficulty that just starts to provoke a sensation of imbalance, to promote compensation (Table 14.2).
  - Customised exercises programme, based on individual's needs and physical condition.
- Psychological assessment—especially when psychological symptoms, such as anxiety, panic attacks, and depression, have developed.
- Medications:
  - In chronic vestibular dysfunction there is no role for anti-emetic drugs.
  - Vestibular sedatives (i.e. cinnarizine), however, may be used in cases of symptom-persistence, to allow the physical exercise programme to be introduced, and then they should be withdrawn to allow a faster compensation process.

Table 14.2 Cooksey–Cawthorne exercises

Eyes	Movements at first slow, then quick: (a) up and down (b) focusing on a finger moving from 90–30cm from face
Head	Check they can stand with eyes closed. Movement first slow, then quick (also with eyes closed): (a) bending forwards and backwards (b) turning from side to side
Trunk	Movement—eyes open and closed, except (d) and (e): (a) bending forwards to pick up objects from the floor (b) bending forwards to pick up ball from floor, and twist body to put ball behind, first to the left, then to the right (c) drop shoulder and head sideways to left and right (d) throwing and catching ball to the side and above head (e) pass ball between legs and above head (f) change from sitting to standing with eyes open and closed, also turning round both ways in between (g) turning on the spot to left and right, with eyes open and closed (will require supervision) (h) walk with another person, throwing and catching ball in a circle and in a straight line (i) with another person's help, walk, eyes open and closed, backwards and forwards, sideways, turning head, looking in all directions to avoid fixating with eyes (j) walking in a circle forwards, and backwards, with the head turned to left and right, eyes open and closed
Lying down	Eyes open and closed: (a) rolling head from side to side, also over edge of bed (b) rolling whole body from side to side (c) sitting up straight, forwards and from side lying

Each exercise should be done about five times with two repeats, 5–10min sessions (including rests), 3–4 sessions a day. **Basically, little and often**.

The external ear

Infection and inflammation of the pinna

- Aetiological factors for infection/inflammation of the pinna may be local (ear piercing, trauma) or the manifestation of systemic conditions (diabetes, immunosupression, autoimmune).
- The infection can be localized or spread to the external ear canal and facial tissues.
- There may be also one or a combination of infectious agents (bacteria, virus. or fungi).

Cellulitis

- Develops most commonly secondary to otitis externa, but also after minor trauma (laceration, piercing, or abrasion) to the pinna.
- Common pathogens are Gram-positive cocci (*Staphylococcus* and *Streptococcus*) and *Pseudomonas* species.
- Systemic risk factors for severe infection of the pinna are diabetes and immunosupression.

Signs and symptoms
Include:
- Red, swollen, hot, and painful pinna.
- It may spread to neighbouring facial tissues and have associated regional lymphadenopathy, although this is uncommon.
- Impetigo (infection caused by *Staphylococcus*) will also present with vesicles on a reddish-purple base. These vesicles will burst producing serous exudates and later crusting.

Treatment
- If infection is localized: remove ear-piercing or insect's sting, and administer oral antibiotics for 1 week. It may be useful to mark the area of cellulitis to monitor progress and review the patient within 48h.
- If there has been no improvement, or the infection has spread beyond pinna or is the extension of an original otitis externa, consider high-dose intravenous antibiotics with antispeudomona cover until resolution of cellulitis, followed by appropriate oral antibiotic cover for 1 week after.

▶ Oral ciprofloxacin has as good systemic absorption as the intravenous form, being also cheaper!

Erysipelas

- Caused by group A β-hemolytic streptococci.
- The cellulitis caused is superficial, fiery-red (St. Anthony's fire) and of well-demarcated margins.
- The systemic symptoms are worse with high fever and general malaise.
- Erysipelas is contagious and should be treated with high-dose of systemic antibiotics.

Perichondritis and chondritis

- Extension of the infection to the underlying cartilage may develop into an abscess with vascular compromise and necrosis of the cartilage (chondritis), and the subsequent loss of the normal pinna architecture (cauliflower ear).

- The treatment must include systemic intravenous therapy (including anti-pseudomonas agent), as well as drainage of abscess and debridement of necrotic tissue but with minimal loss of tissue to prevent further deformity.

Herpes zoster oticus (Ramsay–Hunt syndrome)

- Viral infections of the pinna and external ear are rare.
- Presents in patients with a previous history of varicela-zoster virus infection (chicken pox).
- The virus remains dormant in the geniculate ganglion of the facial nerve and its reactivation during periods of low immunity will manifest as a vesicular rash (of 7–10 days duration) on the skin of the concha and external ear canal corresponding to the area of sensory innervation of a branch of the facial nerve.
- The rash may also spread to areas of vagus and glossopharyngeal nerve innervation (palate, buccal mucosa, hypopharynx).
- The association of the rash, facial nerve palsy (lower motor neuron), with or without concomitant sudden sensori-neural hearing loss, is know as Ramsay–Hunt syndrome.

Treatment

- Oral acyclovir.
- Oral steroids.
- If associated sudden hearing loss (see 🕮 p. 468).
- Post-herpetic neuralgia can have a devastating effect. Steroids are thought to be preventative and tricyclic anti-depressants (amitryptiline) may be necessary.

Allergic or contact dermatitis

- A reactive inflammatory response of the skin of the pinna, secondary to contact with an allergen such as earrings (nickel), cosmetics, or anti-septics (iodine, benzalkonium chloride) and antibiotic drops (neomycin).
- The main clinical feature is itching rather than pain in the pinna.
- Treatment includes recognizing and removing the causative allergen, and applying steroid-based ointment/cream or drops.

Relapsing polychondritis

- This is an autoimmune disease that consists of recurrent episodes of inflammation of cartilage (type II collagen) in different parts of the body.
- It can also affect nasal and laryngeal cartilages (less frequently).
- There may be an association with other autoimmune disorders (e.g. rheumatoid arthritis).
- It may be impossible to distinguish it from infective cellulitis, thus pay careful attention to the history (no trauma and possible evidence of other autoimmnue disease).
- Treatment involves systemic steroids.
- In cases of pinna cellulitis non-responding to antibiotic therapy, administration of steroids may have a diagnostic, as well as a therapeutic, value.

Seborrhoeic dermatitis

- Presents as oily, scaly patches in the post-auricular sulcus.
- Seborrhoea may also be present in the scalp, face, and ear canal.
- Several factors have been implicated in the aetiology of this condition including, neuropsychological and seasonal changes in temperature and humidity.
- Treatment consists of topical steroid preparations.

Eczema

- This inflammatory disorder is characterized by erythema, oedema, pruritus, and vesicles, with later crusting of the skin.
- It may coexist with affectation of the external ear canal (see ▢ p. 334).

Psoriasis

- Dermatological disorder of unknown aetiology that primarily effects the dorsal aspect of the skin on elbows and knees.
- When it affects the skin of the pinna, it presents with the typical silvery flakes over an inflamed base.
- Treatment, like many other dermatological conditions, consists of steroid-based preparations for the acute phase.
- Involvement of dermatologists should be considered for the management of these systemic skin disorders.

Chondrodermatitis nodularis chronica helicis

- Presents as a painful, erythematous papule on the helical rim of the pinna.
- It is thought to be caused by trauma, frostbite, or extremes of temperature.
- The lesion originates in the skin and then involves the perichondrium, treatment involves excising a small wedge of underlying cartilage together with the skin lesion.

Trauma to the pinna

This type of injury is common in contact sports, especially rugby, wrestling, judo and in cases of accidental or deliberate blows to the side of the head.

- Bearing in mind the association with synchronous head injury, find out the force and mechanism of the injury.
- Document the site of injury with a diagram or a photograph.
- Rule out any significant injury to skull, skull base (Battle sign: retroauricular bruising) and neurological deficit (GCS).
- Examine and document the:
  - EAC (look for bleeding, laceration or step in the EAC).
  - Tympanic membrane (with special attention to haemotympanum, perforation, CSF otorrhoea).
  - Facial nerve function.
  - Hearing (perform tunning-fork tests, free field testing, and/or audiogram).
  - Nystagmus.
  - Dizziness.

Lacerations to the skin and/or cartilage

- These are repaired using non-absorbable (absorbable in children) sutures under general or local anaesthetic.
- It is essential to clean the wound thoroughly and debride any necrotic material.
- The closure of the skin must be done with good edge opposition ensure coverage of any underlying cartilage. If there is loss of skin, some of the cartilage edge may be trimmed to allow full cover by skin.
- As in any other laceration, always check the tetanus status and give booster, if necessary.
- Consider antibiotic cover for bite wounds and delayed presentation.

Pinna ring block

- Use a local anaesthetic mixture of 2% lidocaine with adrenaline 1 : 80000.
- Introduce a 23–27 FG needle through the skin at the junction of the superior part of the helix and the side of the face, then infiltrate anteriorly.
- Without taking the needle out of the skin, infiltrate posteriorly in the same way.
- Repeat the same steps inferiorly at the junction of the ear lobe and the face,
- Finally, inject some local anaesthetic to the conchal bowl elevating a small bleb of skin.

Haematoma auris (Fig.15.1a and b)

- This is a collection of blood between the perichondrium and the cartilage of the pinna. If untreated it can lead to chondritis, abscess formation, and 'cauliflower ear' deformity.
- As a general rule, if the size of the haematoma is < 1/3rd of the pinna, treat initially with aspiration with a wide-bored needle and application of compressive head bandage to reduce recurrence.
- If haematoma recurs after aspiration, or size of haematoma is greater than 1/3rd of the size of the pinna, then incision and drainage (under local or general anaesthetic, as for pinna lacerations) is advised, with the addition of through-and-through sutures over dental rolls, to prevent re-accumulation of the haematoma, and a compressive head bandage.
- Antibiotics are required if:
  - Signs of infection (red, painful, swollen, tender ear).
  - Previous aspiration/drainage attempts.
  - Delay in presentation.

Thermal and radiation injuries to the pinna

- First-degree burns can be treated with supportive measures: cool compresses and appropriate analgesia.
- Second- and third-degree burns (blistering and full thickness, respectively) will need also:
  - antibiotic cover (including anti-pseudomonas); and
  - surgical debridement (as necessary).
- Frosbite often affects the auricle (as well as the nose) due to its exposed location:
  - The appearance of the injury is similar to the burn injury, becoming erythematous and developing blisters later.
  - Treatment is by gentle and gradual rewarming. Rubbing the ear will cause more damage.
- Radiation injury is very rare, but most often seen after radiotherapy for ear and temporal bone malignancies:
  - The injury can vary from radiation-induced dermatitis to more severe cartilage necrosis, possibly associated with external ear-canal osteitis.
  - In such a case, treatment may include debridement of necrotic cartilage and bony secuestrae, and consideration for hyperbaric oxygen for severe cases.

Drainage of haematoma auris

- As already mentioned, this usually occurs after trauma to the pinna, especially in the practice of contact sports (rugby, wrestling, judo). If left untreated it may leave a permanent 'cauliflower ear' deformity.
- It is also important not to miss an associated head injury, which may take priority over the ear injury.

Procedure

- The drainage can be done under local anaesthetic (see pinna ring block) or general anaesthesia, if necessary.
- Incise the skin of the pinna along the helical sulcus (see Fig. 15.1b).

- Milk out the haematoma.
- Do not close the wound, as this may cause it to reaccumulate.
- Apply pressure to the ear to prevent recollection, either by packing the contours of the ear with saline or proflavine-soaked cotton wool, and apply a head bandage. Alternatively, use a through-and-through mattress suture tied over a dental roll (or similar, Fig 15.2).
- Review the ear in 4–5 days.
- Surprisingly the ear incision heals without much scarring, as it is under little or no tension.

(a)   (b)

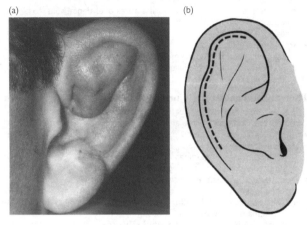

Fig. 15.1 (a) Haematoma of pinna. (b) Incision for drainage.

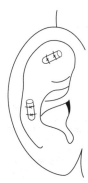

Fig. 15.2 Use of through—and—through mattress suture tied over a dental roll to prevent recollection of pinna haematoma.

Otitis externa

- Otitis externa is an acute or chronic inflammatory reaction of the skin of the external ear canal.
- Approximately 10% of people will be affected by otitis externa at some point during their life.

Local risk factors

- Warm, humid climates.
- Swimming (either in sea or swimming pool water).
- Change in ear canal pH (absence of cerumen).
- Trauma (from hearing aid moulds or foreign bodies).

Systemic factors

- Underlying skin disorders: allergic dermatitis, psoriasis, seborrhoeic dermatitis, eczema.
- Diabetes mellitus.
- Immunosuppression.

Acute diffuse otitis externa (swimmer's ear)

- The most common form of otitis externa. It is a diffuse infection of the external ear canal.

Aetiology

- The organisms most frequently involved are: *Pseudomona aeruginosa*, *Staphilococcus aureus*, and *Bacilus proteus*. This can be confirmed by taking an ear swab before treatment is started.
- Heat and humidity are the main causative local factors (swimmer's ear), but also minor trauma (scratch) to the ear canal.

Clinical features

- Pain is the principal symptom, especially on moving the pinna or the jaw.
- Skin of the ear canal is swollen, red (infiltrative form), itchy, and there may be abundant debri (desquamative form) deeper in the canal and the tympanic membrane intact, but inflamed.
- There may be discharge but mucopus suggests middle ear origin and look for an ear drum perforation. NB: Otitis externa can occur secondarily to middle ear discharge.
- Occasionally there may be spreading cellulitis.

Treatment

- Aural toilet ± insertion of ear wick (small compacted dressing that once introduced in the ear canal expands in contact with ear drops applied onto it).
- Antibiotic–steroid combination drops (preferably anti-pseudomonal).
- Oral antibiotic (if there is no response to initial topical therapy, or spreading cellulitis).
- If the underlying factor/s contributing to acute otitis externa is/are not treated appropriately, recurrence of the episode and even chronicity may develop.
- Recurrent episodes can also lead to stenosis of the external ear canal.

Beware of antibiotic allergy in resistant cases, as the clinical presentation may mimic infection. If no rapid improvement, take a swab from the ear canal, stop the antibiotic drops and review the patient with the results of the microbiology.

Acute localized otitis externa (furunculosis)

Less common form of otitis externa.

Aetiology

- Caused by a Gram-positive bacterial infection (*Staph. aureus*, usually) of a hair follicle of the external ear canal.

Clinical features

- Forms a small abscess (furuncle).
- Extremely painful, localized swelling of the cartilaginous (outer) portion of the ear canal.
- There is no spreading cellulitits.
- Painful pinna to touch.
- Conductive deafness if the ear canal is occluded by the furuncle.
- It may coexist with diffuse otitis externa with accumulation of debri due to occlusion of the external ear meatus.
- May have associated post-auricular swelling (retro-auricular lymphade-nopathy), forwardly pushing the pinna, which may mimic a subperiosteal mastoid abscess, especially if the tympanic membrane is not possible to be assessed.

Treatment

Aural toilet, which may include: incision and drainage of the small abscess (with a 21 FG needle), and/or insertion of a wick (ribbon gauze or pope wick) soaked in:

- Antibiotic-steroid combination drops, or in 10% glycerine-ichthammol solution.
- Oral anti-stapholococcal antibiotic.
- Adequate analgesia (a warm pad may be soothing).

Otomycosis

Aetiology

Resembles acute diffuse otitis externa but the causative agents are fungi: *Aspergillus* species (*niger, flavus, fumigatus*); *Candida albicans*; *Penicillium* and others.

Clinical features

- Itching is a prominent clinical symptom.
- On otoscopy, abundant debri can be visualized, sometimes forming colonies that resemble cotton wool, in the case of *Candida albicans*, or black spores, in the case of *Aspergillus niger*.
- However, in many cases the diagnosis is based on microbiology culture of ear swab, or in failure to treatment after a significant period (3–4 weeks) with antibiotic drops (or orally).

Treatment
- Aural toilet (± insertion of ear wick).
- Antifungal drops (at least for 4 weeks as spores are highly resistant).
- There is no role for systemic antifungals.

Granular and bullous myringitis

- Both can be caused by a group of viruses (influenza and parainfluenza virus), bacteria (*Haemophilus influenza*, *Streptococcus* species, *Moraxella catarrhalis*) and other organisms (e.g. mycoplasma).
- Granular myringitis is a localized form of otitis externa to the tympanic membrane. This appears thickened and inflamed.
- Treatment includes regular aural toilet and topical antibiotic–steroid drops. It can be very refractory to treatment, in which case middle-ear disease must be excluded.
- Myringitis bullosa haemorrhagica (bullous myringitis) is a very painful, self-limited infection of the tympanic membrane.
- As the name indicates, there are serous/haemorrhagic blisters in the tympanic membrane visible on otoscopy.
- The main differential diagnosis is Ramsay–Hunt syndrome.
- Treatment as in other forms of otitis externa, is with topical antibiotic–steroid drops.

Herpes simplex and herpes zoster oticus (Ramsay–Hunt syndrome)

See 📖 p. 327, 444.

Eczema, allergic, and seborrhoeic dermatitis

See 📖 p. 327, 8.

Treatment, once the acute infection has settled, consists of topical steroid preparations (drops, lotions, and ointments) to prevent recurrence.

Necrotizing otitis externa

Also known as malignant otitis externa. This is a rare non-neoplastic, progressive infection of the external ear canal, that develops into osteomyelitis of the canal and spreads along the lateral skull base, causing multiple lower cranial nerve palsies and, in a high percentage of cases, death if not treated promptly.

Aetiology
- It is caused almost solely by *Pseudomona* species.
- Rarely, caused by: *Staph. aureus*, *Aspergillus* and *Proteus*.
- Main contributing factors are diabetes mellitus and/or immuno-compromised patients.

Signs and symptoms
- Severe otalgia, especially in diabetic patients, in whom the pain threshold may be raised due to peripheral neuropathy.
- Granulations on the floor of the canal.
- Spread of the infection can occur into the tympanomastoid suture and tympanic plate to the retromandibular fossa, styloid foramen, petrous apex, jugular foramen, and hypoglossal canal.
- May lead to lower cranial nerve palsies: VIIth, IXth, Xth, XIth, and XIIth. And these can appear even in an almost normal-looking ear canal.
- More rarely involvement of the petrous apex may result in VIth nerve (Gradenigo's syndrome), and also Vth nerve palsy.
- Lateral and cavernous sinus thrombosis, meningitis, and death are likely outcomes if untreated, or if treatment has been delayed.

Diagnosis
- It is mainly based on the history and clinical findings.
- CT ± MRI scan of skull base and brain, which will confirm skull base erosion and intracranial pathology.
- Isotope bone scan.
- Microbiological specimens.

Differential diagnosis
Includes malignant tumours of the temporal bone and infratemporal fossa, granulomatous disorders and Paget's disease. A biopsy of the ear canal may be necessary to rule out malignancy.

Treatment
- Admission for assessment and diabetes control (intravenous insulin on a sliding scale).
- Anti-pseudomonal systemic antibiotics (oral or intravenously) to be continued for 6–12 weeks (discuss with microbiologist).
- Regular aural toilet.
- Topical antibiotic–steroid drops (anti-pseudomonal).
- Surgery only if there is no clinical improvement for surgical debridement and in order to obtain specimen for histology and microbiological studies.

Malignancy of the pinna

- The skin of the pinna is a common site for malignancy to develop (6% of malignant skin lesions), due to its greater sunlight exposure.
- Risk factors are:
  - sun exposure,
  - previous skin cancer,
  - chemical exposure,
  - xeroderma pigmentosum.
- The main types of malignant skin lesions of the pinna are:
  - basal cell carcinoma (BCC),
  - squamous cell carcinoma (SCC) and
  - malignant melanoma.

Basal cell carcinoma (BCC)

- Initially a flat, erythematous lesion that develops a rolled edge with silvery scales and later a central ulcer that may bleed on contact.
- It grows by tissue infiltration. Rarely metastasises.
- There are several subtypes of BCC:
  - Nodular BCC (the most common).
  - Pigmented.
  - Cystic.
  - Micronodular.
  - Superficial.
  - Morpheic.
  - Infiltrative.
- Treatment is by excision biopsy (2–3mm margins).
- Curettage, criotherapy, and radiotherapy can be used but they should need a biopsy to confirm the diagnosis first.

Squamous cell carcinoma (SCC)

- Can be difficult to differentiate from BCC (∴ a biopsy is necessary), although they tend to be more granular with a fresher, ulcerated centre and everted margin, appearance that becomes more obvious as it grows.
- Distant metastases are rare but regional lymph nodes (including intra-parotid nodes) can be involved in up to 10% of cases.
- Treatment is by surgical wide excision (including underlying cartilage, especially if this one is involved, if possible with frozen biopsies control (Moh's micrographic surgery). A margin (5mm) is desirable.
- Radiotherapy may be needed post-operatively or in some cases as the primary modality, depending on the extension of the tumour (no cartilage involvement) and anticipated poor cosmetic result post-excision.

Malignant melanoma

- Rarely seen in the pinna.
- Presents as a rapidly enlarging, nodular, pigmented lesion.
- Regional and distant metastases may occur.
- Treatment is by wide excision, depending on the site, possibly leading to almost total amputation of the pinna and reconstruction with local flap or prosthesis. Treatment of regional lymph nodes is also necessary (consider sentinel node biopsy and interferon treatment).

Wedge resection of the pinna

- Used for excision of medium and large lesions in the upper- and middle-thirds of the pinna.
- The procedure can be perfomed under local or general anaesthesia.

Technique (Fig. 15.3a)

- Consent the patient explaining that the ear will be significantly smaller than the other one.
- Patient is positioned slightly head up, with the head rotated away and the ear canal occluded to prevent blood/liquids trickling into the ear canal.
- The excision wedge is planned and marked on the pinna. Use a ruler to confirm the desired margins.
- The apex of the wedge should be deep enough into the root of the helix or in the conchal bowl, if necessary, to facilitate a free tension closure.
- The lesion is excised full thickness (skin–cartilage–skin), with a size 10 or 15 blade, introducing the tip through the full thickness of the pinna at the apex and then extending the incision peripherally.
- Mark the 12 o'clock margin with a suture to help determine histological margins.
- Secure haemostasis with bipolar diathermy.
- The closure should be tension-free. For this, a pair of Burrow's triangles may be needed. These are triangular pieces of cartilage-only excised at an angle, at either side of the apex of the wound (Fig. 15.3b).
- Use non-absorbable sutures (i.e. 5/0 nylon) to skin.
- Join the sides of the helical rim first (it is really important to get the rim lined-up, although there may be a significant difference in size between both ends).
- Then close the lateral surface of the skin with interrupted sutures.
- Trim/shave any cartilage prominent over the edge of the skin.
- Finally close the medial surface of the pinna.
- Remove sutures in one week.

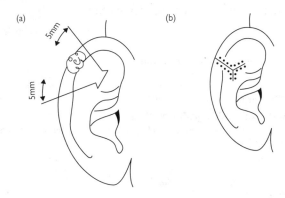

Fig. 15.3 (a) and (b) Diagram of Wedge resection.

Lesions of the conchal bowl

The lesion type, size, and depth will determine the resection and type of reconstruction required.

Healing by secondary intention

A small lesion, involving only the skin of the conchal bowl, can be excised and left to heal by secondary intention. Surprisingly these wounds heal satisfactorily in most of the occasions.

Full-thickness skin graft (Wolfe graft)

Larger lesions involving the skin only (no cartilage) can be reconstructed with a full-thickness skin graft.

Technique
- Check that perichondrium has been preserved in the recipient side (it will not take on bear cartilage!).
- Secure adequate haemostasis in the wound bed.
- A full-thickness skin graft can be harvested from post-auricular, pre-auricular, or neck skin, which provide a similar color and texture.
- Measure the size and shape of your defect (create a template).
- Draw the size of the graft needed in the donor site and extend it to form a complete elipse of tissue, which will then be removed.
- Check the donor site will close directly or with little tension (under-mining may be necessary).
- Take the graft and clean it of any subcutaneous fat (should be as thin as possible).
- Place the graft on the defect and suture it with non-absorbable material. Tie each of the sutures with its 'pair' in the opposite side, over a padding of paraffin dressing or cotton wool soaked in antiseptic (iodine/BIPP), in order to hold the graft securely in place.
- Remove the sutures (preferably yourself) in 10 days time.

Pushed-through post-auricular flap

It can be done only in cases when the lesion excised was full thickness of the concha or middle-third of the pinna.

Technique (Fig. 15.4)
- Measure the size of the defect and mark it on the post-auricular skin, exactly under the defect area itself.
- Incise the skin and elevate slightly the margins, but keep the blood supply from the centre of the local flap.
- Suture the margins of the flap to the edge of the excision.
- Absorbable sutures (especially for the outer/medial margin) may be suitable, as the pinna will usually be medialized, and access to remove sutures in the post-auricular area will be restricted.

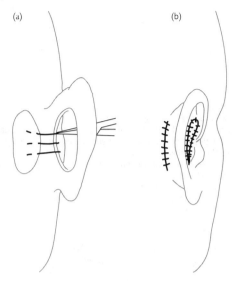

Fig. 15.4 Pushed-through post-auricular flap.(a) Posterior view. (b) Lateral view after closure.

Surgery of the lobule

- Tumours of the lower-third of the pinna or ear lobule can be excised and, if small, can be closed directly, although there will always be a cosmetic change.
- Larger lesions can be closed using the Converse's method of ear-lobule reconstruction.

Technique (Fig.15.5)

- Similar to the pushed-through post-auricular flap, an inferiorly based flap will be created with the skin of the inferior aspect of the ear.
- The skin is incised close to the defect and the edges of the defect are sutured to the margins of the flap (medial to superior, lateral to inferior). After at least 3 weeks (when the defect margin has taken a blood supply), the pedicle of the local flap can then be divided and closed distally to create a new lobule.
- The donor site can be closed directly or with a full thickness skin graft as showed previously.

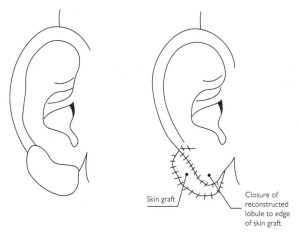

Skin graft

Closure of reconstructed lobule to edge of skin graft

Fig. 15.5 Converse's method of ear-lobule reconstruction.

External auditory canal (EAC) bony abnormalities: congenital

EAC stenosis

- The EAC can be narrow at one point (junction of cartilaginous and bony parts) or in its entire length.
- There may be associated abnormalities of the auricle and middle ear.
- It may not cause any significant symptoms, unless it gets blocked with wax and debri, or suffers recurrent infections which may lead to total closure.

Treatment

- Management requires regular aural toilet to prevent occlusion and otitis externa.
- For more symptomatic cases, a meatoplasty or canalplasty may be indicated (see Chapter 16, 🕮 p. 399, 400).
- There may be an increased risk of cholesteatoma development in cases of a very narrow EAC stenosis. In general this may be dealt with later in childhood age.

EAC atresia

- This is a membrane or bony wall (or both) occluding the EAC.
- Occurs approximately once in every 200 000 births, generally in a sporadic pattern, and it is often associated with malformations of the pinna and middle ear.
- Usually is unilateral and can be graded from mild to severe according to presence of some of the ear canal, total absence of EAC, and abnormalities of the ossicles and middle ear, and finally total absence of EAC, ossicles, and middle ear.

Treatment

- Surgical management may be considered in bilateral atresia to provide adequate hearing and to promote language development.
- Bone-anchored hearing-aids should be considered if the patient cannot wear conventional bone conduction hearing-aids.
- Also consider corrective surgery for any external deformities (see 🕮 p. 714).
- Surgery to open the EAC (not for the fainthearted) is only considered if the prospects of the intervention are considered to be good, based on scores above 6 in Jahrsdoerfer grading system (Table 15.1).

Table 15.1 Grading system for congential atresia*

Anatomical feature	Points
Stapes present	2
Oval window open	1
Middle ear space patent	1
Facial nerve course normal	1
Malleus–incus complex present and normal	1
Pneumatized mastoid present	1
Intact incudostapedial joint	1
Patent round window	1
External ear appearance close to normal	1
Total points	10

* Jahrsdoerfer et al. 1992.

External auditory canal (EAC) bony abnormalities: acquired

Stenosis and atresia

- Can occur secondary to trauma (wounds, burns, radiation) and infection (recurrent acute or chronic otits externa).
- Surgery is indicated for symptomatic cases, and includes meatoplasty and canalplasty.

Keratosis obturans

- Occurs as consequence of defective migration of squamous epithelium in the EAC, which behaves in a similar manner to cholesteatoma in the middle ear with bony expansion (but in this case the tympanic membrane is intact) and at the same time, this inflammatory reaction can cause stenosis of the EAC ('hour-glass' shaped ear canal).
- It can cause deafness and infection of the canal.
- Treatment is by regular microsuction of the EAC (under general anaesthesia, if too painful) and insertion of ear wicks. Severe cases (especially with stenosis) may require canalplasty (see Chapter 16, 📖 p. 400).

Osteoma

- Single, pedunculated, bony (cancellous), benign neoplasm.
- Often arise at the tympanomastoid or tympanosquamous suture.
- Cause hearing loss and/or otitis externa, due to impaction of wax and debri.
- Treatment is permeatal excision by curettage or drilling.

Exostosis (surfer's ear)

- Multiple sessile growths (hyperostosis) of cortical bone in the EAC.
- Associated with exposure to cold water (surfer's ear).
- Small exostosis may be treated conservatively. Large ones will require permeatal excision (Fig.15.6) or canalplasty (see 📖 p. 400).

(a)

(b)

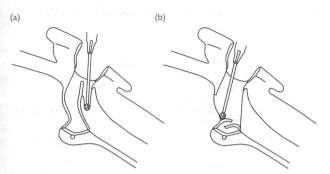

Fig. 15.6 Permeatal excision of exostosis (a) Maximium length of lateral canal skin sleeve is mobilized from canal. (b) Anterior exostosis is 'cored' out.

Malignancy of the external auditory canal (EAC)

Malignancy of the external auditory canal (EAC), either localized or extending to the temporal bone, are rare and a very aggressive type of tumour. It will be more extensively dealt with in the middle ear and mastoid (neoplasia of the middle ear, and skull base chapters). As general introduction it is the most important differential diagnosis in cases of otitis externa, either chronic or refractory to treatment. The great majority are squamous cell carcinoma.

Signs and symptoms
- Severe otalgia.
- Otorrhoea (debri and/or blood).
- Deafness.
- Polypoidal mass in the EAC.
- Cranial nerve palsies: VIIth mainly, but also IXth to XIth nerves.
- Regional lymph node metastasis.

Management
- Obtain deep biopsy (local or general anaesthetic). Repeat biopsy if not sufficient to demonstrate tumour invasion.
- CT scan and MRI scan to assess deeper extent into bone and soft tissues (bone erosion is highly suggestive).
- Discussion in specialized multidisciplinary meeting.
- Treatment ranges from palliation to curative treatment, usually in the form of a combination of surgery and radiotherapy.
- Surgical options (with or without parotidectomy, neck dissection and reconstruction) depending on extent of disease are:
  - Local canal resection.
  - Extended mastoidectomy.
  - Lateral temporal bone resection.
  - Subtotal or total petrosectomy.

Prognosis is rather poor with 2–3 year overall survivals rate around 50%.

The middle ear
and mastoid

Embryology of the middle ear

- The cavity and lining of the middle-ear cleft, Eustachian tube, and mastoid antrum arise from the expansion of the first pharyngeal pouch, with some contribution at the medial end of the second.
- This endoderm expands and is draped over the developing ossicles and associated muscles, tendons, and ligaments, and the labyrinth.
- By week 4, the distal endodermal end lies against the ectoderm of the first pharyngeal groove, forming a sac, the tympanic membrane. In between these two layers, mesenchyme will grow and form a fibrous layer.
- Development of the ossicles (malleus and incus from the 1st arch, stapes superstructure from the 2nd, and footplate from the otic capsule) starts at 4 weeks and ossification is present at 25 weeks.
- Tensor tympani, derives from the 1st arch, thus innervated by the mandibular branch of the Vth cranial nerve (Table 16.1)
- Similarly, stapedius muscle and stapedial artery, when present, are derived from the 2nd arch. The former is ∴ supplied by the VIIth nerve.
- The Eustachian tube and middle-ear space are formed by 8 months, and the attic and antrum at birth.
- The mastoid air cell' may be present at birth, filled with amniotic fluid, and will be 90% aerated by the age of 6.

Table 16.1 Embryology of the middle ear: 1st and 2nd arch derivatives

	Cartilage	Post-trematic nerve	Pre-trematic nerve	Artery
1st Arch Derivatives	(Meckel's) Malleus Incus Mandible Anterior malleolar ligament Sphenomandibular ligament	Mandibular (V)	Chorda tympani (VII)	Maxillary
2nd Arch Derivatives	(Reichert's) Stapes superstructure Styloid process Lesser cornu of hyoid Stylohyoid ligament	Facial (VII)	Tympanic branch IX (Jacoson's nerve)	Stapedial

Anatomy of the middle ear

Tympanic membrane (Fig. 16.1)

- The tympanic membrane measures 9–10mm in diameter, is slightly oval in shape, and lies at 55 degrees to the floor of the ear canal.
- It is divided into:
  - Pars tensa inferiorly, is the largest portion and is attached through the annulus fibrosus to the tympanic portion of the temporal bone. The annulus does not extend to the roof of the tympanic bone, but extends centrally to form the anterior and posterior malleolar folds.
  - Pars flaccida superiorly, immediately above it is the scutum, which is the outer attic wall.
- The tympanic membrane has three layers: outer skin, middle collagen, and inner mucosal layer.

Middle ear

Lateral wall

- Tympanic membrane.
- Scutum.
- Chorda tympani, (that carries the taste fibres from the anterior 2/3 of the ipsilateral tongue and secretomotor fibres to the submandibular gland) enters the middle ear through the junction of the posterior and lateral walls of the tympanic cavity, just lateral to the pyramiddal process. It runs anteriorly between the collagen and mucosal layers of the tympanic membrane (lateral to the long process of incus), and then, in the middle-ear space, medial to the neck of the malleus and from there it disappears into the canal of Huguier, just anterior to the petrotympanic fissure above the Eustachian tube.

Medial wall (Fig. 16.2)

- Promontory: covers the basal turn of the cochlea and contains the tympanic plexus (IX).
- Oval window (fenestra vestibuli), just above and behind promontory, covered by stapes footplate, it measures approximately 1.75 × 3.2mm.
- Round window (fenestra cochleae), below and behind the oval window. It is covered by a membrane and forms part of the floor of the scala tympani of the cochlea. The ampulla of the posterior semicircular canal and the singular nerve are the closest vestibular structures.
- Facial nerve, runs horizontally above the promontory and the oval window in a bony canal (which may be dehiscent) in an anteroposterior direction. It is marked anteriorly by the processus cochleariformis (bony projection that houses the tendon of tensor tympani muscle). Anterior to this there may be a swelling corresponding to the geniculate ganglion (1st genu) from which the greater superficial petrosal nerve runs anteriorly.

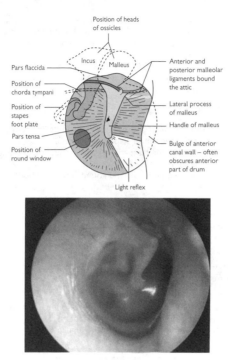

Fig. 16.1 Right tympanic membrane. From the Oxford Handbook of ENT and Head and Neck Surgery. Reproduced with permission by Oxford University Press.

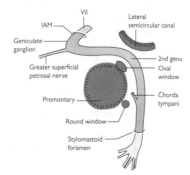

Fig. 16.2 Left middle ear. From the Oxford Handbook of ENT and Head and Neck Surgery. Reproduced with permission by Oxford University Press.

- The facial nerve turns inferiorly (2nd genu) posterior to the oval window and anterior to the lateral semi-circular canal. It then descends in the posterior wall of the tympanic cavity, where it continues to the stylomastoid foramen.
- Lateral semicircular canal (LSCC), whose dome extends a little lateral to the facial canal and is the major feature of the posterior portion of the epitympanum.

Posterior wall (Fig.16.3)
- Aditus ad antrum.
- Fossa incudis (for the short process of incus and its ligament).
- Pyramid (houses the tendon of stapedius muscle).
- Facial recess (between the tympanic membrane and descending portion of the facial nerve).
- Sinus tympani (between the oval and round windows and the pyramid and facial nerve).

Anterior wall
- Eustachian-tube opening.
- Carotid artery.
- Canal for tensor tympani muscle.

Roof
- Tegmen tympani (very thin bony roof that separates the middle ear from the middle cranial fossa dura).

Floor
- Jugular bulb (usually covered by a thin layer of bone, but may be dehiscent in some cases, or abnormally high in others).
- Carotid artery (anterior and medial to the jugular bulb).

Eustachian tube
- Connects the tympanic cavity to the nasopharynx.
- Measures 36mm in the adult.
- Lateral 1/3 is bony and has a 2mm diameter (approximately), the medial 2/3 are fibrocartilaginous.
- Above the Eustacian tube opening into the middle ear lies the tensor tympani muscle and medially is the internal carotid artery.
- The cartilaginous part is fixed to the skull base between the petrous temporal bone and the greater wing of sphenoid.
- Tensor palati muscle forms the upper portion of the front wall of the tube, it converges into a short tendon that turns around the pterygoid hamulus and spreads to the soft palate to meet fibres from the opposite side.
- Levator palate originates from the lower surface of the petrous bone, just in front of the carotid, running inferior and then medially to the tube, and finally spreading out into the soft palate.
- The mechanism of tubal opening is thought to be mainly carried out by tensor palati muscle.

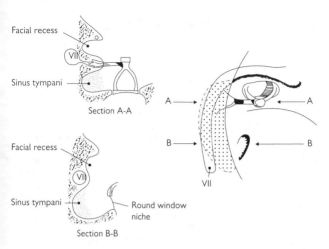

Fig. 16.3 Right ear—posterior wall.

Ossicles, ligaments and folds

- Malleus has a head, neck (where the tendon of tensor tympani muscle inserts medially), anterior and lateral processes, and handle, which is firmly attached to the tympanic membrane. There are superior, anterior, posterior, and lateral malleolar ligaments and folds. The space between the lateral malleolar fold and the pars flaccida of the tympanic membrane is known as Prussak's space, which is of relevance in attic retraction pockets and cholesteatoma.
- Incus has a body that articulates with the head of malleus, a long process to articulate with stapes head (through the lenticular process, and a short process that sits in the fossa incudis (in the posterior wall of the middle ear). There are superior, lateral, and medial incudal ligaments and folds.
- Stapes has a head, neck (where the tendon of stapedius muscle inserts posteriorly), anterior and posterior crura, and a footplate held in the oval window by the anular ligament.

Vascular and nerve supply to middle ear

- Vascular supply is from numerous branches of both internal and external carotid arteries: maxillary (anterior tympanic), posterior auricular and stylomastoid (posterior tympanic), middle meningeal (superior petrosal and superior tympanic), ascending pharyngeal (inferior tympanic).
- Sensory nerve supply is from the IXth cranial nerve (tympanic plexus) with some connexions from the VIth.
- Motor nerve supply from the mandibular branch of the Vth cranial nerve to tensor tympani muscle and from the stapedial branch of VIIth to the stapedius muscle.

Physiology of the middle ear

- The function of the middle ear is to match the impedance of the sound transmission from an air medium to a fluid medium in the cochlea via the oval window.
- The sound is transmitted via three routes to the inner ear:
  - via the ossicular chain movement;
  - via the skull vibration transmitted to the middle ear; and
  - via the skull vibration transmitted to the cochlea.
- Disruption of tympanic membrane and ossicular chain will cause a bone conduction hearing loss, but sound will still reach the cochlea via the 3rd route.
- In a similar way, if routes 1 and 2 are corrected (surgically), the bone conduction thresholds will improve (Carhart effect), more noticeable at 2kHz frequency (Carhart notch) (see 📖 p. 407).
- The surface ratio between the effective vibratory area of the tympanic membrane and the footplate is 14 : 1.
- The conjugated ossicular movement has a lever action with an amplifying sound effect of approximately × 1.3.
- Thus the total transformer ratio of an intact and mobile ossicular chain is 18 : 1.
- A defect in the tympanic membrane will produce a hearing deficit of upto 30dB HL, in a defect of the ossicular chain it will be greater than 40dB HL.

Acute otitis media (AOM)

- Acute supurative otitis media is a very frequent condition affecting almost everyone at some point during their lifetime, and especially children. The peak incidence is in the 1st 12 months of life (23%).
- Acute suppurative otitis media defines inflammation of the middle ear caused by an infective organism.
- Clinically there is a middle ear effusion with other associated signs and symptoms, including otalgia.
- The term 'acute' indicated that this process is <3 weeks of duration.
- If it occurs three or more times in a 6-month period, it is called recurrent AOM.
- Infection lasting more than 3 months becomes chronic suppurative otitis media (CSOM).

Risk factors

- Age <7 years.
- Slightly more common in males.
- Some races are predisposed: American Indians, Canadian Inuits, and Australian Aborigines.
- Presence of upper respiratory infection.
- Bottle feeding.
- Daycare nursery.
- Anatomical abnormalities (cleft palate, craniofacial anomalies).
- Immunological defiencies (Immunoglobulin deficiencies, AIDS, leukaemia, immuno-suppressants).

Aetiology

- Virus (thought to be the commonest cause):
  - Influenza A and B.
  - Rhinovirus.
  - Respiratory syncytial virus.
  - Mumps.
  - Parainfluenza.
  - Adenovirus.
- Bacteria:
  - Streptococcus pneumoniae.
  - Hemophillus influenza.
  - Moraxella (Branhamella) *catarrhalis*.
  - Bacteroides species (uncommon).

Pathophysiology

- AOM, in the absence of complications, is a self-limited condition with tendency to healing and complete resolution.
- There are several stages of AOM (Fig. 16.4).

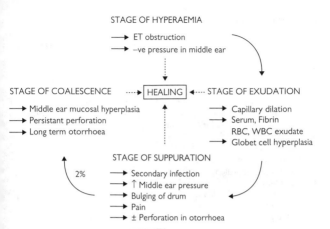

Fig. 16.4 Pathophysiological stages of AOM. From the Oxford Handbook of ENT and Head and Neck Surgery. Reproduced with permission by Oxford University Press.

Signs and symptoms

The initial signs and symptoms usually develop following an upper respiratory-tract infection or barotraumas, and are related to Eustachian-tube obstruction:

- Pressure build-up in the ear.
- Fullness sensation.
- Hearing loss.

At this stage, on otoscopy, there is inflammation and dullness of the tympanic membrane with possibly visible effusion. If the process continues there will be frank suppuration in the middle ear:

- Otalgia.
- Pyrexia.
- On otoscopy the tympanic membrane will be seen bulging or there may be muco-purulent otorrhoea (through a perforation).
- Small children will be irritable:
  - Crying and pulling from the ear.
  - Vomiting and/or diarrhea.
  - Sleepy and lethargic.
  - Febrile convulsions can also occur.

If perforation occurs, there is an improvement of the otalgia.

Secondary otitis externa can supersed the initial middle-ear otorrhoea. The ear canal oedema can make it difficult to see the tympanic membrane and make the correct diagnosis.

In 5% of cases the condition will become complicated with persistence of, or with new signs and symptoms.

Management

- Analgesia and antipyretics.
- Take a swab for culture and microbiological studies and consider topical antibiotic (± steroid) drops.
- There is controversy in the use of oral antibiotics.
  - On one side there are arguments against: not proven reduction of disease process, possible creation of antibiotic-resistent strains.
  - On the other hand in favour of using antibiotics are: a reduction in analgesia during AOM, and a reduction of serious complications, including mortality.
- As the natural history of AOM is to improve in 2 or 3 days (>80% of cases), a sensible option would perhaps be to prescribe antibiotics for any case of complication of AOM or if there is failure of clinical improvement within 24–48h in spite of adequate analgesia and antipyretics.
- In this case the antibiotic of choice would be Amoxicillin 40mg/kg/day for 10 days. If there is failure to respond within 72h then suspect antibiotic resistance and change to co-amoxiclav or another beta-lactamase agent.
- There is no evidence of myringotomy being effective in uncomplicated cases of AOM; however, it may be performed in some cases of severe otalgia or high pyrexia and 'toxic' children, that have poor response to antibiotic therapy.

Complications of acute otitis media 1

Complications of acute (and also chronic) otitis media are rare. They occur as a consequence of spread of the infection via (Fig. 16.5):

- Direct extension through pathological bone defects:
  - fracture lines
  - Osteitis with bony erosion
  - iatrogenic bony defects.
- Spread through normal anatomical channels:
  - oval and round windows,
  - cochlear and vestibular aqueducts.
- Spread through venous channels.

Classification

- Extracranial:
  - Tympanosclerosis.
  - Tympanic membrane perforation.
  - Hearing loss (conductive or sensori-neural).
  - Facial-nerve palsy.
  - Acute mastoiditis.
  - Petrositis.
  - Labyrinthitis.
  - Chronic suppurative otitis media (CSOM).
- Intracranial:
  - Meningitis.
  - Extradural abscess.
  - Subdural abscess.
  - Intracerebral abscess.
  - Lateral sinus thrombosis.
  - Otitic hydrocephalus.

① Mastoidtis
② Labyrinthitis
③ Extradural abscess
④ Sigmoid sinus thrombosis
⑤ Temperal lobe abscess
⑥ Meningitis

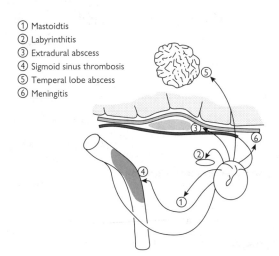

Fig. 16.5 Routes of spread of infection in AOM. From the Oxford Handbook of ENT and Head and Neck Surgery. Reproduced with Permission by Oxford University Press.

Complications of acute otitis media 2: extracranial complications

Tympanosclerosis

- Is a common occurrence after AOM.
- White patches of fibrous tissue (fibroblasts and collagen fibres) with calcification areas form on the tympanic membrane and, rarely, in the middle ear.
- It may be associated with a conductive hearing loss, as it can restrict ossicular chain mobility.
- The great majority do not require treatment. The extensive forms may require excision through a tympanoplasty.

Tympanic membrane perforation

- Usually perforations following AOM heal spontaneously within a few days or weeks.
- Persistent perforation following AOM is uncommon, but can be more likely if there are repeated episodes of infections, leading to CSOM.
- If the perforation remains opened over a period of 3 months, myringoplasty/tympanoplasty should be considered to close it.

Hearing loss

Two types:
- Conductive hearing loss; occurs as a consequence of the middle-ear effusion and this will occur invariably in all cases. The great majority of cases will be a mild conductive hearing loss (30–40dB) and will resolve within a few weeks.
  - In a smaller proportion of cases the infection will settle but the effusion will remain, causing otitis media with effusion (see p. 372).
  - Rarely the acute infection may cause erosion of the ossicular chain (especially the long process of incus due to its poor vascular supply) the hearing loss will be permanent. Treatment is by tympanoplasty with ossiculoplasty.
- Sensori-neural H. loss uses common and caused by acute suppurative spread to the inner ear.
  - Bacterial toxins spread trough the round window into the cochlea.

Facial-nerve palsy

- Approximately 0.5–1.5% of patients can develop facial-nerve palsy following AOM.
- Occurs more commonly in AOM rather than CSOM.
- Infection spreads into the Fallopian canal through congenital dehiscence (present in up to 10% of the population).
- Management is described in the facial nerve chapter (see p. 444).

Acute mastoiditis

- During AOM the mucosa of the middle ear and the mastoid are inflamed; however, progression into an abscess in the mastoid cavity occurs rarely.
- The general view is that antibiotic therapy has reduced this complication compared with the pre-antibiotic era.

- The peak incidence is 6 years.
- Inflammation of the mastoid air cells leads to suppuration and empyema formation within 7–10 days.

Routes of spread of a mastoid abscess
The infection can spread to:
- Mastoid cortex (subperiosteal abscess).
- Zygomatic cells (Luc's abscess).
- Sternomastoid muscle (Bezold's abscess), through the mastoid tip.
- Digastric muscle (Citelli's abscess), also through mastoid tip.
- Petrous apex (petrosistis or Gradenigo's syndrome), via the retrofacial, infra-, retro-, or supra-labyrinthine cells.

Signs and symptoms
- As in developed AOM, but with pain over the mastoid area.
- In cases of subperiosteal abscess the pinna will be pushed forward with a large retro-auricular swelling that is fluctuant and painful to palpation.
- In cases of zygomatic, sternomastoid, and digastric abscess, the swelling will correspond to these areas.

Management
- A CT scan of the brain and temporal bone to rule out an intracranial complication.
- Urgent broad-spectrum intravenous antibiotics (which cross the blood brain barrier well) must be commenced without delay.
- Failure to improve, or worsening in 24h, merit incision and drainage of periosteal abscess, cortical mastoidectomy ± ventilation tube insertion to allow further drainage, topical antibiotic drops, and later ventilation of the middle ear (see 📖 p. 392).
- Masked mastoiditis occurs when the progression of the disease has been altered by the prompt use of antibiotic therapy. There is a slow resolution of the symptoms with persistent otalgia and mastoid tenderness and general malaise.

Petrositis
- Acute petrositis is a rare complication that occurs as the infection spreads into the petrous apex.
- The typical clinical signs and symptoms include those of AOM and specifically a triad known as Gradenigo's syndrome:
  - Pain, deep in the ear and also behind the eye (distribution of the Vth nerve).
  - Otorrhoea.
  - Diplopia (lateral rectus palsy due to involvement of the VIth cranial nerve).
- Treatment as for acute mastoiditis.
- Failure to improve demands surgical intervention by, cortical mastoidectomy and drainage of the petrous apex through infracochlear, supra-, infra-, retro- or trans-labyrinthine approach.

Labyrinthitis and chronic suppurative otitis media (CSOM)
Both of these will be discussed in following sections.

Complications of acute otitis media 3: intracranial complications

- Less common than the extracranial complications.
- When intracranial complications do occur, they are more likely to be secondary to CSOM in adults and to AOM in children.

Meningitis

The mechanism of transmission of infection secondary to AOM is most commonly haematogenous, except where anatomical malformations exist (Mondini).

Signs and symptoms
As for AOM, plus:
- Headache.
- Photophobia.
- Vomiting.
- Restlessness, irritability.
- Nuchal rigidity.
- Kernig's sign.
- Brudzinski's sign.
- Convulsions, coma, and death.

Management
- CT scan of brain and temporal bone to assess associated intra- or extracranial complication.
- Involvement of physicians in the treatment of meningitis.
- Treatment of the AOM or mastoiditis if present as described earlier. Mastoidectomy should be performed in the neurologically stable patient.

Extradural abscess

- A collection occurs between the dura and the temporal bone.
- It is more frequently associated with CSOM than AOM.
- Its presentation can be subclinical, but the presence of headache and pyrexia should alert the clinician.
- CT and/or MRI will assist in the diagnosis.
- Treatment by mastoid exploration.

Subdural abscess

- The infection is localized to the space between the dura and the arachnoid membrane.
- It presents with signs and symptoms of meningitis but with rapid deterioration.
- Treatment is by neurosurgical drainage and surgical exploration of mastoid/middle ear once the patient is stable.
- The mortality rate is high.

Intracerebral abscess

Occurs more frequently in adults than in children, and more as a result of CSOM than AOM.

Signs and symptoms
- Can be minimal for days or weeks.
- The 1st stage is of encephalitis, with:
  - Headache.
  - Pyrexia.
  - Vomiting.
- 2nd occurs localization or encapsulation (asymptomatic period).
- Finally there is an increase in size of the abscess associated with increased intracranial pressure:
  - Lethargy.
  - Other neurological signs:
    — In a temporal lobe abscess:
      – nominal aphasia.
      – quadrantic homonymus hemianopia and later motor paralysis.
    — In a cerebellar abscess:
      – ataxia.
      – nystagmus.

Management
- Investigations with CT scan, which will show a rim-enhanced lesion, and MRI, which is especially useful in cases of subtle cerebritis.
- Repeat scanning days later (even if 1st scan is negative) may be indicated if there is still clinical suspicion.
- Treatment is medical antibiotherapy, neurosurgical drainage of the abscess, and mastoid exploration.
- Mortality rate has been reported to be 10–20% in spite of treatment.

Lateral/sigmoid sinus thrombosis

- This condition is rare.
- The mechanisms involved in its formation are through direct infection of the sigmoid sinus from peri-sinus bone erosion, or spread of infection through small vessels within the temporal bone.

Signs and sypmtoms
- Headache.
- Swinging pyrexia ('picket fence' pattern).
- Associated meningitis.
- Propagation into cavernous sinus thrombosis with:
  - Chemosis.
  - Proptosis.
  - Ophthalmoplegia.
- Otitic hydrocephalus (see next page).
- Distal propagation of the thrombus into internal jugular vein:
  - Painful neck mass along the course of the vein.

Management
- CT and MRI are the main diagnostic imaging methods. MRI offers better soft-tissue discrimination and is able to distinguish early clot formation (intermediate T1-weighted image and hypo-intentse T2), from mature clot (hyper-intense T1 and T2-weighted images).
- MR angiography shows also the thrombus extent.

- Treatment: high dose intravenous antibiotics.
- Anticoagulation only if evidence of cavernous sinus involvement.
- Surgical exploration of the mastoid on the clinically stable patient with decompression of the sigmoid sinus, aspiration of the sinus will confirm the diagnosis of an abscess, and only then should be opened and drained.
- Internal jugular vein ligation is only carried out in cases of septic pulmonary embolisation, or if septicaemia fails to respond to treatment.

Otitic hydrocephalus

- Also a rare complication of AOM.
- The mechanism of pathogenesis is thought to be due to obstruction of the cerebrospinal fluid (CSF) resorption at the arachnoid villus secondary to retrograde thrombophlebitis from the lateral to the sagittal sinuses.

Signs and symptoms

Are of raised intracranial pressure in association with otitis media:

- Headache.
- Vomiting.
- Papilloedema (decrease visual acuity).

Management

- Diagnosis is made with a lumbar puncture to show raised intracranial pressure and MRI scan and angiography to demonstrate sinus thrombosis.
- Treatment to lower the CSF pressure is medical with input from neurologists:
  - Head of the bed elevation to 30 degrees.
  - Mannitol.
  - Endotracheal intubation and mechanical hyperventilation.
  - Systemic steroids?
- Surgical management of the complicated AOM as before.
- The prognosis of otitic hydrocephalus is good.

Otitis media with effusion (OME)

- Otitis media with effusion is an inflammation of the middle-ear mucosa resulting in a collection of fluid in the middle ear.
- Several synonyms have been used to describe this condition, e.g. 'glue ear', serous otitis media, secretory otitis media, catarrhal otitis media.

Epidemiology

- The incidence follows a bimodal distribution with the 1st peak at 2 years of age (up to 40% of children are affected by OME at same time) and at 5 years of age (20% incidence).
- By 6 or 7 years of age the incidence decreases substantially, and by the age of 11 years, the annual incidence is 2%.
- 50% of the episodes of OME last 3 months.

Risk factors

- Age <5 years.
- More common in males.
- Sibling with history of AOM.
- Early 1st episode of AOM.
- Frequent upper respiratory-tract infections.
- Bottle feeding.
- Daycare nursery.
- Parental smoking.
- Atopy.
- Anatomical abnormalities (cleft palate, craniofacial anomalies).
- Physiological abnormalities (Kartagener syndrome, cystic fibrosis).

Pathophysiology

- The mechanisms involved in OME are thought to be:
  - Acute and later chronic inflammatory changes of the middle-ear mucosa, induced by upper respiratory-tract infections, otitis media, and/or allergic response that produce an increase in mucus production in the middle ear.
  - Eustachian-tube dysfunction, either from mechanical obstruction or from physiological interference with mucous clearance.

Signs and symptoms

- Conductive hearing loss.
- Poor speech development in small children.
- Behavioural changes in children.
- Aural pressure, ear popping, or clicking.
- Sensation of imbalance.
- On otoscopy the tympanic membrane is dull, of a yellow/grayish appearance, with/without visible fluid level in middle ear.
- The tympanic membrane may be slightly retracted or bulging, but always immobile to pneumatic otoscopy (Siegel speculum).

Investigations

- Myringotomy and aspiration of middle-ear effusion is the only diagnostic technique 100% accurate.
- Pure-tone audiogram (or age-appropriate audiometry) will show usually a mild conductive hearing loss (20–40dB HL).
- Tunning fork will corroborate the conductive nature of the hearing loss.
- Tympanometry showing a type B curve (flat) with a normal canal volume will have a 96% positive predictive value for OME. However, OME still can be present in C_3 to C_1 curves (see 📖 p. 298).
- In adults with unilateral cases of OME, it is mandatory to examine the post-nasal space with naso-endoscopy to exclude nasopharyngeal tumour.
- Since OME is frequently transient and resolves spontaneously, these investigations should be repeated 3 months apart to confirm the presence of established OME.
- No other investigations are usually necessary. Beware of incidental CT scanning, since OME can be misdiagnosed for CSOM, with or without cholesteatoma, as it has similar appearance of soft-tissue mass in the middle ear/mastoid (except that there is no bony destruction).

Management

It is very important to evaluate the patient in all aspects as the majority of OME sufferers are children. Speech, learning abilities, and behaviour are of main importance in this holistic assessment.

There are three main options in the treatment of OME.

Watchful wait

- The natural history of OME dictates that in 3 months time 50% of children it will resolve spontaneously.
- During the mandatory 3 months watchful waiting period, some parents may ask their child to perform 'auto-inflation', via Valsalva maneovre with/without an assisting device (Otovent®). This is believed to aid resolution in some cases.

Hearing-aid

- To maintain normal hearing until spontaneous resolution occurs.
- Unfortunately many children are poorly compliant with hearing-aids, but they remain a very good alternative to surgery in resistant cases.

Ventilation tubes ± adenoidectomy

The mainstay of treatment is myringotomy and insertion of ventilation tubes. Indications for this are:

- Significant hearing loss (>20dB HL) for at least 3 months.
- Craniofacial abnormalities, neuro-developmental delay.
- Significant speech and language delay
- Recurrent AOM with OME.
- Retraction pockets of the pars tensa.
- The average period of time before grommet extrusion is 9 months.

- Adenoidectomy has also been recognized to reduce the recurrence rate of OME (which is around 20%).
- This may be performed at the same time as the insertion of ventilation tubes.

There is no evidence that tonsillectomy has any beneficial effect in the treatment of OME.

Medical treatment of OME

- Antibiotics. There is no sufficient evidence of benefit for these to be used routinely, although there are some studies that advocate their use.
- Steroids. No proven benefit.
- Decongestants/mucolytics/anti-inflammatories/surfactant. No effect.
- Auto-inflation. Perhaps short-term benefit.

Sequelae of OME or its treatment

- Tympanosclerosis (40% of ears treated with ventilation tubes, and 10% of untreated).
- Atelectatic tympanic membrane (see 📖 p. 388).
- Cholesteatoma formation.
- Tympanic membrane perforation (by OME or by ventilation tubes: 1–2% if tubes extruded <12 months, 40% if tubes lasts 4 years).

Grommet insertion

Indications

Insertion of grommet or tympanostomy tube is indicated in:
- Otitis media with effusion (OME) >3 months of duration.
- Recurrent acute otitis media.
- Complications of acute otitis media (AOM), such as in facial palsy, mastoiditis.
- Occasionally as part of tympanoplasty procedures for chronic suppurative otitis media (CSOM).

Pre-operative checks

- Indication still present (especially if there has been a significant waiting list time). Review recent audiometry and tympanometry.
- Assess the ear canal and middle ear for the presence of active infection, as this may be a relative contraindication.
- If moderate to severe (>50dB HL) hearing loss in OME, counsel patient (or parents) of other possible causes of hearing loss that may also be present and that hearing may not return to normality after tympanostomy tube insertion.

Procedure

- When performed under local anaesthetic, instill 'EMLA' or 'Ametop' anesthetic cream (in a dewaxed ear canal) in contact with the tympanic membrane, using a 2ml syringe with a blunt needle under microscope control. Allow 45–60min for it to work, then removed the cream with microsuction.
- If not fully anaesthetized then inject lidocaine 1–2% (with adrenaline 1 : 80 000 preferably) in the external auditory meatus at the 12, 3, 6, and 9 o'clock. The injection should given be very slowly, between skin and periosteum, without bleb formation.
- Insert an ear speculum.
- Use a myringotome to make a 3–4mm incision radially in the infero-anterior quadrant (to prevent possible damage to middle-ear structures; Fig.16.6a).
- (Tip: Where available use a disposable myringotome, since these are likely to be much sharper and will avoid tearing the tympanic membrane.)
- Other types of incision, such as a marginal incision, are an alternative in some cases.
- Use a size 18 sucker insert to aspirate mucoid or serous fluid from the middle ear as much as possible but without traumatizing the tympanic membrane or causing bleeding 16.6b.
- The grommet is insinuated through the myringotomy incision with crocodile forceps (held from the top, bottom, or waist of the grommet) and then inserted or adjusted with a needle.
- Check the grommet is in place correctly by visualizing middle-ear mucosa through its lumen 16.6c.

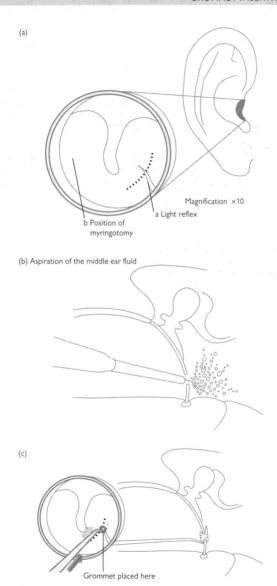

(a)

Magnification ×10

a Light reflex

b Position of
myringotomy

(b) Aspiration of the middle ear fluid

(c)

Grommet placed here

Fig. 16.6 a–c Grommet insertion technique.

Post-operative care
- Day-case, if procedure is performed as a sole procedure or with appropriate considerations with adenoidectomy.
- Antibiotic or steroid drops are advised if bleeding was present during insertion to prevent blockage and/or infection.
- Water precaution with cotton-wool smeared in Vaseline for the 1st 14 days. Thereafter, swimming is not forbidden, although advisable to use ear-plugs and swimming-cap and not to immerse head under the water.
- Post-operative follow up at 6–12 weeks for audiometric assessment.

Complications
- Damage to middle-ear structures e.g. ossicular chain, facial nerve, high jugular bulb) should always be avoided if correct placement of grommet. Suspect high jugular bulb if bluish, inferior aspect of tympanic membrane.
- Otorrhoea, early or late, which usually responds to water precaution, aural toilet, and topical antibiotic drops. If failure of medical treatment, grommet removal may be necessary.
- Tympanosclerosis.
- Atelectatic tympanic membrane.
- Tympanic membrane perforation (more common with long-term tympanostomy tubes).
- Grommet medialization (rare).

Chronic suppurative otitis media (CSOM) without cholesteatoma

Definition
- CSOM without cholesteatoma can be defined as the presence of chronic otorrhoea with a tympanic membrane perforation.
- Prevalence: 0.6% in the adult population.

Pathogens
- Common: *Pseudomona aeruginosa, Staphylococcus aureus, Proteus* species.
- Less commonly: *Escherichia coli, Streptococcus pneumoniae,* and *Bacteroids* species.

Signs and symptoms
- Tympanic membrane perforation (dry if 'inactive disease').
- Recurrent or chronic muco-purulent otorrhoea ('active disease').
- Hearing loss (usually conductive, but a sensori-neural component may coexist).
- Complication signs:
  - facial-nerve palsy,
  - vertigo,
  - intracranial event.
- Aural polyp/granulations.
- Possible associated otitis externa.
- Otalgia is uncommon.

Classification of tympanic membrane perforations (Fig. 16.7)
- The nomenclature can be confusing, since many terms are used in clinical practice to describe the same pathology.
- Pars tensa perforations (also called tubo-tympanic disease):
  - Central: residual membrane or annulus around the perforation. Also called 'safe', because of the low risk of developing cholesteatoma. According to the position in the tympanic membrane can be: anterior/posterior/inferior/subtotal.
  - Marginal: pathological loss of the annulus. (Also called 'unsafe', higher risk of developing cholesteatoma).
- Pars flaccida (also called attico-antral disease).

Management
- Regular aural toilet (ear swab for microbiology studies).
- Topical antibiotic–steroid preparation (precaution with potentially ototoxicity of prolongued or repeated treatment).
- ± Oral antibiotics.
- Surgical repair of tympanic membrane perforation (see myringoplasty).

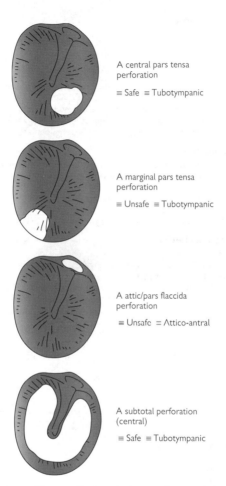

A central pars tensa
perforation

≡ Safe ≡ Tubotympanic

A marginal pars tensa
perforation

≡ Unsafe ≡ Tubotympanic

A attic/pars flaccida
perforation

≡ Unsafe ≡ Attico-antral

A subtotal perforation
(central)

≡ Safe ≡ Tubotympanic

Fig. 16.7 Types of Tympanic Membrane Perforations. From the Oxford Handbook of Ent and Head and Neck Surgery. Reproduced with permission by Oxford University Press.

Myringoplasty

A procedure to repair a tympanic membrane perforation. Also known as
'Type I tympanoplasty' (see 📖 p. 401).

Indications
- Recurrent or chronic otorrhoea in the presence of a tympanic
  membrane perforation.
- Improvement of conductive hearing loss caused by a tympanic membrane perforation in the absence of any other pathology (i.e. ossicular
  fixation or disarticulation, Sensori-neural hearing loss, etc.).

Contraindications
- Eustachian-tube dysfunction (i.e. otitis media with effusion in the
  contralateral ear). In children is advisable to wait until OME resolves
  approximately 9–11 years of age.
- Only hearing ear (relative contraindication).
- Presence of cholesteatoma in the middle ear/mastoid (which will
  require tympanoplasty ± mastoidectomy; see 📖 p. 394, 396, 401).

Pre-operative checks
- Check indications still present.
- Check pure-tone audiometry and tuning-fork testing done not more
  than 3 months prior to surgery (for medicolegal reasons).
- Look for signs of active infection (otorrhoea). If present, treat
  pre-operatively as this is believed to maximize success rate (although
  not proven in any studies, you would not put a skin graft on an
  infected wound!).
- Assess size and site of the perforation, and in particular note if the
  anterior margin of the perforation is visible.
- Clean any wax/debris and exclude any retraction pocket or
  cholesteatoma.
- Assess scar/s position from previous ear operations.

Consent
- Special mention of risks related to the surgery itself (where possible
  quote your own results or those of your unit if these are not available):
- Failure rate (approximately 10–15%).
- Hearing loss (extremely rare).
- Dizziness (possible).
- Tinnitus (possible).
- Facial nerve injury (very unlikely).
- Chorda tympani injury (probably underestimated).

▶ Do not forget to mark the operated ear immediately prior to surgery.

Technique
- Local or general anaesthetic.
- Place patient supine on the table with head resting on a ring and
  turned to the opposite side.
- Prepare the skin and the ear canal with a water-based skin preparation.

- Drape the ear and inspect the ear canal and tympanic membrane with the largest size speculum. Look particularly for the anterior margin of the perforation. If this is not visible permeatally, then a post-auricular approach will be indicated.
- Instill a local anaesthetic—adrenaline mixture (i.e. lignocaine 1–2% with 1 : 80000 adrenaline) in the ear canal at the cartilaginous and bony junction at the 12, 3, 6, and 9 o'clock points. Instill also the incision site chosen for the approach.

Permeatal (transcanal)

- Suitable in a large ear canal with a visible anterior perforation margin.
- A separate incision for the graft will be placed slightly behind tragus to harvest tragal perichondrium ± cartilage, or in the hairline for a temporalis fascia graft.

Endaural (Fig. 16.8)

- If the ear canal is narrow and the anterior perforation margin is visible.
- The incision runs from the eardrum at the 12 o'clock point extending laterally into the inter-cartilaginous groove between the tragus and the helix, and extending in a gentle curve around just in front of the ear and approximately of 2–3cm in length. This extension will facilitate harvesting of temporalis fascia graft.

Post-auricular (Fig. 16.9)

- Also in cases when the ear canal is narrow, but the anterior perforation margin is not visible on examination with an ear speculum.
- The incision in this case runs 1cm behind the post-auricular sulcus, from the mastoid tip to the level of the anterior helix.
- The soft tissues are dissected (including posterior auricularis muscle) until the temporalis fascia/periosteal plane is reached. Gentle traction applied to the pinna with a finger of the other hand in the external auditory meatus (to prevent opening of the meatal skin) may be helpful in this dissection.
- Temporalis fascia is harvested for grafting.
- The soft tissue of the posterior ear canal is separated from the bony ear canal and the posterior flap is elevated. One or two self-retaining retractors are positioned to maintain the view of the ear canl and tympanic membrane.
- Prepare the graft by removing any extra tissue other than fascia or perichondrium on a block or glass slide, and let it air dry or use a press for a quick effect.
- Remove the rolled squamous edge of the perforation, leaving a fresh, bleeding edge where the graft will vascularise and healing will take place.
- This can be done with a Rosen's needle by making a dotted line ('postage stamping') close to the edge and then joining the dots with a sickle knife.
- Raise the posterior tympanomeatal flap at 5–7mm from the annulus. The flap extends at least from 12 to 6 o'clock, but this can be extended if necessary (i.e. large subtotal perforations, very anterior or antero-superior perforations).

- [Tip: Pay special attention not to tear the flap. Use larger instruments (spud, Plester 'D' knife, Rosen's elevator) over as wide area as possible. Take care and time to separate the flap from the tympanomastoid or tympanosquamous sutures].
- Identify annulus in its sulcus and elevate it at 6 o'clock to access the middle ear as at this position there is less risk of ossicular damage (look out for a high jugular bulb present!).
- Use an elevator (Hughes's, Beale's, Rosen's elevator) or curved needle to elevate the annulus, against the bony sulcus rather than lifting the fibrous annulus, as this may tear the flap.
- When elevating annulus superiorly, chorda tympani must be visualized and preserved (a needle may be helpful for this) and care must be taken not to damage the incudostapedal joint, which may be visible under chorda itself (Fig. 16.10).
- Assess the ossicular chain integrity and mobility (by checking for the 'round-window reflex').
- Place the graft 'underlay' (the graft lies under the annulus and resting on the bone of the posterior ear canal wall), ensuring good contact at the anterior margin of the perforation (support it if necessary with absorbable material, i.e. gelfoam, placed in the middle ear).
- Alternatively an 'onlay' technique can be used, in which the outer squamous epithelium layer of the tympanic membrane is elevated, leaving annulus *in situ*, and the graft is then placed over the perforation and the rest of the tympanic membrane layers, keeping it in position solely with dressing material in the ear canal.
- Check the graft is stable and applied to the under-surface of the tympanic membrane. View of the anterior perforation margin is essential to check the graft is in good position and in direct contact all the way around.
- Apply in the ear canal, directly onto the tympanic membrane and graft, an absorbable dressing (i.e. gelfoam) or a piece of fine silastic (0.25mm thickness), followed by either BIPP ribbon gauze (2–3 small pieces) or an expandable Merocel® dressing with antibiotic ear drops.
- Absorbable or non-absorbable sutures to close the incision can be used.
- An otological head bandage can be used if an endaural or post-auricular approach has been used (although not all surgeons favour this).

Post-operative period
- Water precautions to ear.
- Hair can be washed in 2–3 days, but advisable to cover the ear (paper cup) while someone else washes the patient's hair.
- Dry thoroughly but gently (hairdryer).
- Remove the dressings from the ear canal at 2 weeks.
- Gentle microsuction post-operatively, and steroid or antibiotic-steroid drops for 3–5 days to prevent infection and facilitate healing.
- Avoid flying for 6 weeks (suggested by most surgeons, although there is no hard evidence to support this).

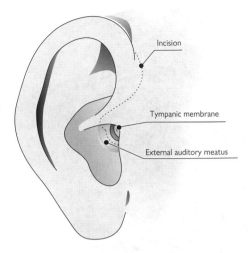

Fig. 16.8 Endaural approach.

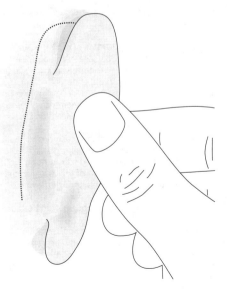

Fig. 16.9 Post-auricular approach.

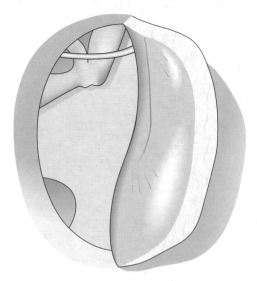

Fig. 16.10 View of right middle ear after elevating the tympanomeatal flap.

Complications
- Failure of graft (approximately 10–15% of cases). A common area where the graft fails is the anterior edge of the perforation. Some surgeons create a small pocket outside the anterior margin of annulus to secure an anterior tail made in the graft.
- Graft lateralization is not common in 'underlay' grafting (as annulus help to maintain the graft and tympanic membrane in its anatomical position), but it may occur if the graft is placed 'onlay', where the graft is not held in place by annulus.
- Cholesteatoma 'pearls' can occur if any squamous epithelium is left under the graft, also more common in onlay grafting technique.
- Hearing loss in the high frequencies (8kHz) can rarely occur. This may be due to excessive manipulation of the ossicular chain.
- Dizziness and tinnitus can also occur, although they tend to be temporary.
- Facial nerve injury is very unlikely, although could be caused by post-operative oedema.
- Chorda tympani injury (changes in taste and sensation of the lateral anterior 2/3 of the tongue) may be caused more often than thought, although in the majority of cases the patient may recover or compensate quickly, and therefore may not be reported unless specifically asked for.

Chronic suppurative otitis media (CSOM) with cholesteatoma

- A simple definition of cholesteatoma is 'skin (or keratin) in the wrong place', i.e. in the middle ear. The literal meaning of cholesteatoma implies it is a cholesterol containing neoplasm, but neither statement is true.
- Microscopically cholesteatoma is a benign keritinizing squamous cell cyst, with keratin in the centre, sorrounded by several layers of squamous cells (up to 15 layers), and surrounding all this, inflamed connective tissue.
- The prevalence of cholesteatoma in the Western World has been estimated as 6 cases per 100 000 of population, with slightly higher figure for children.

Classification of cholesteatoma

- **Congenital cholesteatoma** results from an abnormal focus of embryonic squamous epithelium in the middle-ear space (anterior epitympanum), that can spread into the middle ear or into the petrous portion of the temporal bone.
- **Acquired cholesteatoma** results from evolution of retraction pockets or perforations in the tympanic membrane (thought to be due to Eustachian-tube dysfunction). It can also occur from implantation of squamous epithelium into the middle ear (posttraumatic or iatrogenic).

Grading of pars flaccida retraction pockets

Tos classification (see Fig. 16.11):
- Grade 1: dimple or retraction of pars flaccida but not in contact with malleus neck.
- Grade 2: pars flaccida retraction in contact with malleus neck.
- Grade 3: erosion of scutum.
- Grade 4: pocket with keratin, not self-cleaning (= cholesteatoma).

Staging of pars tensa retraction pockets

Sadé classification (see Fig. 16.12):
- Stage 1: mild retraction, the annulus is stretched.
- Stage 2: retraction onto incudostapedial joint (not adherent).
- Stage 3: retraction onto promontory (but not adherent to it).
- Stage 4: adhesion of pars tensa to promontory.

Pathophysiology of acquired cholesteatoma

- The squamous epithelium of the tympanic membrane migrates laterally (outwards) in normal conditions, but in an established retraction pocket becomes misdirected, producing accumulation of keratin within it.
- Superadded infection stimulates activation of osteoclasts and release of lytic enzimes which leads to bone destruction and expansion of the cholesteatoma 'sac'.

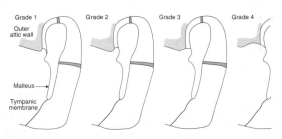

Fig. 16.11 Tos classification of pars flaccida retraction pockets.

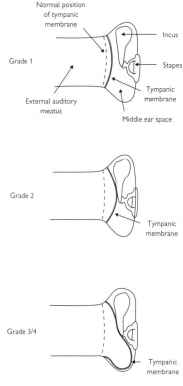

Fig. 16.12 Sade classification of pars tensa retraction pockets.

Signs and symptoms

As for CSOM without cholesteatoma.

Management

Retraction pocket

- Controversial.
- Ventilation tubes favoured by many surgeons to prevent progression of retraction pockets.
- Improve nasal and Eustachian-tube function.
- Regular aural toilet to remove/clean debris in the pocket.
- If symptomatic (recurrent/chronc otorrhoea, hearing loss) may need surgery: tympanoplasty (± cartilage reinforcement ± grommet insertion).
- If pocket is not possible to be cleaned, then the continuation of the pathophysiological changes will lead to the formation of an established cholesteatoma.

Established cholesteatoma

- Aural toilet while awaiting surgery or for cases in which surgical treatment is contraindicated.
- Audiometry to establish a pre-operative baseline.
- CT scan of the temporal bone.
- It is optional in the management of cholesteatoma, as the diagnosis is clinical.
- Some surgeons do not require pre-operative CT scan, while others argue that CT is useful because:
  - Confirms the diagnosis by demonstrating bony erosion, particularly of the scutum in attic cholesteatoma.
  - Helps to assess the lateral semicircular canal, integrity of ossicular chain, middle or posterior cranial fossa plate defects, and relation of the cholesteatoma with the facial nerve.
  - Assists in deciding surgical approach, by assessing the degree of pneumatisaton of mastoid.
  - To exclude petrous cholesteatoma.
- Generally CT scan is recommended for revision procedures or for the presence of complications of CSOM.
- Surgery to erradicate cholesteatoma can be performed via one of two approaches (see 📖 p. 394–8):
  - Canal wall-up (or close technique).
  - Canal wall-down (or open technique).
- In either case regular follow-up is necessary to exclude residual/recurrence of cholesteatoma.

Middle ear and mastoid surgery 1

Surgical approaches to the middle ear

The three main approaches have been described on p. 383. In mastoid surgery, usually endaural and post-aural approaches are used, the latter always for canal wall-up procedures, whilst both (endaural and post-aural approach) can be used for canal wall-down procedures.

How to use an otological drill?

- Otological surgery drills can be powered by pressurized air or electrical current (more common nowadays).
- The handpiece can be straight or angled; the latter one for when working down the ear canal or when delicate, fine work is required (less pressure required).
- The burs texture determines whether they are used for cutting or polishing. In 'cutting burs', the fewer number of teeth they have the more they cut. Polishing burs can have either a large number of teeth or they can be covered with a diamond paste ('diamond burs').
- When drilling, use the largest size bur possible, as this is safer. A small bur will create a narrow hole with poor visualization and greater risk of damaging structures.
- Irrigation is essential to prevent tissue damage from overheating (especially close to the facial nerve), as well as suctioning to evacuate excess fluid that may obstruct the view over the drilling surface.
- Familiarize yourself with the equipment before you start (it is not good to start drilling in reverse!).
- When removing bone with the drill do it in layers from superficial to deep, gentle (applying little pressure) but firm, long strokes of the handpiece, and use the side of the cutting bur (not the tip) to remove the bone.
- Identify 1st your landmarks (i.e. middle cranial fossa dura, sigmoid sinus, and posterior canal wall for a cortical mastoidectomy) and stay close to them, that way you will preserve them and achieve as wide exposure as possible (not digging into a dark deep hole!).
- When drilling you may start without the microscope, using it later when closer to more delicate areas (i.e. mastoid antrum). Change the microscope position and/or rotate the operating table in order to obtain optimal visibility.
- Change burr size and texture as often as required when you work in smaller areas. Protect soft tissues as they can be damaged with the burr.

Middle-ear and mastoid surgery 2: cortical mastoidectomy

- The cortical bone of the mastoid is removed from lateral to medial until reaching the mastoid antrum, leaving the posterior canal wall intact.

Indications

- Acute mastoiditis and drainage of subperiosteal abscess.
- Jointly with a myringoplasty in cases of CSOM without cholesteatoma (when suspected reservoir of infection in the mastoid).
- Canal wall-up technique (combined approach tympanoplasty) for CSOM with cholesteatoma.
- Surgery for Ménière's disease (saccus decompression, labyrinthectomy).
- Middle-ear and cochlear implantation.
- Extended cortical mastoidectomy for vestibular nerve section, trans labyrinthine removal of acoustic neuromas.

Pre-operative checks

- Check pure-tone audiometry and tuning-fork testing not more than 3 months prior to surgery (for medicolegal reasons).
- Treat active infection (antibiotics: drops/oral).
- Assess scar/s position from previous operations in the ear.
- Mark the ear pre-operatively.
- Review imaging (if perfomed).

Consent

Special mention of risk related to the surgery itself:

- Hearing loss.
- Dizziness.
- Tinnitus.
- Facial nerve injury.
- Chorda tympani injury.
- CSF leak, meningitis, intracranial complications.

Technique

- Prepare the patient and infiltrate local anaesthetic in the standard way for major ear operations (see 📖 p. 383).
- Apply electrodes for facial nerve monitor and test it is working in good order (see 📖 p. 438).
- Proceed to incision according to the selected approach. Usually for a cortical mastoidectomy, a post-auricular approach is the most commonly used.
- Elevate a superiorly, inferiorly, posteriorly, or anteriorly-based periosteal flap exposing from mastoid tip to zygomatic line, and use self-retainer retractor/s to keep these soft tissues out of the surgical field.
- Choose a large (6mm) cutting burr to drill the cortical bone. Start by delineating landmark structures (middle fossa dura, posterior canal wall, and sigmoid sinus). Stay close and follow them to ensure you can see them at all times in order to prevent any damage (hole in dural plate, dura, or sigmoid sinus).

- Layer by layer remove the cortical mastoid bone with good wide exposure and avoid creating a narrow tunnel.
- The most important landmark as the drilling continues medially is the mastoid antrum, recognizable by visualizing the LSCC in its medial wall and the fossa incudis (for the short process of incus in its lateral wall).
- At this point, the size of the drill may have been changed to a 3–4mm burr.
- The reflection of the short process of the incus on the irrigation fluid during drilling may be visible before reaching it, and special care must be taken not to touch the short process of incus with the drill, as this may cause irreversible damage to the ossicular chain and inner ear.
- Open all the air cells to ensure disease is cleared (i.e. granulations, cholesteatoma, or cholesterol cysts).
- Irrigate any bone dust away with saline or water.
- Close in layers: periosteal flap, subcutaneous tissue, skin.
- Otological head bandage (for 24h) to prevent haematoma.
- Similar post-operative instructions to myringoplasty.

Middle-ear and mastoid surgery 3: combined approach tympanoplasty (CAT)

Also known as 'canal wall-up' procedure or closed-technique mastoidectomy.

Indications
- CSOM with cholesteatoma.

Pre-operative checks and consent
As for cortical mastoidectomy, plus mention in the consent the need for further (stages) surgery and the possibility of residual disease and recurrence (approximately 15–30%).

Technique
- The technique includes the steps of a cortical mastoidectomy and a myringoplasty, with the addition of clearing cholesteatoma from the middle ear and/or mastoid.
- If the cholesteatoma sac is medial to the incus and head of malleus, these will most likely need to be removed in order to achieve clearance of disease.
- With an intact incudostapedial joint, disarticulate this with a small double-angled knife or small right-angle hook. Remember the joint is between the lenticular process of incus and head of stapes, in a slightly more medial position than initially suspected. (If the ossicular chain has been eroded this will facilitate the work of removing the sac).
- Remove incus by using a curved needle or right-angle hook to separate the malleo-incudal joint and remove the incus either via the middle ear or mastoid antrum.
- The malleus head can be excised at the level of the neck with the use of the malleus nipper forceps (with care not to damage stapes).
- The tendon of tensor tympani muscle can be divided with an angled knife, sickle knife or microscissors, and the tympanic membrane reflected further anteriorly for inspection of anterior mesotympanum and Eustachian-tube opening.
- Cholesteatoma around stapes may be difficult to remove. Do this by using an angled needle, peeling off the cholesteatoma sac in the direction of the stapedius muscle tendon from the pyramidal process to the stapes itself, as this tendon will offer anchoring to the stapes. If available, an Argon or KTP laser can be very useful for this task (being careful of the facial nerve).
- At the level of the facial nerve canal (Fallopian canal) the cholesteatoma sac must be very carefully dissected, as this bony canal may be dehiscent in an approximately 10% of cases.
- If the sac extends into sinus tympani and facial recess, it can be cleared with the help of a 40° endoscope and endoscopic instruments, and/or a posterior tympanotomy (excision of the facial recess). To create a posterior tympanotomy use a 2–3mm diamond burr to remove a triangle of bone from the posterior canal wall. This triangle is bounded

by the facial nerve chorda tympani and fossa incudis (Fig.16.13). Plenty of irrigation during drilling is essential to prevent thermal injury to the nerves. Visualization of the nerve (or accompanying vessels) is a good method of avoiding accidental damage to it. A good view of the stapes is also obtained with this approach. However, the sinus tymapni may still be out of sight, and 30–45-degree endoscopes can help to view this area better.

- Cholesteatoma sac extension to mastoid antrum and beyond can be easily removed, but again care must be taken with the lateral semicircular canal beware unsuspected erosion/fistula.
- The anterior epitympanum is a difficult area to inspect, as access is sometimes restricted. To maximize access to this area, one must drill anteriorly to the antrum from lateral to medial (being careful as middle fossa dura is lower laterally than medially at this point), until the head of malleus is completely seen and free of disease (If involved with cholesteatoma, then it should be excised, as described earlier).
- Once all disease is cleared, temporalis fascia ± cartilage graft (either tragus or conchal cartilage) is used to reconstruct and reinforce the attic and/or postero-superior aspect of the pars tensa.
- Place underlay fascia graft 1st, then the cartilage between the fascia and the bony edge of the postero-superior canal wall (to prevent retraction of the fascia and cartilage graft) and pack as in myringoplasty procedure.
- Closure in layers.

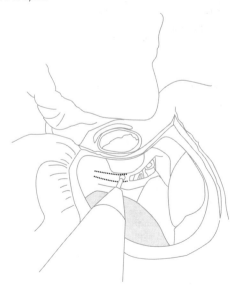

Fig. 16.13 Creation of a posterior tympanotomy (left ear).

Middle-ear and mastoid surgery 4: modified radical mastoidectomy and atticotomy

Also known as 'canal wall-down' procedure or open-technique mastoidectomy.

Indications
- CSOM with cholesteatoma.

Pre-operative checks and consent
As in closed technique, during the consent explain there might be need for further surgery for recurrence of cholesteatoma or for recurrent/chronic infections of the mastoid cavity itself (up to 30% of cases, approximately), as well as the required need for follow-up.

Technique
- The patient is positioned and prepared as previously described.
- Endaural or post-aural approach.
- There are two distinctive approaches to eradicate cholesteatoma from the mastoid and middle ear:
  - Front to back.
  - Back to front.

'Front to back' approach
- The cholesteatoma sac is followed from the middle ear/attic into mastoid antrum and its extension into the mastoid bowl further posteriorly.
- Drilling starts with a 4–5mm cutting burr at the level of the outer attic and posterosuperior canal wall. Following a medial to lateral direction, the bone is removed to facilitate exposure of the cholesteatoma sac. The bony defect created is ∴ no larger than the sac.
- Always try to widen the exposure during drilling by creating an inverted cone with the apex at the attic/posterior canal wall, but take care not to damage the middle fossa dura, since it is lower laterally and so at risk when removing the drill from the ear.
- If the disease is limited to the attic there is no need to drill further backwards into the mastoid. The resulting cavity will be covered with fascia or cartilage (as previously described) resulting in a fairly small attic defect (atticotomy).
- A small cavity has the advantage of more often being selfcleaning and easy to manage. If the ossicular chain was intact (cholesteatoma lateral to it) the hearing results can be very good. If removal of the cholesteatoma necessitates disruption of the ossicular chain this can be reconstructed either later at a second procedure or primarily, however if primary reconstruction is to be considered, you must be sure that all cholesteatoma has been cleaned.
- If the disease extends posteriorly beyond mastoid antrum, then a mastoid cavity will result.

'Back to front' approach

- Removal of the cortical mastoid bone (as described in the cortical mastoidectomy section), and then the posterior canal wall is taken down, as low as possible over the facial nerve to allow clearance of middle-ear cholesteatoma. The resulting bony divide is known as 'the facial ridge'.
- The cholesteatoma sac is approached from behind and as a result the surgical cavity created may be larger than the sac itself.
- The ossicles involved or eroded by cholesteatoma are removed (incus and malleus head).
- A temporalis fascia graft is placed under the tympanic membrane and lies in contact with the stapes suprastructure (if remaining) creating a type 3 tympanoplasty (see 📖 p. 401) and also covering the rest of the mastoid cavity (modified radical mastoidectomy; Fig. 16.14). This type of reconstruction can lead to very good hearing results 25–30dB HL threshold.
- When all middle-ear structures are removed (except stapes suprastructure or footplate alone), as well as the posterior ear canal wall and the mastoid air-cell system as far as the sigmoid sinus and middle cranial fossa dura, the resulting cavity is termed a 'radical' mastoidectomy.
- To minimize the size of the cavity a periosteal or temporalis muscle and fascia local flap (superior or inferiorly-based) can be dropped into the cavity, and covered with fascia. However this local flap can hide residual or recurrent cholesteatoma, and some surgeons only perform this on revision surgery cases when there is no cholesteatoma in the mastoid cavity.
- Adequate meatoplasty (see 📖 p. 399) must be performed to allow aeration of the cavity, promote cavity self-cleaniness, and good visualization during follow-up inspection.
- Closure as before, leaving the packing for 2–3 weeks.

Table 16.2 Summary of pros and cons of canal wall-up/down techniques

	Pros	Cons
Canal wall-down (open technique)	• One procedure only. • Safer in most hands. • Small self-cleaning cavity if good surgical skills (but cavity size dictated by size of cholesteatoma sac).	• Resulting cavity may need long-term care. • Prone to infections if swimming. • Revision surgery if cholesteatoma recurrence or infected cavity.
Canal wall-up (close technique)	• Maintains middle-ear/ mastoid anatomy and physiology. • Self-cleaning ear. • Swimming as normal. • Allows preservation of ossicular chain or its reconstruction at 2nd stage.	• Two or more procedures. • Technically challenging (especially if intact ossicular chain). • May form retraction pocket and recurrent or cholesteatoma.
Both techniques	• Hearing results can be similar when ossiculoplasty (closed technique) or type 3 tympanoplasty (open technique).	• Both need follow-up to detect residual or recurrent cholesteatoma.

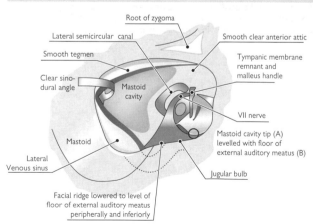

Root of zygoma

Lateral semicircular canal

Smooth clear anterior attic

Smooth tegmen

Tympanic membrane remnant and malleus handle

Clear sino-dural angle

Mastoid cavity

VII nerve

Mastoid

Mastoid cavity tip (A) levelled with floor of external auditory meatus (B)

Lateral Venous sinus

Jugular bulb

Facial ridge lowered to level of floor of external auditory meatus peripherally and inferiorly

Fig. 16.14 Right modified radical mastoidectomy.

Middle-ear and mastoid surgery 5: meatoplasty

Definition: Surgical enlargement of the cartilagenous external auditory meatus.

- It is performed when a narrow meatus impedes self-cleaning of the ear canal, or the access necessary for adequate examination of the ear during the post-operative follow-up.

Indications

- CSOM with cholesteatoma, as part of modified radical or radical mastoidectomy.
- EAC stenosis or atresia (jointly with canalplasty if bony EAC involved).

Pre-operative checks and consent

- In ear canal stenosis or atresia a CT scan of the temporal bone will confirm the presence of middle-ear cleft, ossicles, tympanic membrane, and depth of the stenosis.

Technique

- Following preparation and infiltration as in a modified radical mastoidectomy.
- The meatoplasty is probably best done at the start, as it will avoid excessive bleeding at the end of the mastoidectomy (just when the graft has been placed and minimal disruption is desireable).
- Several flaps can be used to enlarge the external auditory meatus (EAM):
  - single-flap (inferior or posteriorly-based),
  - two-flaps (Köner: anterior and posterior flaps,
  - three or five-flaps (Portman technique).
- In all these techniques there are some common steps:
  - Incise skin with a size 11 blade from the ear canal outwards to allow increase of EAM size (approximately until you can pass the tip of the little finger).
  - Undermine skin of the flap and excise underlying conchal cartilage to prevent the flap from springing back into natural position.
  - The flaps can be sutured to the subcutaneous tissues to keep in position.
  - Pack with a BIPP for 3 weeks in order to splint open the new wider EAM.

Middle-ear and mastoid surgery 6: canalplasty

- Surgical enlargement of the bony ear canal.

Indications
- EAC stenosis or atresia.
- Exostosis.

Technique
- Same soft tissue work as meatoplasty for the cartilaginous part of the canal.
- Elevate the skin of the deep ear canal (there may not be any available in atresia or deep stenosis) and excise any scar tissue, if present.
- Drill the bony canal placing a silastic or a foil paper (i.e. a silk suture packet) to protect the ear canal skin and tympanic membrane. If necessary use a diamond drill, as this will cause less damage to the skin, and drill from medial to lateral to widen the canal in its full length.
- Take care anteriorly not to enter the capsule of the temporomandibular joint or posteriorly mastoid air cells.
- If there is a small skin defect in the ear canal, the underlying bone can heal by secondary intention or be covered with temporalis fascia.
- If the skin defect is large, a split skin graft (harvested from skin of the arm or thigh) can be applied in longitudinal strips from medial to lateral over the temporalis fascia to improve graft take.
- Pack the ear canal with silastic sheeting (to prevent adherence to dressing material) and Bismuth Iodine Parafin Paste (BIPP) or an ear wick for 3–4 weeks.
- Dress the donor site with a non-adherent dressing for 7–10 days.

Middle-ear and mastoid surgery 7: tympanoplasty

- An operation to eradicate disease in the middle ear and reconstruct the hearing mechanism.
- The aims of tympanoplasty are to achieve a disease-free, stable and fuctional ear. This may be achieved through a combination of tympanic membrane grafting and mastoid surgery.
- The principles of tympanoplasty are:
  - Intact TM.
  - Mobile and unobstructed oval/round window.
  - Mechanism to link TM and oval window.
  - Ventilated middle ear.

Indications

- CSOM with or without cholesteatoma.

Classification of tympanoplasty[1]

This is based on what normal structures remain after clearance of disease.

- Type 1: tympanic membrane perforation. Reconstruction of the tympanic membrane (in the presence of intact ossicular chain).
- Type 2: absent malleus handle. Tympanic membrane reconstructed over malleus remnant to lie onto long process of incus.
- Type 3: absent malleus and incus. Myringostapediopexy: tympanic membrane reconstructed with strut to head of stapes (recreating a columella effect as seen in bird hearing mechanism).
- Type 4: only remains a mobile stapes footplate (all other ossicles absent). Footplate will be exteriorized into the mastoid cavity and round window will be covered by draping the tympanic membrane superiorly onto promontory to create a round window baffle.
- Type 5: only remains a fixed-stapes footplate (all other ossicles absent). Fenestration of the lateral semicircular canal is performed (or more commonly now a stapedotomy).

---

1 Wullstein (1953). *Proceeding of the Fifth International Congress of Oto-Rhino-Laryngology.* Amsterdam. pp. 104–18.

Complications of mastoid surgery and chronic suppurative otitis media (CSOM)

- The complications of CSOM are very similar to the complications of acute otitis media (see 📖 p. 364–70).
- For mastoid surgery there are some specific complications to mention.

Facial nerve injury

- Rarely reported (0.5–1%). Good anatomical knowledge and surgical technique are essential to prevent accidental damage.
- Early injury: may be due to the effect of the local anaesthetic infiltration too close to the mastoid tip. In this case the palsy is immediate after surgery and should resolve within a few hours, if it doesn't, then immediate re-exploration of the ear should be considered.
- Delayed injury: as a consequence of post-operative oedema. In this case systemic steroids are advisable to decrease oedema and removal of tight ear-canal packing (in open technique).
- If there is obvious damage during surgery, decompression of the nerve ± grafting (if transected nerve) may be necessary (see Chapter 17).
- The most common site of injury is the horizontal portion, where it may be dehiscent (15%). Cholesteatoma or any granulations over this area may contribute to the injury. A facial-nerve monitor may prove helpful, but is not a substitute for careful dissection technique.

CSF leak, meningitis, and intracranial complications

- The position of the dura depends greatly on the level of pneumatization of the temporal bone. A low, middle fossa dura is more at risk.
- A defect in the dural plate or dura can be repaired with bone dust, temporalis fascia, and collagen tissue glue.
- The use of prophilactic antibiotics is arguable as some consider antibiotics lead to resistant forms of meningitis, whereas others believe it to be preventative.

Hearing loss

- A conductive hearing loss will result from disarticulation of the ossicular chain, often required in order to clear cholesteatoma (this is not a complication *per se*, but a side-effect of surgery).
- Sensori-neural hearing loss can be due to excessive manipulation of the ossicular chain or to a lateral semicircular canal perylymph fistula.

Dizziness

- Dizziness can also occur from excessive manipulation of the ossicular chain.
- Fistula in the lateral semicircular canal is usually caused by advanced disease or previous mastoid surgery. The patient may have a positive fistula sign (vertigo and nystagmus induced by intermittent compression of the tragus of the affected ear).

- To prevent dizziness, care must be taken when dissecting cholesteatoma sac from the LSCC or cochlea.
  - If open technique is perfomed, the matrix of the sac can be left *in situ* with temporalis fascia tucked under the margins and left to epithielize the mastoid cavity.
  - In close-technique surgery, the matrix can be carefully removed (leave this until the end of the procedure) and the fistula covered with temporalis fascia, or the matrix can be left intact and a 2nd stage scheduled to assess and remove residual cholesteatoma (present in only 50% of cases).

Tinnitus
- Usually a hearing loss has also occurred.
- The majority tend to be temporary, but permanent in some (see Chapter 18, 🕮 p. 462).

Chorda tympani injury
- Chorda tympani injury may occur purposely if sacrified during surgery when involved in cholesteatoma.
- The patient may experience changes in taste ('metallic taste') during several weeks, which generally returns to normal in the long term.

Haemorrhage
- Intra-operatively a high jugular bulb or an anteriorly placed sigmoid sinus can be inadvertently damaged.
- Pre-operative CT scan may be of help to identify abnormal anatomy.
- Bleeding from the jugular bulb can be controlled with pressure using absorbable gelfoam or sugical.
- Sigmoid sinus bleeding can be dealt by:
  - Packing with gelfoam.
  - Consider bone removal over sinus to allow adequate compression.
  - Ligate sinus, but ensure patent contra-lateral sinus exists.
  - Abandon operation (pack and close).
- Post-operative reactionary bleed:
  - On return to normal blood pressure at the end of hypotensive anaesthesia.
  - An otological head bandage may prevent a haematoma.
  - Some recommend the use of a drain for 24h.
  - Haematoma may require incision and drainage (can be performed under local anaesthesia).

Post-operative infection
- Unusual.
- Not enough evidence to justify the routine use of prophylactic antibiotics in mastoid surgery.

- Occasional infection of a mastoid cavity is a common, late complication that can occur as a result of cavity-specific problems (high facial ridge, poor self-cleaning ability, small meatoplasty, tympanic membrane perforation). It usually responds to medical therapy (aural toilet + antibiotic/steroid drops ± systemic antibiotics).
- If otorrhoea is chronic (approximately 1/3 of mastoid cavities) or resistant to medical therapy, then revision surgery may be necessary.

Residual and recurrent cholesteatoma

- In closed technique there is a risk of 'invisible' disease left behind in the mastoid, ∴ in up to 30% of cases in closed-technique procedures, but can also occur in open procedures.
- Closed technique: risk of 'invisible' disease in closed mastoid, ∴:
  - 2nd look (stage) operation at 9–12 months.
  - Consider MRI scanning, but may miss small volume disease.

Otosclerosis

- An osseous dyscrasia of the temporal bone affecting mainly the ottic capsule and ossicles.
- Hereditary autosomal dominant transmission with incomplete penetrance.
- The inciting event is unknown:
  - Endocrine?
  - Metabolic?
  - Infective?
  - Vascular?
  - Autoimmune?
  - Hormonal?

Epidemiology

- Prevalence 1 in 100 000.
- 0.3% of the population have clinical manifestation of the disease.
- 6.4% of temporal bones have evidence of otosclerosis post-mortem.
- Affects women more commonly.
- Bilateral in 70% of patients.
- 50% of patients have a family history of otosclerosis.

Pathophysiology

A pleomorphic replacement of normal bone with spongiotic or sclerotic bone, which progresses in two stages:

- Active (otospongiosis phase):
  - Bony resorption and replacement with new spongiotic bone.
  - Osteoclasts appear at the leading edge of the lesion, and sheets of connective tissue replace bone.
  - The result is disorganized bone, increased population of osteocytes, and enlarged marrow spaces containing vessels and other connective tissue.
- Mature (sclerotic phase):
  - Formation of dense sclerotic bone with marrow vasculature and few recognizable haversian systems in areas of previous resorption.
- Pleomorphism: coexistence of both stages of otosclerosis in any single temporal bone.

Most common involved sites are:

- The fissula ante fenestram at the anterior oval window (80–90%).
- Stapes: fixation results when the annular ligament calcifies or stapes footplate becomes involved. When both are involved it is known as an obliterative footplate (3% of cases).
- Round window niche.
- Cochlea and labyrinth (8%). Resulting in sensori-neural hearing-loss thought to be caused by toxic metabolites, decreased blood supply, or by direct extension into cochlea and degeneration of the organ of Corti.

Sign and symptoms

- Slow progressive conductive hearing loss (bilateral in 70% of patients), usually beginning in the patient's 20s or 30s.
- Tinnitus (75% of patients).
- Dizziness can occur in up to 25% of patients.
- Paracusis of Willis: Improved hearing in the presence of background noise. It occurs also in other causes of conductive hearing-loss. It is due to the reduction of background volume that occurs in conductive hearing-loss, which improves the ability to hear someone who is speaking directly to the patient with a higher volume to overcome the background noise.
- Otoscopy: normal tympanic membrane or in 10% of cases a 'flamingo pink' blush of the tympanic membrane (Schwartze's sign), due to the increased vascular supply to the otospongiotic focus.

Investigations

- PTA: conductive hearing-loss with a Carhart's effect, which is an increase of the bone-conduction thresholds at the middle ear's resonant frequency (i.e. the frequency at which system vibrates most efficiently) between 650 and 2000Hz. Raised bone-conduction thresholds of the Carhart's effect are most evident at 2kHz: Carhart's notch (Fig. 16.15).
- ▶ This is an artefact, it is not representative of cochlear reserve, and it disappears after successful surgery.
- Tuning-fork test will confirm the conductive hearing-loss and in bilateral cases, may help in deciding which ear has the greater conductive loss at a different range of frequencies (useful to decide which ear is operated 1st).
- Tympanometry shows normal middle-ear pressure curve and absent stapedial reflex.
- Speech audiometry. Ensure maximum speech discrimination score >70%, as this will improve hearing quality.
- CT scan can help in the differential diagnosis:
  - excluding anatomical anomalies,
  - assessing ossicular discontinuity,
  - measuring the density of the otospongiotic focus (<1400 Hounsfield units).

Differential diagnosis

- Paget's disease:
  - Diffuse involvement of the bony skeleton (e.g. frontal bossing).
  - Elevated alkaline phosphatise.
  - CT scan shows areas of 'washed-out' appearance in the temporal bone due to demineralization.
- Osteogenesis imperfecta (Van der Hoeve syndrome).
  - Blue sclera.
  - History of multiple bone fractures.
- Congenital stapes fixation.
- Ossicular fixation (malleo-incudal joint) and discontinuity (incudo-stapedial joint).

If surgery is perfomed, the diagnosis is confirmed by assessing fixation of the stapes footplate.

Treatment

- Non-surgical.
- Observation. In the early stages.
- Hearing-aid. Trial for 6–12 months recommended before contemplating surgery.
- Fluoride therapy. It has been propose since the discovery of areas of low fluoride content in water had a higher prevalence of otosclerosis. However, there is no proven benefit of this treatment. The usual dose is 20mg daily in adults and it may be useful in cases with sensori-neural hearing loss, vestibular sysmptoms, or evidence of active otosclerotic focus (Schwartze sign).

Surgery

- Stapedotomy (see 🕮 p. 410).
- Bone Anchored Hearing Aid (BAHA) (see 🕮 p. 420).

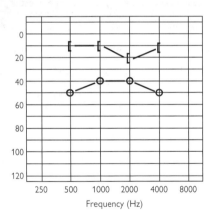

Fig. 16.15 Conductive hearing loss with Carhart's notch at 2khz. (Typical of otosclerosis).

Stapedotomy

- An operation to replace a fixed stapes with a prosthesis to improve hearing.
- Stapedotomy has superseded other operations for otosclerosis, such as stapedectomy (where the entire footplate is removed, as opposed to a small hole in stapedotomy), stapes mobilization, and lateral semicircular canal fenestration. All of which had poorer results and higher complications rate.

Indications
- Otosclerosis. Favourable cases are those with a large air–bone gap, with a bone-conduction threshold not worse than 30dB HL.

Contraindications
- Active external ear or middle ear infection.
- Poor speech discrimination (<60%).
- If the patient will still need to use a hearing-aid after the operation (i.e. mixed hearing loss where even the closure of bone gap will not achieve a satisfactory hearing result according to the 'Belfast 15/30dB rule of thumb' (see 📖 p. 824).
- Severe vertigo after 1st stapedotomy/ectomy in the contralateral ear. It is a relative contraindication. Vestibular function tests should be carried out to evaluate the vestibular reserve function before surgery is offered in the 2nd ear.
- Only hearing ear. Surgery in the 2nd ear should be delayed for at least one year (as there may be a small risk of late hearing loss).

Consent
- Dead ear (usually quoted in the literature between 0.5 and 1%).
- Incomplete closure of air–bone gap (approximately 5% cases).
- Abandon the procedure (persistent 'large' stapedial artery, abnormal facial-nerve trajectory, wrong diagnosis, otosclerosis obliterating round window, coexisting ossicular fixation of malleus/incus, congenital stapes anomaly).
- Vertigo.
- Tinnitus.
- Alteration of taste.
- Facial-nerve palsy.

Technique
- Usually under general anaesthesia (hypotensive anaesthesia is vital for this as for many other middle-ear procedures), although local anaesthesia is preferred by some surgeons.
- The preparation and positioning of the patient is as described on myringoplasty (see 📖 p. 382). Some surgeons prefer a slight tilt of the table away from the surgeon in order to have a more vertical approach to the ear.

- A small superficial vein graft can be harvested form the dorsum of the hand through a small incision. The graft is then opened to form a small rectangle of approximately 5–7mm of length, and is placed on a cutting block (adventitia side down) and allowed to dry at room temperature while the rest of the procedure is carried out.
- Permeatal approach, but a small endaural incision can help in narrow canals.
- The tympanomeatal flap is raised (from 12 to 6 o'clock) about 6–8mm form the annulus, elevated, and middle ear entered at 6 o'clock. Chorda tympani is identified and preserved.
- The posterosuperior canal wall/outer attic wall is removed using a curette (always in the direction away from the facial nerve to prevent damage), until a good view of the footplate, facial nerve and pyramidal process is obtained (Fig.16.16).
- Confirm the diagnosis, by checking the fixation of stapes, if necessary by dividing the incudo-stapedial joint with an angled knife, and by applying gentle pressure in the head of stapes. Look for movement of stapes and for the resulting round-window reflex.
- Also check for fixation of ossicles (malleus ankylosis is present in 0.6% of cases, and more frequently in children).
- Check that facial nerve is in its normal position and for dehiscence of the Fallopian canal. Also check for the presence of an abnormal stapedial artery.
- Divide stapedius tendon with micro-scissors or with laser (KTP or Argon laser).
- Divide the posterior crus of stapes with the laser or microdrill, avoiding the facial nerve. Then repeat the procedure with the anterior crus (this one may no be so easily visible). Remove remnant of stapes superstructure.
- Before drilling the hole in the footplate, use a measuring instrument to assess the distance between footplate and long process of incus, and choose the appropriate size prosthesis. In cases of thick or obliterative otosclerotic involvement of footplate, then repeat the measurement once the fenestra has been made. Usual piston length varies from 4 to 5mm. Diameter between 0.4 and 0.8mm.
- Cut the prosthesis to correct length (Teflon piston or bucket-handle prosthesis) and open the loop of the piston to ease later insertion.
- Prepare the vein graft for insertion.
- With a laser on 0.5W make a rosette on the footplate and/or use the microdrill (usually 0.6–0.7mm diameter; i.e. 0.2mm larger than the piston width). With very gentle pressure make the stapedotomy. Start the drill before making contact with the footplate as the drill may jump or oscilate and cause injury.
- Once the stapedotomy has been made, avoid any suction onto it as this may cause irreversible damage to the cochlea and vestibule. If necessary, use a small cotton-wool or ball with adrenaline to achieve haemostasis.
- Place the vein graft (to prevent perilymph leak) onto stapedotomy.

- Place piston onto graft covering the stapedotomy (Fig.16.17) and with the use of two double-angled hooks place the piston loop on to the long process of the incus, and then use a crimping forceps to tighten it.
- Check the piston is in place by pushing the shaft of the piston anteriorly, and this will make it bow a little.
- Replace the tympanomeatal flap (check there are no perforations).
- Pack the ear canal with one or two small pieces of BIPP or a wick. Remove the pack in seven days.
- Hearing can be checked then, but more reliably at 6 weeks.

Complications

Intra-operative

- Facial nerve injury:
  - Dehiscent Fallopian canal and facial nerve overhanging the footplate: Consider using a facial-nerve monitor or even abandon the procedure to prevent injury to the facial nerve.
  - The heat generated by the laser and/or microdrill may be responsible for thermal injury to the nerve.
- Floating footplate:
  - During stapedotomy (or more commonly during stapedectomy) when the footplate dislodges from the surrounding oval window niche.
  - The use of the laser to create the stapedotomy may reduce this complication.
  - If it occurs, one solution is to leave the fragment of footplate in place, and place the vein graft onto it with the piston on top as usual.
  - Attempts to remove the floating footplate may result in further damage.
- Obliterative otosclerosis:
  - It is not a complication as such, but makes surgery more difficult, thus more risk of complications.
  - When the otosclerotic focus is very large and affects the whole of the footplate (3% of cases), the excess bone should be very carefully removed using a laser and/or microdrill.
- Perilymph gusher:
  - A rush of perilymphatic fluid coming from the stapedotomy hole as soon as this is made. It is thought to be associated with patent cochlear aqueduct.
  - This raises the risk of sensori-neural hearing loss:
  - Raise the head of the patient, place the vein graft and piston on top as normal and apply gelfoam on to the graft to maintain its position and stop the perilymph leak.

Post-operatively

- Sensori-neural hearing loss:
  - In experience hands it should be less than 1% of cases.
  - It can be caused by:
    — reparative granuloma,
    — perilymphatic gusher/leak,
    — suctioning of perilymph from fenestra,
    — medial displacement of the piston.

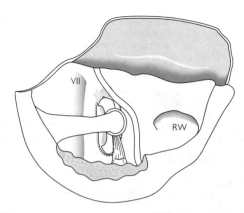

Fig. 16.16 Required exposure for stapedotomy (Right ear). Reproduced from *Diseases of the Ear* (Harold Ludman and Tony Wright), with permission of Edward Arnold (Publishers) Ltd ©1997 Arnold.

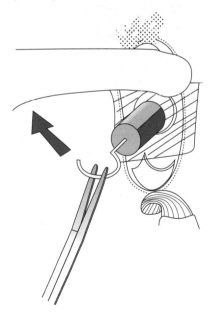

Fig. 16.17 Piston and vein graft placement (Right ear).

- Dizziness:
  - This may occur as a consequence of damage to the saccule during the stapedotomy (place the stapedotomy posteriorly to prevent this).
  - Perilymphatic fistula will cause fluctuating sensori-neural hearing loss and tinnitus. Exploration of the ear should be carried out and the fistula patched.
- Reparative granuloma:
  - Incidence is 1–2% of cases. Typically the patient has initial good hearing but develops a drop in hearing, and can be associated with tinnitus and vertigo.
  - Treatment is by exploration and removal of the granuloma that usually surrounds the piston and ossicles (the laser may be very helpful).
- Conductive hearing loss:
  - In experience hands the air bone gap is closed to within 5dB HL in over 90% of cases.
  - Failure to close the air bone gap can be due to:
    — ossicular fixation (or ankylosis).
    — too short piston.
    — displacement of the piston (spontaneous or trauma).
    — avascular necrosis of the long process of incus (delayed).
    — revision surgery may be necessary.

Ossiculoplasty

Is an operation to reconstruct the ossicular chain to improve hearing.

Indications
- Conductive hearing loss due to ossicular fixation or discontinuity.

Contraindications
- Active infection of external or middle ear.
Relative contraindications:
- Only hearing ear.
- High risk of cholesteatoma recurrence.

Pre-operative checks
- Recent pure-tone audiogram (within 3 months) showing air-bone gap.
- If bilateral hearing-loss, assess the status of non-operated ear and apply the Belfast rule of thumb (or Glasgow benefit plot) to see if surgery is worthwhile pursuing (see 🔲 p. 824).
- Tympanogram is helpful to assess middle-ear ventilation and Eustachian-tube function. Poor ET function = poor prognosis.
- Assess contralateral ear for evidence of disease or hearing loss.

Consent
- Failure to completely close air–bone gap.
- Dead ear.
- Sensori-neural hearing loss.
- Facial nerve and chorda tympani injury.
- Vertigo and tinnitus.

Technique
- Choose approach and raise tympano-meatal flap (as described in myringoplasty 🔲 p. 382).
- Assess ossicular chain and mobility by checking for the round window reflex.
- Several types of ossiculoplasty can be undertaken, depending on the ossicular findings.

Ossicular prosthesis
Depending on the graft donor
- Autograft: tissue from the same individual (preferred option).
- Allograft: tissue from another individual (same species).
- Isograft: tissue from genetically identical individuals.
- Xenograft: tissue from different species.

Depending on the material used
- Bone autograft: usually the remains of an ossicle (usually incus), or a piece of cortical bone harvested from the squamous portion of the temporal bone.
- Cartilage: from tragus or concha.
- Plastics: Teflon (used in stapedotomy pistons), polyethylene and silastic.

- Bioceramics: hydroxylapatite prosthesis (HA) can become mineralized and incorporated to bone. Extrusion through the tympanic membrane may be a less common complication of this type of synthetic material.
- Metals: stainless steel, platinum, and titanium can form all or be part of the prosthesis. If combined with HA head will reduce the prosthesis extrusion rate.
- Ionomeric glass: a cement used to bridge partial defects of ossicles (i.e. eroded long process of incus). They are very effective, but one must protect facial nerve or chorda tympani, as this compound is neurotoxic during its application.

Depending on the ossicular defect to be restored
- Partial ossicular reconstruction prosthesis (PORP): when stapes superstructure is present. The prosthesis sits on the stapes head and it is placed under the tympanic membrane or malleus handle.
- Total ossicular reconstruction prosthesis (TORP): when stapes superstructure is missing. The prosthesis stands on the footplate and under tympanic membrane or malleus handle.

Erosion of long process (LP) of incus

- If the rest of the ossicular chain is mobile, good results can be achieved with the use of ionomeric glass cement joining the LP remnant and head of stapes, or with the use of a ceramic preformed prosthesis (Applebaum type).
- If the ossicular chain is fixed elsewhere (i.e. malleo-incudal joint, malleus head), then incus can be removed, reshaped, and repositioned between the stapes head and the malleus handle (Fig. 16.18). Alternatively, a PORP can be fitted from stapes head to malleus handle, or directly to tympanic membrane. In this latter case, cartilage may have to be used to reinforce the tympanic membrane and prevent extrusion.

Erosion of stapes superstructure

- A TORP must be used.

Erosion of malleus handle

- Less commonly the handle of malleus is eroded, in such a case, a PORP or TORP can be placed directly under the tympanic membrane. Cartilage reinforcement may be necessary to help prevent extrusion.

Complications

- Sensori-neural hearing loss.
- Facial palsy.
- Chorda tympani injury.
- Failure to close air–bone gap. In ossiculoplasty a post-operative air–bone gap of 20dB HL is considered to be a good result.
- Prosthesis extrusion: cartilage interposition between prosthesis and tympanic membrane helps, as does hydroxylapatite prosthesis.

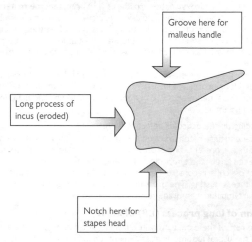

Fig. 16.18 Preparation of an incus autograft ossicular prosthesis.

Osseointegration and bone-anchored hearing-aids (BAHA)

The insertion of a titanium fixture into the temporal bone/skull was developed as an offshoot of osseointegrated dental implantation, where the properties of titanium to osseointegrate with the living bone were 1st applied.

Osseointegrated fixtures can also be used for prosthetic implants in the reconstruction of congenital or surgical defects in the ear, nose, eye, palate and other.

Indications of BAHA

Audiological indications

- Unilateral or bilateral conductive hearing-loss, with bone-conduction thresholds better than 45dB HL (measured at 0.5, 1, 2, and 3kHz).
- A maximum speech discrimination score >60%.
- If the hearing loss is symmetric, bilateral BAHA leads to binaural hearing.

Patient's indications

Inability to use a conventional air-conduction hearing-aid, in:

- Congenital ear-canal atresia or acquired meatal stenosis.
- CSOM and infected mastoid cavities.
- Bilateral recurrent or chronic otitis externa, also where hearing-aid cause otorrhoea.
- Otosclerosis.

Contraindications

- Bone-conduction thresholds worse than 45dB HL.
- Poor speech discrimination (<60%).
- Severe eczema on the implant area.
- Poor hygiene. The skin around the abutment must always be clean.
- <5 years of age, the skull thickness may not be adequate.

Technique

One-stage procedure

- Measure placement of a 'dummy' BAHA in the post-auricular area, approximately 50–55mm from the external ear meatus, and at a 45-degree angle with the tragus.
- Inject a mixture of local anaesthetic and adrenaline to reduce pain and provide tension under the skin flap area.
- Create a superiorly (or inferiorly) based skin flap (3 x 4cm approximately) with the dermatome at 2000–3000rpm.
- Excise subcutaneous tissue down to periosteum. The edges of the skin flap should be bevelled for better contact of the flap with the periosteum.
- The periosteum at the fixture site should be incised and removed.
- Drill a 3mm-deep hole (with spacer kept on) in the skull. If adequate bone thickness, then continue to 4mm depth by removing the spacer on the burr. Use plenty of irrigation as heat can damage the bony tissue and jeopardize osseointegration.

- Widen the hole with a countersink drill.
- Insert the self-tapping fixture with the pre-mounted abutment at low-speed setting (40rpm; Fig. 16.19). It is essential to use a low speed during insertion to achieve a stable position that allows full osseointegration of the fixture. There should be no irrigation at this point until the 1st grooves of the fixture are well within the bone, then abundant irrigation can be used.
- Use the hand key to tighten the fixture, if necessary.
- Suture the skin flap to the scalp with absorbable or non-absorbable sutures.
- Punch a hole in the skin overlying the abutment and push it through the skin (Fig.16.20).

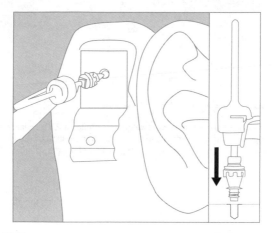

Fig. 16.19 Insertion of self-tapping fixture with pre-mounted abutment.

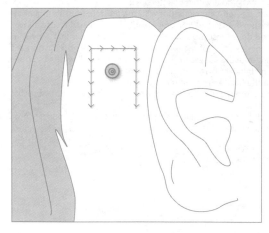

Fig. 16.20 Abutment pushed-through the skin flap.

- Place non-adherent dressing between the skin flap and the healing cap.
- Change dressing at 5–7 days and regular outpatient care of the flap.
- Allow at least 3 months for osseointegration before the sound processor is fitted.

Two-stage procedure

Here osseointegration of the fixture occur under the skin flap. The second stage involves making a hole in the skin, through which the abutment is secured to the fully osseointegrated fixture.

Complications

- Skin-flap haematoma and/or infection.
- Granulations and localized infection around the abutment. This usually responds to regular cleaning and dressing with antibiotic-soaked gauze placed under the healing cap. Occasionally oral antibiotics are needed.
- Abutment mobility suggests failure of osseointegration, and requires replacement of the implant.

Cochlear implantation

Cochlear implant is an electrical device that transforms sound into an electrical signal which stimulates the ganglion cells and cochlear nerve. This is used for profoundly deaf people who cannot obtain useful hearing with a conventional hearing-aid.

The implant consists of two parts (Fig. 16.21):
- External component formed by a:
  - Microphone.
  - Sound processor.
  - Transmitter coil (transcutaneous).
- Internal component (surgically inserted):
  - Internal receiver–stimulator.
  - Electrode array (1–24 electrodes).

Indications
Audiological criteria
- Profound sensori-neural hearing-loss with pure-tone thresholds >100dB HL at 2kHz and above, (aided thresholds >50dB) with speech discrimination scores less than 30%.

Patient factors
- In post-lingual deafness there is no upper age limit but the ability of the central nervous system to adapt to learn a new task (neuronal plasticity) is reduced with advancing age.
- In post-meningitis patients, the implantation must occur within a few weeks i.e. before extensive fibrosis and ossification of the cochlea jeopardize the electrode insertion.
- In pre-lingual deafness, the timing of implantation is important to achieve good speech and communication skills—ideally at the age of 2 or 3.

Contraindications
- Deafness due to central and auditory nerve pathology.
- Long duration of profound deafness is a poor prognostic indicator of implantation.
- Active CSOM (with or without cholesteatoma).
- Presence of a mastoid cavity. The cavity should be obliterated 1st.
- Patient unfit for general anaesthesia.

Pre-operative checks
- Check there is a normal cochlea and IAM contents with CT/MRI.
- Pneumococcal vaccination pre-operatively to minimize the risk of meningitis after surgery.
- The patient and/or parents must have adequate motivation to complete the rehabilitation programme.

Consent

- Meningitis and other intracranial complications.
- Facial-nerve injury.
- Chorda tympani.
- Dizziness.
- Infection and healing problems of the scalp flap.
- Undesirable electrical effects of the implant (pain, tinnitus, facial-nerve stimulation).
- Implant failure (need for further surgery).

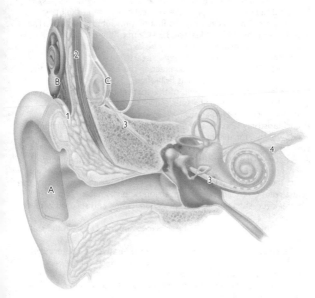

Fig. 16.21 How do we hear with a cochlear implant system? Image Courtesy of Cochlear Limited 2008.

The cochlear implant system has both external and internal parts; sound processor (A) with coil (B) is worn behind the ear; and implant (C) is placed just under the skin, behind your ear.

1. The sound processor captures sound and converts it into digital code.
2. The sound processor transmits the digitally coded sound through the coil to the implant just under the skin.
3. The implant converts the digitally coded sound to electrical signals and sends them along the electrode array, which is positioned in the cochlea.
4. The implant's electrodes stimulate the cochlea's hearing nerve fibres, which relay the sound signals to the brain to produce hearing sensations.

Technique

- The patient is prepared and positioned as for major ear surgery. Use a facial-nerve monitor.
- Broad-spectrum antibiotics are given intravenously at induction and continued for 24h.
- The incision must be placed at least 2cm away from the position of the implant.
- Soft tissue and periosteum are elevated in one or two separate flaps.
- A limited cortical mastoidectomy is performed (small cavity, without opening the sino-dural angle, and not exposing the sigmoid sinus).
- Using a drill create a trough in the cortical bone of the skull posterior to the cortical mastoidectomy. To fit a dummy internal implant. The anterior end should lie at least at 3.5–4.5cm of the ear canal.
- In thin skulls (children) the dura may be exposed and may be depressed slightly by the device if necessary.
- A groove in the cortical bone connecting the cortical cavity and the bed of the receiver-stimulator is fashioned.
- Drill holes in the posterior end of the cortical cavity or the groove to allow placement of retaining sutures to anchor the implant.
- Create a posterior tympanotomy (see 📖 p. 394, 5).
- A cochleostomy is made at the anteroinferior margin of the round-window niche, for the insertion of the electrode array in the scala tympani (Fig. 16.22).
- Alternatively, the electrode array can be inserted directly through the round window.
- Insert the electrode array with the help of a claw and, if necessary, use gentle rotation to facilitate the insertion (approximately 2cm).
- The receiver–stimulator is then placed in its bed and secured with sutures.
- The implant reference electrode is placed superiorly within the soft tissue.
- Before closure the implant is tested intra-operatively to determine thresholds and to estimate discomfort levels, which will be very helpful for the switching on procedure.
- Close in layers. The periosteum may be tight to close and a 2nd layer of soft tissue should overlap it.
- A head bandage is placed for 24h.

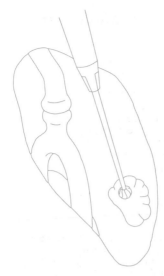

Fig. 16.22 Cochleostomy—right ear.

Post-operative period and rehabilitation

- A transorbital X-ray (Stenver's view) is undertaken the day after surgery to confirm the position of the electrode array in the cochlea.
- The device is switched on at 4–6 weeks with a close rehabilitation follow-up.
- Generally it may take 6–12 months to realize the full benefit of the implant.
- In pre-lingual children under the age of 4, results are encouraging, with approximately 2/3 going to mainstream education by the age of 5–6 years (half developing open set listening with good speech intelligibility, the rest requiring additional educational aid).

Complications

- Haemorrhage and haematoma.
- Skin-flap infection and wound breakdown, which can lead to device extrusion.
- Facial-nerve injury (most at risk during the posterior tympanotomy).
- Chorda tympani injury (as above).
- Perilymph fistula can cause temporary dizziness, or in more permanent cases, may require plugging of the cochleostomy.
- Meningitis after surgery or complicating an episode of acute otitis media (early antibiotic therapy recommended).
- Rarely, intracranial complications (i.e. intracranial haemorrhage).
- Implant failure.
- Malposition of the electrode array, requires reinsertion.

Trauma to the middle ear

- Tympanic-membrane injury (perforation).
- Ossicular injury (discontinuity, fixation).
- Tympanic-cavity injury (barotraumas, haemotympanum).
- Facial-nerve injury (temporal bone fracture).

Tympanic membrane injury

Common injury, usually due to:
- Sudden air or fluid compression (as it occurs in a hand-slap to the side of the face/ear, or ear syringing).
- Direct trauma from a foreign body (cotton-bud).
- Skull-base fracture, when the fracture line involves the tympanic ring.

Signs and symptoms
- Otalgia.
- Hearing loss (conductive in type, unless temporal bone fracture involving inner ear).
- ± Tinnitus.
- ± Dizziness.
- ± Otorrhoea (bloody initially, purulent if infection supervenes. Also CSF otorrhoea in temporal bone fracture).
- Otological examination will reveal a pars tensa perforation with bleeding or bruised edges (if recent injury).
- Look also for signs and symptoms of head injury in severe cases.

Treatment
- 1st: management of any associated head injury.
- Hearing assessment using free field testing, tuning fork and/or pure-tone audiometry. To confirm conductive hearing loss, if sensori-neural loss, suspect temporal bone fracture.
- If otorrhoea is present: swab for microscopy, culture, and sensitivity, and if purulent treat with topical antibiotics. If CSF is suspected clinically (typically the fluid leaves a 'halo effect' on a white tissue paper), aspirate a sample (if collected on a swab, wash with a small amount of normal saline) and send it in a universal container (frozen) to analyse for $\beta2$-transferrin (some biochemistry labs also require a clotted blood sample of the patient to compare the electrophoresis patterns of $\beta1$ and $\beta2$-transferrin).
- Water precautions.
- If failure to heal within 3 months then consider myringoplasty.

Ossicular injury

Caused by head injury with or without temporal bone fracture.

Ossicular discontinuity
- Usually dissrupting the incudo-stapedial joint, which is the most exposed part of the ossicles (the rest are 'shielded' by the scutum).
- Conductive hearing-loss (air–bone gap >50dB HL) with a high type A tympanogram.

Ossicular fixation
- As a consequence of ossicular dislocation, ligament rupture, or fracture line through the temporal bone.

- These injuries may require different types of ossiculoplasty.
- In incudo-stapedial joint dislocation, simple repositioning of the joint may suffice.

Tympanic cavity injury

Barotrauma
- It is caused by rapid increase of extratympanic pressure (e.g. non-pressurized airplane descent or rapid diving ascent: 'Caisson disease') middle-ear pressure compensation fails. A critical locking pressure (80mmHg) prevents Eustachian tube opening.

Signs and symptoms
- Otalgia (severe).
- Hearing loss (conductive in type, but in severe cases sensori-neural hearing loss can occur).
- Tinnitus.
- Dizziness.
- Tympanic membrane may be injected, retracted, with evidence of a middle ear effusion, or haemotympanum or perforation.
- May resolve spontaneously within days or weeks, or may progress into persistant otitis media with effusion (OME).

Treatment
- Prophilactic use of nasal vasoconstrictor/decongestant and otoinflation may be helpful.
- Treat infection, if present.
- Pain control.
- Otoinflation (with Valsalva maneouvre, or Otovent® device).
- If failure to resolve middle-ear effusion: myringotomy with or without grommet insertion (for longstanding and recurrent cases).

Facial-nerve injury

Caused almost exclusively by temporal bone fractures (see Chapter 18).

Neoplasia of the middle ear

Classification
- Benign
- Malignant:
  - Primary.
  - Secondary.

Benign tumours of the middle ear

Glomus tumours
Most common (see Chapter 19).

Adenoma
- 2nd most common.
- Presents (as glomus tumours) with a conductive hearing-loss and tinnitus.
- Otoscopy: a pink/red mass behind the tympanic membrane.
- CT and MRI scan are helpful to assess, extend, and exclude glomus tumours.
- Treatment: surgical excision via transcanal or transmastoid depending on the size of the tumour.

Facial nerve schwannoma
- Presents as a lower motor neurone facial-nerve palsy, recurrent or slowly progressive, or a previously misdiagnosed Bell's palsy that fails to show signs of recovery (usually within 3 months).
- Hearing loss and tinnitus are less common.
- The most common site is the region of the geniculate ganglion. CT scan will show expansion of this portion of the nerve.
- MRI scan to assess intracranial involvement.
- Surgical excision is carried out only when the facial paralysis is advanced, as results after surgery are usually poor (at best grade 3 in the House–Brackmann classification; see Chapter 17).

Others
- Meningioma (Very rarely results as an extension of a petrous apex or cerebellopontine angle meningioma).
- Haemangioma.
- Glioma.

Malignant tumours of the middle ear
- Primary malignancy of the ear and temporal bone is rare and very aggressive.
- Incidence: 1–6 cases per million.
- It is estimated that 1 case of primary middle-ear carcinoma occurs for every 5000–20 000 cases of benign middle-ear disease (CSOM).
- The commonest histological type is squamous cell carcinoma.
- These tumours spread mainly by direct invasion into the temporal bone and neighbouring structures (parotid, infratemporal fossa, dura, and brain).
- Metastatic disease is rare.

Signs and symptoms
- Chronic otorrhoea (bloody or purulent) and/or ear canal polyp.
- Otalgia (usually deep-seated otalgia, disproportionate to clinical findings).
- Hearing loss (mainly conductive).
- Facial-nerve weakness (and other lower cranial nerve injury if tumour spreads to involve the skull base).
- Lymphatic metastases are uncommon (10% to parotid nodes and neck) and distant spread extremely rare.

Diagnosis and staging
- Deep biopsy.
- CT and MR are complementary and play a vital role in staging and prognosis.
- The most commonly used staging system for SCC of the temporal bone is the University of Pittsburgh (Box 16.1).

Treatment
- Multidisciplinary assessment and treatment.
- In general lesions localized to the external auditory canal (EAC), (T1 lesions) are treated with a 'limited' resection (i.e. local resection, radical mastoidectomy).
- More advanced lesions (T2–T4) are treated by '*en bloc*' resection (lateral temporal bone resection, subtotal petrosectomy, total petrosectomy).
- Radiotherapy is advocated as an adjunct to surgery, or for palliation, rather than a curative treatment in itself.
- Survival rates are good for T1 and T2 lesions (50–100%), but poor in for T3 and T4 tumours (0–50%).

Box 16.1 University of Pittsburgh TNM staging system for tumours of the ear and temporal bone

T status

T1: tumour limited to the external canal without bony erosion or evidence of soft tissue involvement.

T2: tumour with limited external auditory canal bone erosion (not full thickness) or limited (0.5cm) soft-tissue involvement.

T3: tumour eroding the osseous external auditory canal (full thickness) with limited (<0.5cm) soft-issue involvement or tumour involving the middle ear and/or mastoid.

T4: tumour eroding the cochlea, petrous apex, medial wall of the middle ear, carotid canal, jugular foramen or dura, or with extensive soft-tissue involvement of the temperomandibular joint or styloid process, or evidence of facial paresis.

N status

Involvement of lymph-node metastases is a poor prognosis finding: any node involvement should automatically be considered as advanced disease, i.e. T1N1 = stage III and T2, T3, T4 N1 = stage IV.

M status

Distant metastases indicate a very poor prognosis and should be considered as stage IV disease.

In the absence of metastatic lymph nodes or distant metastases, T status of the tumour defies the clinical stage.

433

The facial nerve

Anatomy

- The facial nerve is derived from the second branchial arch and contains motor, sensory, and parasympathetic fibres.
- The motor fibres have their bodies in the facial motor nucleus, situated in the pons. It receives some fibres from the superior salivatory nucleus.
- The nerve exits the brainstem at the cerebellopontine angle.
- Motor fibres supply the muscles of facial expression, buccinator, platysma, stapedius, stylohyoid, and posterior body of digastric muscle.
- Sensory fibres (nervus intermedius) carry taste via the chorda tympani nerve from the anterior 2/3 of the tongue, and via the palatine and greater petrosal nerves.
- Secretomotor preganglionic parasympathetic fibres to the submandibular and sublingual salivary glands, and lachrymal, nasal and palatine mucosa glands.

The course of the facial nerve can be divided into three portions (Fig. 17.1).

CPA

- 23–24mm long.
- Between brainstem and IAM.
- VIIth lies anterior to VIIIth, also anterior to anterior-inferior cerebellar artery and its branch the labyrinthine artery.

IAM

- 8–10mm long.
- Within the IAM.
- VIIth lies in the anterosuperior compartment of the IAM, anterior and superior to VIIIth (Fig. 17.2). Important relationship in acoustic neuroma surgery.

Intratemporal

- Labyrinthine segment:
  - 3–5mm long.
  - Between the IAM and the geniculate ganglion.
  - It is the narrowest portion.
  - At the geniculate ganglion, gives the first branch: greater superficial petrosal nerve.
- Tympanic segment:
  - 12–13mm long.
  - Between the geniculate ganglion and second genu.
  - Passes horizontally across the medial wall of the tympanic cavity within a bony canal (Fallopian canal), which may be dehiscent in up to 15% of cases.
  - Its anterior landmark in the tympanic cavity is the processus cochleariformis, from where the tendon of tensor tympani is directed to the malleus.
  - Posteriorly the nerve lies between the oval window (inferiorly) and the lateral semicircular canal (superiorly).

- Mastoid segment.
  - 15–20mm long.
  - From the second genu to the stylomastoid foramen.
  - Here it lies in front and lateral to the ampulla of the posterior semicircular canal, and medial to the tympanic annulus.
  - The nerve to stapedius muscle (also known as the descending segment of VII) and chorda tympani leave and join, respectively.
  - The digastric ridge just posterior to the stylomastoid foramen is an useful landmark.

Extratemporal portion

From the stylomastoid foramen the nerve passes inferiorly and laterally around the styloid process and enters the parotid gland, here it divides into two main trunks and then five branches (with anatomical variations):

- temporal,
- zygomatic,
- buccal,
- marginal mandibular, and
- cervical.

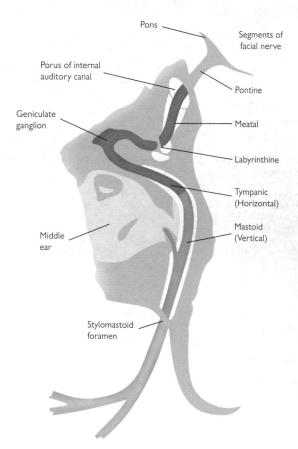

Fig. 17.1 Course of left facial nerve.

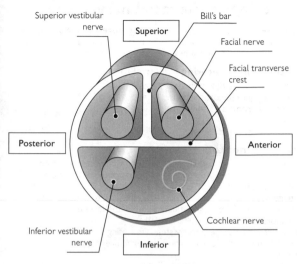

Fig. 17.2 Lateral view of right IAM.

Monitoring of the facial nerve

The purpose of using a nerve monitor during surgery is to aid surgeons in the identification and monitoring of the nerve at risk during surgery, but it is not a replacement for experience in surgical decision-making.

Indications for monitoring the facial nerve

- Mastoid surgery (either primary or revision).
- Revision surgery for otosclerosis.
- Acoustic neuroma surgery.
- Parotid surgery.
- Submandibular gland surgery.

Facial-nerve monitor

- The instrument gives audible interpretation of muscle movement, sensed by electrodes placed in the muscles controlled by the nerve/s to be monitored.
- Activity near neural fibres will cause the muscles to contract and the instrument will emit a distinctive sound, the level of which is proportional to the stimulus applied.
- The nerve may also be directly stimulated using a small current via a 'stimulation probe' (i.e. to confirm the structure in question as facial nerve).
- Muscle contractions are only possible if limited or no neuromuscular block is used by the anaesthetist.
- The instrument consists of:
  - main unit,
  - sensing electrodes, and
  - stimulation probe.
- The position of the electrodes varies depending on the monitor used and the type of surgery carried out.

Testing of the facial nerve

Facial-nerve palsy can be evaluated: clinically, audiometrically, radiologically, and also with the use of electrophysiological tests.

Clinical function tests

These tests will help to confirm the degree of disability and can aid in determining the site of the lesion.

Testing facial movement

- Will distinguish between upper motor neurone (forehead moves normally) and lower motor neurone (the entire face is affected, including the forehead).
- The well-recognized classification system for clinical grading of facial-nerve palsy is the House–Brackmann classification (Table 17.1).

Blink test

- There is a delay in blinking on the affected side when tapping on the patient's glabella with the examiner's finger.

Schirmer test

- Lacrimation can be measured using a folded strip of blotting paper placed in the lower conjunctival fornix of both eyes for 5min.
- Where abnormal test, the lacrimation is decreased by 75% compared to the other normal side bilateral when less than 10mm of paper is soaked on each side after 5min.
- ▶ Unilateral geniculate ganglion lesion can produce bilateral reduction of lacrimation).
- Positive test = lesion at geniculate ganglion.

Stapedial reflex test

- This test is discussed in Chapter 14.
- Positive test = lesion proximal to the nerve to stapedius muscle.

Taste testing

- Either clinically tasting for salt, sweet, sour, and bitter in the lateral aspect of the anterior 2/3 of the tongue.
- Or with electrogustometry, where the same area of the tongue is stimulated electrically, increasing the current until a metallic taste is perceived. The threshold of the affected side (increased) is compared to the other side (normal 1mA).
- Positive test = lesion at or proximal to the root of the chorda tympani.

Salivary-flow testing

- The flow of saliva in the cannulated submandibular gland duct is measured following salivatory stimulation (6% citric acid solution). The affected side will show a reduction of 25% compared with the normal side.
- Positive test = lesion at or proximal to chorda tympani.

Table 17.1 House–Brackmann classification of facial-nerve palsy

Grade	Characteristics			
	Gross	Motion		
		Forehead	Eye	Mouth
I	Normal function			
II	Slight weakness	Moderate to good function	Complete closure without effort	Slight weakness on maximum effort
III	Obvious weakness but not disfiguring Normal symmetry at rest	Slight to moderate function	Complete closure with effort	Slight weakness on maximum effort
IV	Obvious weakness and disfiguring asymmetry	No function	Imcomplete closure	Asymmetric on maximum effort
V	Barely perceptible motion Asymmetry at rest	No function	Imcomplete closure	Slight movement
VI	No movement at all			

Topognostic testing (see Fig. 17.3)

Electrophysiological tests

Most often used to predict the prognosis of a facial nerve injury.

Minimal nerve excitability test

• This test determines the minimal electrical (DC) current necessary to stimulate muscle contraction. It compares the normal and affected sides of the face.
• A difference of 3.5mA or > is significant and suggests nerve degeneration.

Maximal stimulation test

• Is similar but this time it determines the maximal stimulation current that the patient can tolerate.
• The response is compared to the normal side.
• The test has no value in the 1st 72h following the injury, as it can still show normal values.

- After this period a total lack of excitability will correspond to nerve degeneration. Neuropraxia will have a normal threshold, and partial degeneration will show raised thresholds compared to the normal side.

Electroneurography (ENoG)

- It is the most accurate of all the tests. It measures the amplitude of the stimulated muscle action potential ('evoked electromyography', EEMG), by placing an stimulating electrode in the skin over the stylomastoid foramen and recording electrodes on the skin over facial muscles (nasolabial fold).
- The stimulus is increased until there is no further increase in the amplitude of the response.
- The affected and the normal sides are compared. The result of the paralysed side is expressed as a % of the normal side.
- A <90% degeneration value will have complete recovery.
- Values over this figure will have a lower chance of recovery, and may be candidates for surgical decompression.

Electromyography (EMG)

- This test measures the electrical activity in the facial muscles.
- A needle electrode is inserted into the muscle and electrical activity is recorded at rest and during voluntary muscle contraction.
- Evidence of muscle denervation takes 2 weeks to present from the time of the injury, by way of spontaneous electrical activity (fibrillation potentials). The test is best used after this period of time.
- Re-innervation potentials can be demonstrated 4–12 weeks prior to clinical improvement is noticed, and are ∴ predictors of recovery.
- The presence of some motor unit potentials during muscle contraction implies that some nerve fibres are intact.
- All these electrophysiological tests, although useful, are of limited value during the immediate period following injury (4–14 days).

Magnetic stimulation

- For proximal nerve evaluation (intra temporal/brainstem).
- Magnetic stimulation of motor cortex corresponding to facial territory (experimental).

Radiological tests

CT scan

- Delineates the bony architecture of temporal bone.
- Especially useful in trauma and tumours.

MRI

- Visualizes the facial nerve itself.
- Especially useful for intra-temporal inflammation and also tumours (perineural invasion/spread).

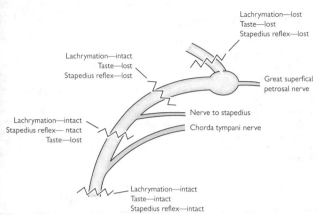

Fig. 17.3 Diagram of topognostic testing of the facial nerve. Reproduced From *Diseases of the Ear* (Harold Ludman and Tony Wright), with permission of Edward Arnold (Publishers) Ltd ©1997 Arnold.

Facial-nerve palsy

Causes of facial-nerve palsy

Idiopathic/Bell's palsy

- Unknown aetiology, although highly suspected to be viral (herpes virus). Viral prodrome.
- Common: estimated incidence 15–40 cases per 100 000 population.
- ♂ = ♀, 1 : 1.
- It is recurrent in approximately 10% of patients.
- Damaged caused by oedema followed by ischaemia due to compression against the bony canal.
- Recovery usually quick, but can take up to 12 months.
- Incomplete recovery in 13% cases.

Trauma

- Temporal bone fractures and facial wounds.
- Iatrogenic during otological, acoustic neuroma and parotid surgery.

Bacterial

- Acute otitis media (dehiscence in the facial nerve canal).
- Cholesteatoma.
- Malignant otitis externa.
- Lyme disease:
  - Caused by the spirochaete *Borrelia burgdorferi*, transmitted by tick bite.
  - Clinically also with fatigue, headache, neck stiffness, arthralgia, and skin rash (Erythema migrans).
  - Serological tests (IgM, IgG) are necessary to diagnose this disease.

Viral

- Herpes zoster oticus/Ramsay–Hunt syndrome:
  - 3–12% of causes of facial-nerve palsy.
  - Clinically severe pain and vesicles in the ear canal, pinna and face (within 24–48h).
  - VIIIth cranial nerve involvement: sensori-neural hearing loss and vertigo.
  - Diagnosis with rise in antibodies titres to the varicella–zoster virus.
  - Worse prognosis than Bell's (30–50% persistent palsy).
- HIV.

Tumours

- Parotid tumours (adenoid cystic, mucoepidermoid).
- Facial neuroma.
- Acoustic neuroma.
- Meningioma.
- Intraosseus haemangioma.
- Arachnoid cyst.

Inherited

- Myotonic dystrophy: progressive muscle weakness and mental impairment.
- Albers–Schoenberg disease: osteopetrosis of bony canals for cranial nerves causes blindness, deafness and facial palsy.

Congenital
- Möbius syndrome:
  - Unilateral or bilateral VIth and VIIth palsy.
  - Also III, IV, V, VIII, X, and XIIth cranial nerves can be affected; malformation of extremities and abscence of pectoralis muscle can be present.
- CHARGE syndrome.
- OAV (Oculo-auriculo-vertebral syndrome): unilateral hypoplasia of maxilla, mandible, and ear, 1st and 2nd branchial arch derivatives.
- CULLP (Congenital Unilateral Lower Lip Palsy) or hypoplasia of the depressor anguli ori muscle, associated also in some cases with congenital heart defects.

Systemic disease
- Sarcoidosis.
- Mononucleosis.
- HIV.
- Leukaemia.
- Guillain–Barré syndrome.
- Multiple sclerosis.

Other
- Melkersson–Rosenthal syndrome.
  - Recurrent unilateral or bilateral facial-nerve palsy.
  - Unknown cause.
  - Associated with facial oedema and fissured tongue.
- Brainstem cerebrovascular accident.
- Petrous cholesteatoma.

Assessment of facial palsy
- Take a detailed history.
- Test each branch:
  - Wrinkling of the forehead when looking up.
  - Tightly closing the eyes.
  - Wriggling the nose.
  - Blowing the cheeks.
  - Smiling or showing the upper teeth.
- Grade and document the palsy using House–Brackmann classification.
- Bell's phenomenom: the eyeball is rolled upwards to protect the cornea when the eyelid cannot close completely.
- Check for lachrymation, taste and salivation.
- Also examine:
  - Ear (trauma, CSOM with/without cholesteatoma, herpes zoster vesicles, malignant otitis externa).
  - Parotid gland (neoplasm).
  - Rest of cranial nerves (specially Vth in acoustic neuroma).
  - Hearing.

Management of facial palsy

General

- Eye care:
  - Ophthalmology review to assess ocular damage (corneal abrasion/ ulceration) if present.
  - Wear glasses for eye protection.
  - Close the eyelid at night with the help of an eyepad and/or tape across the eyelid.
  - Prescribe artificial tears.
  - If long-term care needed, consider tarsorraphy or upper eyelid gold weight prosthesis.
- Facial massage and exercises.

Medical treatment

- Bell's palsy/Ramsay–Hunt:
  - Oral steroids (i.e. prednisolone 60mg initially –1mg/kg body weight, reducing dose over a period of 10–14 days).
  - Oral antivirals (i.e. aciclovir 400–800mg five times a day for 1 week).
  - Adequate analgesia (i.e. carbamazepine, amytriptiline).
- Acute otitis media/mastoiditis:
  - Treated with oral steroids and systemic antibiotics.

Surgical treatment

- Bell's palsy: some surgeons advocate that a >90% degeneration value in ENoG predicts a poor prognosis and ∴ surgical decompression should be considered, however this has not shown significant benefits compared to medical treatment.
- Acute suppurative otitis media/mastoiditis: myringotomy ± ventilation tube and/or cortical mastoidectomy.
- Chronic suppurative otitis media: mastoidectomy and facial nerve decompression.
- Iatrogenic post-ear surgery:
  - Immediate facial-nerve palsy after otological surgery may be due to the effect of local anaesthetic (wait and re-assess).
  - Once this has been ruled out, if the surgeon is entirely confident that the nerve has not been transected, i.e. the epineurium is intact, a conservative approach in the management can be taken with the use of high-dose steroids.
  - ENoG should be carried out within 1 week and the ear re-explored if >90% degeneration.
  - Otherwise urgent re-exploration and decompression or nerve-grafting must be considered and by another more experienced surgeon, if necessary.
  - Delayed palsy can be due to pressure from an over-tight mastoid packing (in open technique), which should be removed.
  - Post-operative oedema and infection can compress the nerve and are treated with high-dose steroids and antibiotics.
- Temporal bone fracture:
  - Immediate and total facial-nerve palsy requires facial-nerve decompression by a neurotologist (as soon as the patient's medical condition allows it, preferably within 2–3 weeks of injury).

- If the palsy was not immediate or the diagnosis delayed due to loss of consciousness use ENoG degeneration value of >90% as an indicator of poor recovery and surgical exploration is indicated.
- Topognostic testing will help to dictate the surgical approach:
  — Impaired lacrimation and complete sensori-neural hearing-loss: translabyrinthine approach.
  — Impaired lacrimation but no sensori-neural hearing-loss: middle-fossa approach.
  — Intact lacrimation and no sensori-neural hearing-loss: transmastoid approach.

Facial-nerve grafting

The facial nerve can be damaged by trauma or tumour from the level of the cerebellopontine angle to the extratemporal individual motor branches. At any of these points, surgical repair, either direct suture or interpositon nerve-grafting. can be carried out.

Several donor nerves can be used, depending on the length of nerve needed for grafting:

- Greater auricular nerve (can be found in the upper-third of the posterior border of sternomastoid or at Erb's point and trace superiorly).
- Sural nerve (found approximately 2cm posterior and proximal to the lateral malleolus, running parallel to the small saphenous vein, and can be traced proximally through a step ladder incisons to provide a longer graft).

Technique (Fig. 17.4)

- Neural repair is performed using microsurgical techniques.
- The nerve endings must be mobilized, cleanly transected,and opposed without tension.
- The bundles of fascicles (or perineurium) are aproximated and sutured with 10/0 nylon.
- The nerve sheath is also be approximated in similar fashion.
- Just two or three sutures may be enough to maintain nerve continuity while minimizing foreign-body reaction.
- If the injury occurred in the Fallopian canal, the anastomosis may not require suturing if the nerve endings are stable.
- An alternative to suturing is placing a vein graft secured with glue (more suitable for anastomosis at the cerebellopontine angle).

(a)

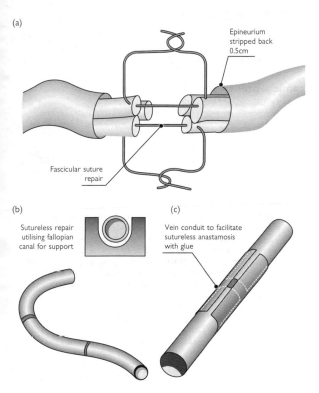

Epineurium
stripped back
0.5cm

Fascicular suture
repair

(b)

Sutureless repair
utilising fallopian
canal for support

(c)

Vein conduit to facilitate
sutureless anastamosis
with glue

Fig. 17.4 Techniques of facial nerve repair.

Facial re-animation

The objective of facial reanimation is to restore the static (facial symmetry, resting tone) and, if possible, the dynamic (movement) characteristics of the face following facial-nerve damage.

There are several steps in the re-animation 'ladder'.

Dynamic procedures

- Primary repair (direct anastomosis).
- Cable/interposition nerve grafting (as described).
- Nerve substitution (if the proximal end of facial nerve is unavailable for anastomosis):
  - Facial-hypoglossal anastomosis (Fig. 17.5a):
    — Through an extended parotidectomy incision into the neck.
    — The hypoglossal nerve is identified deep to the posterior belly of digastric.
    — The nerve is dissected proximally to provide adequate length for a tension-free anastomosis.
    — The facial-nerve trunk is exposed 1cm deep to the tragal pointer as per parotidectomy, and divided proximally.
    — The hypoglossal nerve is passed under posterior belly of digastric to a tension free anastomosis with VIIth.
    — A variation using the greater auricular nerve to join a partially transected (50% of its diametre) hypoglossal nerve with the distal stump of the facial nerve preserves XIIth function. (Fig. 17.5b).
  - Cross-facial grafting: a two-stage procedure:
    — 1st stage: harvest and place a tunnelled sural nerve conduit from the normal VIIth to the paralysed VIIth. The growth of axons is followed clinically with Tinel's sign (tingling sensation caused by tapping the growing end of the nerve).
    — Second stage: performed once regeneration has occurred. The sural nerve graft is then anastomosed to the stump of the paralysed VIIth.
- Muscle transfer:
  - Regional-temporalis muscle.
  - Provides tone and some dynamic movement of the oral commissure.
  - Approach: through a rhytidectomy incision.
  - An inferiorly based temporalis muscle flap elevated and reflected inferiorly and sutured to orbicularis oris muscle (Fig. 17.6).
  - Free muscle transfer (gracilis, latissimus dorsi), with neurovascular anastomosis.

Static procedures

- Fascia lata sling:
  - Useful to address unsightly asymmetry due to poor tone.
  - Fascia lata graft anchored from temporalis muscle and periosteum of zigoma to orbicularis and nasolabial tissue.
  - An eyebrow lift may complement this procedure.

(a)

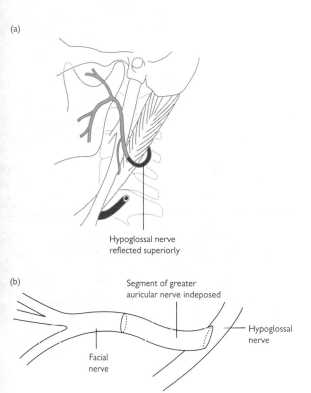

Hypoglossal nerve
reflected superiorly

(b)

Segment of greater
auricular nerve indeposed

Facial
nerve

Hypoglossal
nerve

Fig. 17.5 Facial-hypoglossal anastomosis: (a) classic procedure, (b) modification.

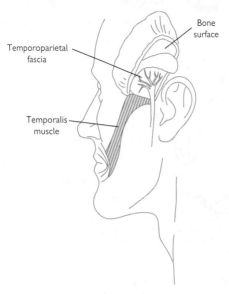

Fig. 17.6 The repositioned temporalis muscle is swung down and attached to the tissues of the corner of the mouth.

The inner ear

Embryology and anatomy of the inner ear

Embryology

The membranous labyrinth

- In the 3rd week of development, the 'otic placode' (thickening of ectoderm) is formed in the first occipital somite on each side of the skull.
- At 30 days, an enlarging 'otocyst' is developed. This will form the endolymphatic duct medially and the utriculosacular chamber laterally.
- At 35 days, three ridges are formed at right-angles of each other (the semicircular canals), and the ridge centre will be replaced by the surrounding mesoderm.
- Certain thickened epithelial areas give rise to the neuroepithelium of the macula (14–16 weeks), cristae (23–24 weeks), and organ of Corti (25 weeks).

The bony labyrinth

- The mesoderm surrounding the labyrinth forms the bony otic capsule and the perilymphatic spaces of the inner ear.
- The ossification takes place from the 15th to the 21st week, from up to 14 centres.
- The interior of the bony labyrinth communicates with the outside through 7–8 channels:
  - IAM, subarcuate fossa.
  - vestibular aqueduct.
  - cochlear aqueduct.
  - fissula ante fenestram.
  - fissula post fenestram (incostant).
  - oval window and round windows.

Anatomy

The inner ear can be divided into two parts: the cochlea and the vestibular system (Fig. 18.1).

The cochlea

- Organ of sound transduction, encased in the petrous temporal bone.
- The cochlear duct spirals 2.5 turns. Its base measures 9mm, height is 5mm and length 29–40mm. It has a triangular section and contains the 'organ of Corti' (Fig.18.2).
- The modioulus (central cone), contains canals that accommodate the bipolar ganglion cells of the spiral cochlear ganglion.
- The osseous spiral lamina arises from the modiolus and divides the cochlea into 'scala vestibuli' and 'scala tympani', these communicate at the apex (helicotrema).
- The scala vestibuli opens into the vestibule with the fenestra vestibuli (oval window) and the stapes footplate very close to it.
- The scala tympani is a blind-ending tube that has in its base at the fenestra cochleae (round window).

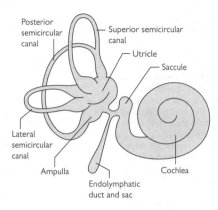

Fig. 18.1 Diagram of the inner ear. From the Oxford Handbook of ENT and Head and Neck surgery. Reproduced with permission by Oxford University Press.

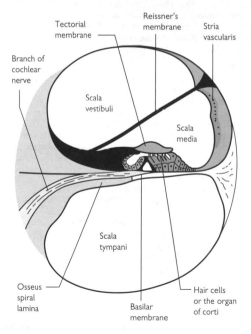

Fig. 18.2 Cross section of the cochlea. From the Oxford Handbook of ENT and Head and Neck surgery. Reproduced with permission by Oxford University Press.

The vestibular system

- It is situated behind the cochlea, the utricle lies posteriorly, and the saccule anteriorly (underneath stapes footplate). Both are connected by their corresponding ducts, which together will form the endoly mphatic duct, this passes through a bony canal (the vestibular aqueduct), and expands into a flattened endolymphatic sac, blending into the posterior cranial fossa dura.
- In the utricle and saccule there is specialized sensory epithelium called 'macula' (in the horizontal plane in the utricle, and vertical plane in the saccule). The macula forms part of the 'otolithic organ' (Fig. 18.3a).
- The bony semicircular canals (superior, lateral, and posterior) are placed at right-angles of each other, the lateral one is inclined 30 degrees to the horizontal plane and the superior and posterior canals 45 degrees to the sagittal plane. The canals of both sides are orthogonal to each other.
- Each has a dilated portion anteriorly (ampulla) and a non-ampullary end that is joined to the superior and posterior canals ('crus comune').
- The ampulla contains vestibular sensory epithelium, 'crista' (Fig. 18.3b).
- The sensory cells in the macula and crista contain stereocilia, graded in height, with the tallest closest to the kinocilium. The kinocilium has a 9 + 2 arrangement of microtubule doublets.
- Deflection of stereocilia towards the kinocilium results in an increase in the firing rate of the afferent neuron.
- Deflection away causes a decrease in the firing rate.

Blood supply

- Mainly from the internal auditory artery, branch of the anterior-inferior cerebellar artery (AICA) or from the basilar artery.
- The internal auditory artery divides into:
  - The common cochlear artery (supplying the cochlea, and inferior portion of utricle and saccule, and posterior semicircular canal).
  - The anterior vestibular artery (supplying the superior portion of the utricle and saccule, superior and lateral semicircular canals).

Innervation

Central auditory pathway

- Afferent pathway (ECOLI mnemonic):
  - E—8th (cochlear) nerve (approximately 30 000 fibres)—1st-order neurone.
  - C—cochlear nucleus in the pons—2nd-order neurone.
  - O—superior olive, ipsi-, and contra-lateral side via the trapezoid body—3rd-order neurone.
  - L—lateral lemniscus to the …
  - I—inferior colliculus to the medial geniculate body—4th-order neurone.
  - From here the fibres go to the auditory cortex via the internal capsule.
- Efferent pathway—from auditory cortex to the cochlear nuclei (with additional contributions from the superior olive, bilaterally), continuing into the superior division of the vestibular nerve and terminating in the outer hair cells.

Central vestibular pathway
- Afferent fibres:
  - The superior-vestibular division (nerve) carries the fibres from the superior and lateral semicircular canals and the utricle.
  - The inferior-vestibular division (nerve) carries the fibres from the posterior semicircular canal (singular nerve) and saccule.
  - The vestibular nerve enters at the lower border of the pons, separated from the facial nerve by the acoustic nerve, the intermediate nerve, and usually AICA.
  - Afferent fibres terminate in the vestibular nuclei: superior, lateral, medial and descending, all in the floor of the fourth ventricle.
- Efferent fibres from the vestibular nuclei to:
  - Contra-lateral vestibular nuclei.
  - Motor nuclei of III, IV, and VI cranial nerves.
  - Cerebellum.
  - Spinal cord.
  - Autonomic nervous system.
  - Temporal lobe cortex.

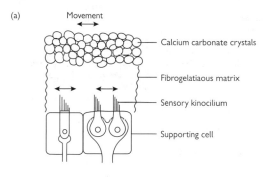

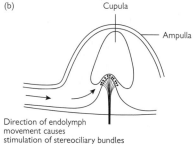

Fig. 18.3 Ultrastructure of sensory epithelium of: (a) utricle and saccule, (b) semicircular canals. From the Oxford Handbook of ENT and Head and Neck surgery. Reproduced with permission by Oxford University Press.

Physiology of the inner ear

Physiology of hearing

- Tonotopic representation: different areas of the cochlea are frequency-specific.
- The sound transmitted to the oval window creates a wave in the basilar membrane. High-frequency sound vibrates this membrane with greater amplitude at the base of the cochlea, whilst the low tones stimulate more the apex.
- This is the principle of the 'cochlear travelling wave' postulated by von Békésy, whose work on the physiology of hearing was awarded the Nobel Prize in 1961.
- The movement caused by the wave leads to a shearing force between the basal and tectorial membranes. This leads to movement of stereocilia of the hair cells, ions flow across the cell membrane, and IHC depolarizes with release of neurotransmitters at its base, which generates an action potential in VIIIth nerve fibres.
- Each fibre has a frequency of stimulation for which it is most sensitive.
- As the stimulus intensity is increased, so is the activation of IHC and ∴ the firing rate of the auditory nerve fibres, but this is in a non-linear manner.
- The role of the OHC is to generate the mechanical amplification of the basal membrane vibration.
- The activity of the OHC produce the cochlear microphonics (used in electrocochleography) and also they are responsible for otoacoustic emissions (OAEs) (see 🕮 p. 302).
- Most cochlear sensori-neural hearing-loss is due to loss of the amplification mechanism by the OHC.
- This loss of OHC also is responsible for the 'recruitment' effect (see 🕮 p. 293).

Physiology of balance

- The vestibular system is formed by five distinct organs: 3 semicircular canals (superior, lateral and posterior), and 2 otolith organs (utricle and saccule).
- It is important not to forget that the vision and proprioception organs have also a very important role in balance function.
- The semicircular canals sense angular acceleration, whereas the otolithic organs sense linear acceleration (the utricle in the horizontal plane, the saccule in the vertical one).
- Ampullopetal flow (towards the ampulla) of endolymph is excitatory in lateral canals, but inhibitory in the superior and posterior canals.
- Ampullofugal flow (away from the ampulla) has the opposite effect.
- The effect of the canals is paired: right and left lateral canals, right superior with left posterior, and left superior with right posterior. This explains how compensation is possible after unilateral vestibular loss.

Vestibulo-ocular reflex

- One of the functions of the vestibular system is to maintain optical fixation during head movement, this is the vestibulo-ocular reflex.
- The membranous labyrinth moves with head movement, but the endolymph remains static, thus causing relative motion, e.g. if your head turns to the right, whilst continuing to read this passage:
- The motion stimulates the sensory neuroepithelium of your right canal (the cupula on the right lateral canal is deflected towards the utricle causing increase of the firing rate), resulting in stimulation/contraction of the right medial rectus and the left lateral rectus muscles, and inhibits the opposite side (cupula in the left deflects away from the utricle causing a decrease in the firing rate), resulting in inhibition/relaxation of the right lateral rectus and left medial rectus muscles.
- ∴ the eyes remain fixed on the target, in this case the text on the page.

Vestibulospinal reflex

- Senses head movement and position relative to gravity.
- Projects to antigravity muscles via three pathways: lateral and medial vestibulospinal, and reticulospinal tracts.

The physiology of the otolithic organ is explained on 📖 p 456. More information of vestibular function can be found on 📖 p. 310 & 322.

Presbyacusis

- This term describes 'age-related' or 'degenerative' hearing-loss.
- Affects men (over 60 years of age) more than women.
- Pathophysiology: a reduction in the number of spiral ganglion cells as well as hair cells.

Signs and symptoms

- Bilateral, progressive, symmetrical sensori-neural hearing loss, with no history of noise exposure.
- The patient may have worse speech discrimination than expected when reviewing the audiogram.
- Normal findings on otoscopy.

Investigations

Pure-tone audiogram shows the typical 'ski slope' curve (Fig. 18.4).

Types of presbyacusis

Based on the shape of the audiogram and the site of loss, and can be subdivided as follows:

- Sensory presbyacusis:
  - Steep, sloping audiogram above speech frequency.
  - Speech discrimination preserved.
  - Results from degeneration of the organ of Corti.
- Neural presbyacusis:
  - Shows a down-sloping, high-frequency loss.
  - Flatter audiogram than sensory presbyacusis.
  - Thought to be 1st-order neurone loss.
  - Disproportionate poor discrimination score.
- Strial presbyacusis:
  - Has a flat audiogram.
  - Good discrimination.
- Cochlear conductive/indeterminate presbyacusis.
  - Down sloping audiogram.
  - Increasing stiffness of basilar membrane.
- Central presbyacusis:
  - Loss of GABA in inferior colliculus.

Management

- There is no reversal of the hearing loss. Management is directed at coping with the hearing disability:
- Hearing-aid.
- Hearing therapy (environmental aids, lip reading).

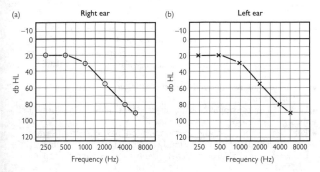

Fig. 18.4 Pure-tone audiogram of presbyacusis ('ski slope' curves for (a) right ear and (b) left ear). From the Oxford Handbook of ENT and Head and Neck surgery. Reproduced with permission by Oxford University Press.

Tinnitus

- Tinnitus is an auditory perception that can be described as the experience of sound, in the ear or in the head, in the absence of external acoustic stimulation (not heard by anyone else) ∴ subjective.
- It can be also objective: body sounds, vascular anomalies, palatal myoclonus.
- The term tinnitus is derived from the Latin word 'tinnre', which means to ring or tinkle.
- Up to 18% of the population are affected by tinnitus, the majority mildly.
- Between 0.5 and 3% of the adult population may suffer from severe chronic tinnitus, which can seriously affect their normal lives by producing mood disorders, anxiety, depression, or altered sleep patterns.

Aetiology

- Tinnitus can occur as an isolated symptom without a recognizable cause or in association with a middle- or inner-ear disorder, such as:
  - Sensori-neural hearing loss.
  - Sudden deafness.
  - Presbycusis.
  - Otosclerosis.
  - Ménière's disease.
  - Glomus tumour.
  - Acoustic neuroma.
- Many environmental factors can also cause tinnitus, such as:
  - Acute acoustic trauma.
  - Exposure to occupational noise.
  - Exposure to recreational and amplified music.
- Iatrogenic factors causing tinnitus include drug-induced ototoxicity caused by:
  - Amynoglycosides antimicrobials.
  - Cysplatin.
  - Quinine.
  - Aspirin and NSAIDs.
  - Xylocaine.
- Other general causes include:
  - Cardiovascular disease.
  - Haematological disorders (anaemia).
  - Endocrine (thyroid dysfunction, uncontrolled diabetes).
  - Neurological disorders (migraine, multiple sclerosis).
  - Alcohol intoxication.

Pathophysiology

There are several theories:
- Tinnitus arises not in the ears but in the brain, suggesting that 'abnormal connections' in the central auditory system may play a role in tinnitus perception.
- Genetic origin for tinnitus.

- The 'neurophysiological model for tinnitus' (Jastreboff) proposes that tinnitus results from the abnormal processing of a signal generated in the auditory system. This abnormal processing occurs before the signal is perceived centrally. This may result in 'feedback', whereby the annoyance created by the tinnitus causes the individual to focus increasingly on the noise, which in turn exacerbates the annoyance and so a 'vicious cycle' develops (Fig. 18.5).
- There is a strong relationship between the symptom of tinnitus and the activity of the prefrontal cortex and limbic system (which mediates emotions).

This is of great importance in understanding why the sensation of tinnitus is, in many cases, so distressing for the patient.

- When symptoms are severe, tinnitus can be associated with major depression, anxiety, and other psychosomatic and/or psychological disturbances, leading to a progressive deterioration of quality of life.

Diagnosis

- History, including the relevant otological (pulsatile, progressive, associated with imbalance), general, and family history.
- General examination and also focusing on the ears, teeth, neck, and scalp muscles.
- Pure-tone audiometry.
- Tympanogram.
- Tuning-fork testing.
- MRI of the internal auditory meatus and brain is recommended in persistent, unilateral tinnitus, to exclude acoustic neuroma or other lesions, such as glomus tumours, meningiomas, adenomas, and vascular lesions.

Treatment

At present no specific therapy for tinnitus is acknowledged to be satisfactory in all patients.

- Hearing-aid. Many patients who complain of tinnitus and who also have a significant hearing impairment will benefit from a hearing-aid. Not only will this help their hearing disability, but also the severity of their tinnitus may be reduced.
- Drugs: tricyclic anti-depressants have been shown to improve tinnitus-related disability in people with or without depression and chronic tinnitus. Other pharmacological agents used with less beneficial results include:
  - anti-epileptics.
  - Baclofen (skeletal muscle relaxant and central nervous system depressant).
  - benzodiazepines.
  - cinnarizine (a cerebral vasodilator and vestibular sedative).
  - nicotinamide (vitamin B group).
  - zinc.
  - ginkgo biloba.

- Lidocaine and tocainide (local anaesthetics and anti-arrhythmics that act by stabilizing hair-cell membrane and cochlear nerve fibres) have also been used in the treatment of tinnitus with no significant benefit but with reported adverse reactions (gastrointestinal upset, dizziness, mouth dryness, rash, and tremor).
- Other interventions:
  - Tinnitus retraining therapy (see 📖 p. 320).
  - Psychotherapy (including cognitive-behavioural therapy).
  - Tinnitus masking devices ('white-noise generators').
  - Biofeedback.
  - Hypnosis.
  - Acupuncture.
  - Electromagnetic stimulation.
  - Low-power laser to tympanic membrane.

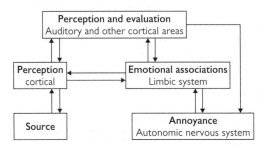

Fig. 18.5 Neurophysiological model for Tinnitus (Jastreboff). From the Oxford Handbook of ENT and Head and Neck surgery. Reproduced with permission by Oxford University Press.

Noise-induced hearing loss

- Damage to the inner ear caused by exposure to loud noise.
- There is a relationship between the volume of sound and its duration:
  - 8 hours of exposure to a sound level of 85dB during several years usually causes damage.
  - Louder sounds will cause damage at shorter exposure times.
  - Sounds >180dB cause acute acoustic trauma.

Pathophysiology

- Loud sound pesented to the cochlea causes a temporary threshold shift (TTS) that will recover after a rest period.
- If this loud stimulus continues, the TTS will become permanent, due to irreversible damage to the cochlea, in particular the outer hair cells of the basilar turn (thus high frequencies affected first), then also affecting the inner hair cells and degeneration of the spiral ganglion cells.
- Hearing loss is greatest in 3–6kHz region of the cochlea.
- <2kHz the acoustic reflex is protective.
- External ear-canal resonant frequency is 1–4kHz, so energy delivered to the middle ear at these frequencies is greatest.
- At present there is no evidence of hair-cell regeneration in humans.

Signs and symptoms

- Bilateral and symmetrical sensori-neural hearing loss.
- In cases such as riffle shooting, the hearing loss can be unilateral, corresponding to the ear closest to the end of the gun barrel (the left ear in a right-handed person).
- There may be an initial noise-induced TTS that recovers after a rest period.
- The patient also may have difficulty hearing in background noise or may have tinnitus.
- Otoscopy is normal.

Investigations

- Pure-tone audiometry: 3–6kHz dip (Fig. 18.6).
- Tympanometry: normal.
- Tuning-fork testing: Rinne positive, Weber lateralized to the opposite ear.

Management

Prophylactic measures:
- Health and safety at work.
- Provision of ear defenders.
- Routine hearing screening for occupations at risk.

In established hearing loss:
- Hearing-aid.
- Hearing therapy.
- Compensation may be sought (1975 Social Security Act).
- The percentage disability is calculated by taking the average hearing thresholds at 1, 2, and 3kHz and adjusting (using tables) for age, sex, and exposure duration.

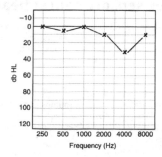

Fig. 18.6 Pure-tone audiogram of noise-induced hearing loss (3–6kHz dip). From the Oxford Handbook of ENT and Head and Neck surgery. Reproduced with permission by Oxford University Press.

Acute onset sensori-neural hearing loss

- Sudden onset sensori-neural hearing loss is an emergency.
- The term acute refers to the onset: instantaneously, or over hours, although the time of presentation to the ENT department for treatment may have been delayed by days or even weeks.

Aetiology

- Idiopathic (the commonest cause).
- Infective (bacterial/viral, e.g. measles, mumps, rubella, varicella-zoster; labyrinthitis, meningitis, syphilis).
- Trauma (iatrogenic, temporal bone fracture, perilymph fistula-barotrauma, acoustic trauma).
- Tumours (acoustic neuroma).
- Ototoxic drugs (see 🕮 p. 472).
- Neurological (brainstem cerebrovascular accident, multiple sclerosis).
- Autoimmune (see 🕮 p. 470).
- Other (Ménière's disease, diabetes, sarcoidosis, non-organic hearing loss) (see 🕮 p. 474–84).

Assessment

- Full drug history.
- Exclude head or acoustic trauma.
- Exclude ear wax.
- Exclude middle-ear effusion.
- Tuning-fork testing:
  - Rinne positive in the affected ear (AC > BC).
  - Weber lateralized to the opposite ear.
- Pure-tone audiogram confirms sensori-neural hearing loss with no air–bone gap.
- Laboratory investigations: FBC, ESR, U&Es, glucose, cholesterol, triglycerides, viral titres (and repeat at 6 weeks), angiotensine converting enzyme (ACE) level, antinuclear antibodies (ANA), anti-neutrophil cytoplasmic antibodies (ANCA), anti-endothelial cell antibodies, anti-phospholipid/anticardiolipin antibodies, anti-thyroid antibodies, syphilis serology, and urinalysis.
- Plain CXR to exclude mediastinal sarcoidosis.
- MRI to exclude acoustic neuroma or other central pathology.

Management

- Without treatment approximately 50–60% of the patients will recover their hearing loss.
- There is little evidence to support the current treatment strategies in acute sensori-neural hearing loss. The effects carefully and shlould however, are often permanent and the disability great, ∴ the decision must be taken involve discussion between clinician and patient.
- A frequently used regime:
  - Admission for bed rest.
  - Oral steroids (prednisolone, starting at a dose of 60mg daily and then reducing gradually over a period of 10–14 days).

- Oral acyclovir (500–800mg five times a day for 7 days).
- Oral betahistine (16mg three times a day for 10–14 days).
- Carbogen gas (a mixture of 5%CO_2 and 95%O_2 given as inhalation for 10min every hour, resting at night, for 48h).
- Daily audiograms to monitor progress.
- If there is improvement in the hearing at 48h, continue with the treatment. If not, discharge on a reducing course of prenisolone, and retest hearing within one to two weeks.
- Hearing-aid is to be considered if enough hearing disability.
- Hearing therapy referral.

Autoimmune ear disease

May be organ specific, or systemic.

Organ-specific

Vestibulo-auditory autoimmunity or evidence of cell mediated immunity against inner ear antigens.

Systemic disease

Part of a recognized systemic autoimmune disease:

Polyarteritis nodosa
- Necrotizing vasculitis of small and medium vessels.
- Mucosal ulceration, retinal haemorrhages, pericarditis, and renal affectation.

Cogan's syndrome
- A non syphilitic interstitial keratitis with vestibuloauditory dysfunction.
- It presents with photophobia and lacrimation 1–6 months before vertigo and hearing loss develop.
- In atypical Cogan's, the interstitial keratitis develops 1–2 years before.

Wegener's granulomatosis

- A necrotizing granulomatous vasculitis of the lower and upper respiratory tract, which also affects the kidneys causing focal necrotizing glomerulonephritis.
- 90% of patients have a sensori-neural hearing loss and 20% have a conductive loss due to OME.

Relapsing polychondritis

- This giant cell arteritis and systemic vasculitis cause recurrent episodes of inflammatory necrosis.
- Raised ESR and a false-positive VDRL.
- Rheumatoid arthritis.
- Very common condition with characteristic arthropathy.

Systemic lupus erythematosus

- Anti-nuclear antibodies and immunocomplex deposits in the basement membrane of blood vessels.
- Characteristic butterfly rash on the face, and also affects the heart, lung and kidneys.

Signs and symptoms

- Bilateral unexplained sensori-neural hearing loss.
- The hearing loss can be rapidly progressive over days or weeks.
- There may be also fluctuant dizziness or Meniere's-like syndrome with aural fullness.
- May also be associated with VIIth nerve palsy.
- Coexisting systemic immune disease (which may be undiagnosed).
- Normal otoscopic examination.

Investigations and treatment
- As for acute onset sensori-neural hearing loss.
- Once the diagnosis has been established, treatment should be given under the guidance of a rheumatologist.
- The initial treatment consists of oral steroids (Prednisolone 1mg/kg).
- Oral steroids are likely to be required in the long term, but need to be tritrated to the lowest possible dose that achieves symptom control.
- Alternatives are steroid-sparing medications (although these are not without significant side-effects either): cyclophosphamide and methotrexate.

Ototoxicity

- Drugs can damage the cochlea and vestibular system.
- Audiovestibular symptoms (tinnitus, hearing loss, and vertigo) are usually bilateral and occur a few days (3–4) after starting the drug treatment.
- It is important to take a careful drug history, as a wide range of drugs can be ototoxic:

Antibiotics

Aminoglycosides

- There are numerous aminoglycosides, including:
  - Gentamicin.
  - Streptomycin/Dihydrostreptomycin.
  - Neomycin.
  - Kanamycin.
  - Tobramycin.
  - Amikacin.
- These antibiotics have a narrow therapeutic index and can cause damage to the inner ear.
- They enter the perilymph, then slowly the endolymph, remaining for days.
- Damage occurs to the sensory hair-cell: the outer hair-cells first affected, followed by the inner hair-cells.
- Damage also occurs to the crista and the macula of the vestibular system.
- The plasma level of these antibiotics should be monitored closely during therapy, taking into account also renal function, as these are excreted by the kidneys.

Topical administration

- Antibiotics drops are commonly used for otitis externa and CSOM, as the bacteria targeted are usually sensitive to them (*Pseudomona*, *Proteus*, etc.).
- Theoretically there is a risk of ototoxicity in cases of CSOM, where the antibiotic, passing through a tympanic membrane perforation, reaches the round window and diffuses through its membrane into the inner ear.
- This risk has not been quantified, but it is thought to be low, because of the lower concentration used in the topical preparation. However, prolonged courses (>2 weeks) should be avoided.
- The risk of hearing loss due to no treatment must also be considered.
- **Other ototoxic antibiotics**:
  - vancomycin.
  - erythromycin.
  - polymyxin B.

Loop diuretics
- Frusemide, bumetanide, and ethacrynic acid cause hearing loss and tinnitus.
- Their effect is usually reversible, but may be permanent in a small number of cases.

Salicylates
- An overdose of aspirin causes high-frequency tinnitus and hearing loss in all frequencies.
- No vestibular symptoms.
- OHC are affected.
- The effects are reversible.

Propranolol
- The sensori-neural hearing loss caused by this beta-blocker can be reversible.

Quinine
- It is an antiprotozoal, but also used to be prescribed to treat night cramps.
- The sensori-neural hearing loss caused can be permanent.

Cisplatin
- High-frequency sensori-neural hearing loss.
- Reversible.

Phenytoin
- The use of this anticonvulsant can cause vertigo.
- Its level should be monitored.

Anti-depressants
- 5-Hydroxytryptamine (5-HT) agonists and Imipramine have an effect on the central auditory pathway.

Non-organic hearing loss

- Also known as pseudohypacusis.
- There is a discrepancy between the patient's claim of hearing loss and the audiological test results.
- Usually occurs in children, and more in females than males.

Clinical presentation

- Example 1: a child having difficulties at school or home who presents with a very poor hearing-test result. However, the hearing loss documented on the pure-tone audiogram seems out of keeping with the child's responses during the consultation.
- Example 2: a patient who is pursuing a claim for damages as a result of a hearing loss.
- In such cases, the audiologists may raise concerns about inconsistent responses.

Investigations

- Pure-tone audiometry (inconsistent responses; poor repeatability).
- Tuning-fork test—Stenger test (see Chapter 14).
- Stapedial reflex testing (suggests lower threshold than on PTA).
- Speech audiometry (discrepancy between PTA and speech audiogram).
- Delayed-speech feedback: the patient reads aloud and their speech is played into the affected ear. The playback is slightly delayed, which will cause the patient to hesitate or stutter if they can hear.
- Oto-acoustic emissions (transient evoked OAE's are useful to check threshold).
- Auditory brainstem response and cortical electrical audiometry (ABR and CERA are the gold standard in litigation cases, but they requires patient's cooperation).

Management

- Careful handling of non-organic hearing-loss is required. It may be wise to suggest to affected children that you know their hearing is better, but without being confrontational.
- Repeat audiogram at another outpatient appointment may be necessary and often may reveal an improvement in the hearing.
- One must also be aware of psychological disorders and involve the appropriate team in the management of the patient.
- Litigation claims need more tact and multiple investigations (see above) before any confrontation.

Assessment of the patient with dizziness

As stated earlier, in Chapter 14, balance disorders can result from peripheral (visual, proprioceptive, or vestibular system) or central nervous system pathology. The origin of dizziness ∴ can be multifactorial: neurological, vascular, otological, etc. (Table 18.1).

Clinical assessment history

- Much can be gained from the history, both general medical history (cardiovascular, neurological, ophthalmological, rheumatological, drug history) and the history of dizziness.
- Patients may describe dizziness as a sensation of light-headedness, fainting, or imbalance, or less commonly as 'true' rotatory vertigo (hallucination of movement: room or patient rotating).
- The patient may continue explaining his/her symptoms in a random manner for some part of the consultation, but it is essential to explain to the patient that there are key questions that need to be answered as accurately as possible.
- It is useful to enquire about the 1st episode the patient experienced dizziness, which may be several months or even years earlier, although they didn't seek specialized advice at the time.
- This 1st episode or attack may give important clues to the true diagnosis, as subsequent attacks may represent de-compensation episodes of an original peripheral or central pathology.
- Important details on the history are:
  - Is it rotatory vertigo?
  - How did it start (waking up, while at work, walking, seating, etc.)?
  - How long did the episode last (seconds, minutes, hours, or days/weeks)?
  - Any predisposing or precipitating factors (URTI, head/neck movement, head injury, etc.)?
  - Any associated symptoms (hearing loss, tinnitus, palpitations, breathlessness, black-outs, blurred or temporary loss of vision, disarthria, limb weakness, seizures, headaches, among others)?
  - Were there other episodes/attacks, and if so were they different in terms of presentation, duration, or different characteristics, pattern of presentation?

Examination

General medical examination

- Cardiovascular (special attention to changes in systolic BP lying/standing >10%, heart murmurs, carotid bruit).
- Ophtahmological (ocular movement, nystagmus, fundoscopy looking for papilloedema).

Neurotological examination

- Otoscopy.
- PTA and tuning-fork tests.
- Fistula test.

Table 18.1 Common causes of balance disturbance/dizziness

	History	Examination	Diagnosis	Page
True Vertigo	Positional Lasts seconds	Dix–Hallpike test +ve	BPPV	480
	Recurrent attacks Lasts hours Aural fulness Tinnitus	PTA (fluctuating hearing loss)	Ménière's	484
	Single attack Lasts days Unwell for 1 week	PTA (normal) Romberg's and Unterberger's +ve	Labyrinthitis = vestibular neuronitis = vestibular failure or CVA	478
Disequilibrium	Constant (elderly patient)	PTA and Vestibular function tests normal	Multifactorial causes	—
	Intermittent (previous vertigo attack)	PTA normal	Decompensation after a resolved vestibular failure episode	—

- Dix–Hallpike test.
- Cranial nerves examination.
- Smooth pursuit.
- Vestibulo-ocular reflex (by turning the head to one side, while asking the patient to keep their gaze straight and observe for saccadic movement of the eyes).
- Cerebellar testing (rapidly pronating and supinanting one hand over the other for dysdiadochokynesis and finger–nose pointing for past-pointing).
- Heel/toe gait (walking putting one foot in front of the other, heel to toe).
- Romberg (standing with the feet together and eyes closed).
- Unterberger tests (walking on the spot with the eyes closed, arms stretched, and palms facing upwards). +ve test = patient rotates on the spot over 30–60 seconds.

Investigations

- Most patients will need no investigations, apart from suspected general disease (cardiovascular, anaemia, diabetes, thyroid dysfunction, etc.).
- Depending on the nature of the symptoms, specialized investigations may be needed: in order to exclude serious pathology or confirm a vestibular cause.
- Vestibular function tests (see 🔲 p. 310).
- MRI of IAM and brain, to exclude acoustic neuroma or central pathology.

Labyrinthitis

- Synonyms: vestibular neuronitis, acute (or sudden) vestibular failure.
- Presents as a sudden episode of vertigo in a previously well person.
- ♂ : ♀, 1 : 1; common age of onset 30–40 years.
- There may be a prior upper respiratory-tract infection.
- Single or multiple attacks may last 1–2 days and improve over a period of weeks due to central compensation.
- Rarely, both vestibular systems may be affected.

Aetiology and physiopathology

- Suspected viral aetiology, i.e. rubella, herpes simplex virus, reovirus, cytomegalovirus, influenza and mumps.
- Axonal loss: endoneurial fibrosis and atrophy of the vestibular nerve.

Signs and symptoms

- Hearing usually normal.
- Nystagmus present (fast component beating away from the affected side).
- Positive Romberg's and Unterberger's test.
- Rest of neurological examination is normal.
- Normal otoscopy.

Investigations

- Most cases will resolve, but recurrent cases will need investigation:
- Pure-tone audiogram.
- ENG and calorics.
- MRI to exclude central pathology or acoustic neuroma (if neurological suspicion, persistence of symptoms and/or significant asymmetry in vestibular tests).

Treatment

- Vestibular sedatives for the acute attack (prochlorperazine po, im or buccal).
- Oral steroids if SNHL (prednisolone 1mg/kg).
- Vestibular rehabilitation (Cawthorne–Cooksey exercises).

Benign paroxysmal positional vertigo (BPPV)

- The most common cause of true rotary vertigo.
- Usual age of onset: 40–60 years.

Pathophysiologylogy

It is thought to occur as a result of stimulation of the posterior semicircular canal by otoconia from the otolith organ that have disloged and deposited on the cupula ('cupulolithiasis theory') or in the canal ('canalolithiasis theory').

Signs and symptoms

- Seconds of rotatory vertigo brought on by head movement, in particular looking up and rolling over in bed.
- Presentation:
  - Acute episode <3 months duration.
  - Intermittent episodes.
  - Chronic episodes lasting years.

Investigations

- Full neurotological examination.
- Pure-tone audiometry (hearing normal).
- Normal otoscopy.
- Positive Dix–Hallpike test:
  - Position the patient: sitting up on a couch/bed with the head turned 30 degrees to one side.
  - The patient is then placed lying down with the head extended over the edge of the couch/bed, 30 degrees below the horizontal.
  - Rotatory nystagmus and vertigo sensation will develop after a few seconds (latency period).
  - The nystagmus is clockwise beating, when the right ear is being tested, and anticlockwise when the left ear is being tested. It does not change direction on repetition of the test.
  - The nystagmus lasts 20–40s and it is fatigable (decreased responses) if the test is repeated.
  - Frenzel glasses can be of help to observe nystagmus as they prevent optic fixation and magnify eye movements.
  - The test is repeated to the opposite side to test the contralateral ear. BPPV may be present in both ears.
  - If the features are atypical, then an acoustic neuroma or a central origin of the vertigo must be excluded (MRI).

Treatment

Fatiguing vestibular exercises (Fig. 18.7)

- Brandt–Daroff exercises, help to produce central adaptation by provoking the attacks repeatedly.

Epley's manoeuvre (Fig. 18.8)

- It can bring relief in 90% by repositioning the displaced otoconia. This manoeuvre may need to be repeated.

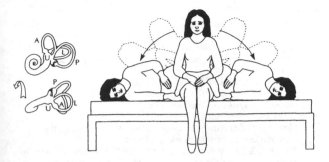

Fig. 18.7 Brandt-Daroff exercises.

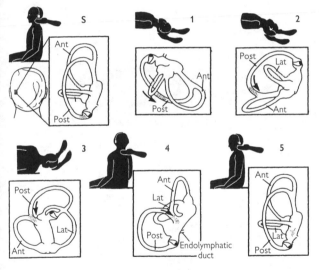

Fig. 18.8 Epley's manoeurve. From the Oxford Handbook of ENT and Head and Neck surgery. Reproduced with permission by Oxford University Press.

Surgery
- Posterior ampullary nerve section:
  - This nerve (singular nerve) carries the afferent fibres from the ampulla of the posterior semicircular canal.
  - The nerve can be accessed by drilling into its channel just below the round window.
  - There is a high risk of sensori-neural hearing loss.
- Vestibular nerve section: can be achieved via a retrosigmoid approach to the IAM, and has a 1% mortality risk.
- Posterior canal occlusion:
  - Movement of otoconia can be prevented by compressing the membranous posterior semicircular canal.
  - The procedure is peformed via a mastoidectomy approach and the posterior semicircular canal is 'blue-lined', bone wax or bone dust is inserted to compress the membranous canal.
  - 5% risk of sensori-neural hearing loss.

Ménière's disease 1: syndrome and disease

- Described in 1861 by Prosper Ménière.
- Definition: A disease of the membranous inner ear consisting of vertigo associated with tinnitus and reduced hearing, which has it's pathological correlate of endolymphatic hydrops.
- Incidence: 50–150 cases/100 000 population.
- More common in females.
- Occurs usually 35–40 years old.
- 30–50% of patients have bilateral symptoms within 3 years of presentation.

Aetiology

- Ménière's syndrome: same symptoms as Ménière's disease, but secondary to other diseases of the middle and inner ear, e.g.:
  - Post-traumatic: head injury or ear surgery.
  - Post infection, i.e. measles and mumps.
  - Late-stage syphilis.
  - Cogan's syndrome and atypical Cogan's.
- Ménière's disease: when the endolymhatic hydrops is idiopathic (i.e other causes have being excluded).

Pathophysiology

Saccin theory

- Endolymphatic hydrops is due to deficient absorption of the endolymph. The endolymphatic duct becomes temporarily obstructed and induces the secretion of proteins and a hormone in the endolymphatic sac (saccin), which increase the endolymph production.
- When a critical volume/pressure of endolymph is reached, the obstruction is overcome and it flows into the endolymphatic sac, causing the episode of vertigo.
- As a consequence of this endolymphatic hydrop, the scala media and saccule are most affected, and the utricle and semicircular canals to a lesser extent.

'Dark-cell' theory

- Suggests there is malfunction of 'dark cells' (normally present in the periphery of the macula and utricle and in the crista of the semicircular canals), leading to the excess production of endolymph.

Signs and symptoms

- Typically: aural fullness, vertigo, tinnitus, and hearing loss. The attack lasts from 20min to 6h.
- Associated nausea and vomiting.
- Horizontal or horizonto-rotatory nystagmus is always present.
- The patient may experience dysequilibrium after an attack for several days.
- A fluctuating low-frequency sensori-neural hearing loss, which recovers after an attack is found in the early stages of the disease.
- Later the hearing loss becomes permanent also affecting the high frequencies.

Natural progression

A gradual reduction of the severity and frequency of attacks but at the cost of a 50–60dB hearing loss over 5–10 years:

- Stage I: classical symptoms, hearing is normal between attacks.
- Stage II: hearing loss is established (low-frequency SNHL), but it can still fluctuate. Episodes of vertigo reach a maximum then start to recede. Up to 50% of patients will develop bilateral disease.
- Stage III: hearing loss is more severe (50–60dB SNHL) and is now the primary disability. There is no episodic vertigo, but a residual unsteadiness.
- From every stage 50% of patients will progress to the following stage.

Variants of Ménière's disease/syndrome

Lermoyez syndrome

- The symptoms occur in the reverse order: increasing aural fullness, tinnitus, and hearing loss, which are relieved by the vertigo attack (physiopathology is unclear).

Vestibular hydrops

- Vertigo only. 20% will develop classical Ménière's disease.

Cochlear hydrops

- Hearing loss and tinnitus only. 80% will develop classical Ménière's disease.

Crisis of Tumarkin

- Affects 2% of Ménière's patients. The patient has drop attacks without warning, vertigo, loss of consciousness, or paralysis.
- Thought to be caused by undefined sudden change in the otolithic organs. This variant has implications on safety while driving vehicles (see 📖 p. 832).

Investigations

There is no single diagnostic test:

- Neurotological examination.
- Pure-tone audiometry—Initially normal between attacks in early phase.
- Characteristic low-frequency sensori-neural hearing loss and eventually thresholds >60dB.
- MRI scan to exclude an acoustic neuroma.
- Laboratory investigations as per sudden onset hearing loss (see 📖 p. 468) and rule out autoimmune hearing loss (see 📖 p. 470).
- Electrocochleography (EcoG). An increase ratio of the summating potential compared to the action potential >30% suggests hydrops (Fig. 18.9).
- Calorics. Canal paresis is the commonest finding, but also a directional preponderance to the normal ear, or a combination of both can be found.
- Glycerol dehydration test. Improvement of the hearing on PTA, speech audiometry and ECoG after a solution of glycerol (or mannitol) is given orally or intravenously. This drug has an effect of lowering the plasma osmolality.

American Academy of Ophthalmology and Otology (AAOO) classification and guidelines for the diagnosis and evaluation of therapy in Ménière's disease. Used in clinical practice and research to evaluate efficacy of treatment and progression of disease (📖 p. 812):

- Class A: vertigo controlled, hearing improved.
- Class B: vertigo controlled, hearing unchanged.
- Class C: vertigo controlled, hearing worse.
- Class D: uncontrolled vertigo.

Diagnostic scale

Staging of hearing

Mean thresholds at 0.5, 1, 2, and 3kHz on PTA:

- Stage I: <25dB.
- Stage II: 26–40dB.
- Stage III: 41–70dB.
- Stage IV: >70dB.

Functional impairment and disability

- Dizziness does not affect activities.
- Have to stop what you are doing during an attack. Still drive and do most activities without changing them.
- Have to stop what you are doing during an attack. Some changes to lifestyle.
- Work, drive, and look after the family with great effort. Barely managing.
- Unable to work, drive, or take care of the family.
- Disabled for >1 year, and/or receiving compensation.

Box 18.1 Criteria for reporting results (vertigo) of treatment

$$X/Y \times 100$$

X = average of spells/month during 18–24 months post-treatment
Y = average of spells/month during 6 months pre-treatment

Score	Class
0	A
0–40	B
41–80	C
81–120	D
>120	E
2nd treatment	F

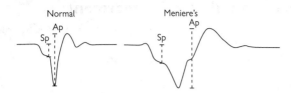

Fig. 18.9 Electrocochleography. SP/AP >30% in Meniere's.

Ménière's disease 2: treatment

Remember: there is a spontaneous remission rate of vertigo in between 60 and 80% of cases.

Medical treatment of Ménière's disease
Supportive
- Reassurance, counselling (Ménière's society).
- Vestibular rehabilitation.
- Hearing-aid.
- Tinnitus rehabilitation.

Vascular
Aim to improve middle ear blood flow:
- Betahistine.
  - Synthetic histamine analogue.
  - Causes capillary vasodilatation.
  - Little evidence that it modifies the disease process.
  - Smoking cessation, caffeine reduction, regular exercise.

Vestibular sedatives
Paradoxically both histamine agonists and antihistamines can be used to treat Ménière's:
- Antihistamines, such as prochlorperazine, cyclizine, and cinnarizine are useful vestibular sedatives.

Electrolyte balance
- Dietary salt restriction (<2g/day) as for hypertension control.
- Fluid restriction.
- Diuretics (bendrofluazide): Little evidence of benefit.

Immunological
- Intratympanic and/or systemic steroids.
- Cytotoxic drugs.
- Plasmapheresis.

Surgical treatment of Ménière's disease (see Table 18.2)
- Only after medical treatment failure.
- Two categories: hearing preservation and non-preservation procedures.

Hearing preservation procedures
Grommet insertion
- This treatment is based on the supposition that endolymphatic hydrops is secondary to negative middle-ear pressure acting on the round window.
- It probably has a placebo effect.
- The Meniett® low-pressure pulse generator (Medtronic Xomed Inc.) can be used once a grommet has been inserted. This device it is thought to work by transmitting pressure pulses into the middle ear and then acting on the round window to displace the perylymphatic

fluid, which in turn, stimulates the flow of endolymph and results in a reduction of endolymphatic hydrops.
- The use of Meniett® is thought to be a safe option after medical therapy failure, before other more radical surgical treatments.

Intratympanic gentamicin
- Aim is to produce chemical ablation of the vestibular system and hence the censation of episodic balance disturbance.
- A solution of 2ml of Gentamicin (40mg/ml) + 0.5ml of 8.4% sodium bicarbonate + 0.5ml of water is injected into the middle ear with a fine-bore needle under microscopic guidance, and the patient is asked to performe Valsalva manoeuvre to encourage the solution to enter the middle ear. The patient is then lying onto the injected side for a few minutes.
- Gentamicin diffuses through the round-window membrane into the perilymph of the cochleovestibular system. Its effect is mainly vestibulotoxic, but at high concentration can be cochleotoxic as well.
- The procedure may need to be repeated several times until symptom control is achieved.
- Vertigo control occurs in 85% of patients.
- Hearing loss in 5%.

Endolymphatic sac decompression
- The basis for this procedure is that decompression of the endolym-pahtic sac may encourage drainage or resorption of endolymph so as to reduce its pressure.
- The procedure is carried out through a cortical mastoidectomy, exposing the endolymphatic sac, which usually lies at or below 'Donaldson's line' (prolongation of the axis of the lateral semicircular canal towards the posterior fossa dura).
- The sac may be left exposed but intact, opened into the mastoid cavity or a shunt (between the sac and the mastoid caivty) may be created by inserting a valved tube.
- Results claim 40–70% vertigo improvement. Hearing loss <5%.
- These results are comparable to cortical mastoidectomy alone, as demonstrated in a double-blind, control trial 'sham study', in which patients receiving a cortical mastoidectomy alone had similar results in vertigo control.

Vestibular nerve section
- This technique is effective for control of vertigo of peripheral vestibular origin, Meniere's or other.
- Several approaches can be used by the neurotologist: middle fossa, retrolabyrinthine, and retrosigmoid approach.
- Results.
  - Symptom control in 90%.
  - Hearing loss <5%.
  - Facial-nerve injury 3%.
  - CSF leak 6%.

Others

Rarely employed:

- Cochleostomy: creating a fistula between the endolymphatic scala media and the perylymphatic scala tympani.
- Cochlear dialysis: use of osmotic agents to reduce the inner ear electrolyte imbalance.
- Cervical sympathectomy: increasing blood flow to the labyrinth.
- Vestibular ultrasonic ablation: destruction of the lateral semicircular canal by ultrasonic radiation.
- Cryosurgery: destruction of the lateral semicircular canal by the application of a cryoprobe.

Non-hearing preservation procedures

Labyrinthectomy

Via a transtympanic or transmastoid approach:

- A cortical mastoidectomy is perfomed.
- The semicircular canals are skeletonised and then are drilled out (including their ampulla) being careful not to damage the facial nerve, especially close to the lateral semicircular canal (use facial-nerve monitor).
- The vestibule is opened posteriorly and the utricle and saccule are removed.
- Results are of vertigo control in 85%, but with total hearing loss.

Table 18.2 What procedure should be performed in failed medical therapy?

Unilateral	Good hearing	—endolymphatic sac decomp
		—vestibular nerve section
	Poor hearing	—intratymphanic gentamicin
		—labyrithectomy
Bilateral	Vertigo caused by better hearing ear	—endolymphatic sac decomp
	Vertigo caused by worse hearing ear	—endolymphatic sac decomp
		—labyrithectomy

Vascular causes of inner ear dysfunction

Posterior inferior cerebellar artery occlusion
- Due to thrombosis of one vertebral artery, leading to severe vertigo.
- Numbness of the ipsilateral face and a sensory loss (pain and temperature) in the contralateral side of the trunk and extremities. VIth, VIIth, and Xth cranial nerve palsies may be present and Horner's syndrome.

Basilar migraine
- Spasms of the posterior cerebellar artery cause areas of ischaemia in the occipital cortex.
- There is visual aura followed by vertigo, tinnitus, dysarthria culminating in an intense headache.

Vertebrobasilar ischaemia
- Due to hyperextension or rotation in patients with aterosclerotic narrowing of these vessels.
- Symptoms are of vertigo, blurred vision/hemianopia, dysphasia and even hemiparesis.

Occlusion of the labyrinthine artery
- Sudden onset of vertigo and hearing loss.
- The patient may have a prior history of transient ischaemic attacks (TIAs). Up to 62% of TIA patients have episodic vertigo.

Occlusion of anterior vestibular artery
- Causes hearing loss and vertigo (BPPV-like symptoms).
- Recurrent vestibulopathy/vascular loop syndrome.
- As a result of an abnormally placed blood vessel (AICA) impacting upon the vestibular nerve in the IAM.
- Age of presentation 35–55 years old; ♀: ♂, 2 : 1.
- Affects approximately 7% of vertigo patients and 50% have high-frequency hearing-loss.

Other vascular causes
- Vasculitis, such as polyarteritis nodosa and Wegener's.
- Embolization after cardiac surgery.
- Thrombosis in hypercoagulation states (polycythaemia).
- Hypoxia, from any systemic cause.

Investigations
- Full neurotological examination.
- PTA.
- MRI/MRA.

Treatment
- Vasodilators and steroids for occlusion and spasm.
- Treatment of TIA when suspected.
- Microvascular decompression for vascular loop syndrome.

Temporal bone fractures

- A consequence of blunt trauma to the head.
- Management of head injury has priority over the management of the temporal bone fracture itself.
- Usually delayed referral to the otololaryngologist.

Types of temporal bone fractures (Fig. 18.10)

According to the direction of the fracture line in relation to the long axis of the temporal bone, can be classified into:

- Longitudinal (70–80%):
  - Fracture line along the temporal bone longitudinal axis, extending from the squamous portion of the temporal bone, medially along the external auditory canal into the roof of the middle-ear cleft and then into the petrous apex. It can occur bilaterally.
  - The mechanism of the injury is a lateral blow to the side of the head.
  - Symptoms usually related to the middle ear.
- Transverse (10–20%):
  - Fracture line lies across the longitudinal axis, through the labyrinthine capsule.
  - The mechanism of the injury is a blow to the front or back of the skull.
  - Symptoms usually related to the inner ear.
- Mixed (10%).

Signs and symptoms

- Local haematoma/ bruising of the skin:
  - 'Battle sign': post-auricular bruising.
  - 'Raccoon sign': extensive periorbital bruising, due to the fracture line running from front to back of the skull base.
- Otorrhagia: blood in the external ear canal, and a laceration of the skin, or a step in the bony canal are often seen in the longitudinal fractures.
- Haemotympanum, if the fracture involved the middle-ear cleft. More common in longitudinal fractures.
- CSF effusion into the middle ear occurs if the tegmen and the middle cranial fossa dura were breached (10–25% of cases):
  - CSF otorrhoea, if there is a disruption of the tympanic membrane.
  - CSF otorhinorrhoea, if the drainage of CSF occurs via the Eustachian tube into the nasopharynx/nose (more common in the transverse fractures).
- Hearing loss can be:
  - Conductive hearing loss due to middle-ear effusion, blood in the external canal or ossicular damage.
  - Sensori-neural hearing loss is more common in the transverse fractures and can be total.

- Facial nerve injury:
  - Lower motor neurone type.
  - More common in transverse fractures.
  - Most often immediate.
- Dizziness is common but mainly temporary.

Investigations and management

- Manage the head injury and/or other associated injuries.
- Neurological examination, with special attention to the facial nerves.
- Tuning-fork tests are easily done at the bedside of a conscious patient.
- Pure-tone audiogram.
- Examination of ears and, if possible, careful microsuction of blood clots in ear canal.
- If CSF otorrhoea, send a sample for β_2-transferrin analysis (see 📖 p. 428). Conservative treatment (bedrest with head elevation) will be adequate in most cases, leaving surgical closure for persistent leaks and recurrent meningitis.
- The role of prophylactic antibiotics is controversial.
- CT scan of skull base and temporal bone (fine cuts with bony algorithms) will delineate the fracture line and involved structures.
- If clear history of immediate and total facial-nerve palsy, consider facial-nerve decompression by neurotologist (see 📖 p. 446).

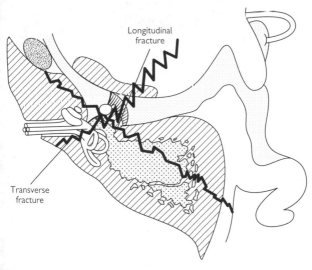

Fig. 18.10 Temporal bone fractures.

The skull base

Anatomy

The skull base is a complex anatomical region that is technically challenging for surgeons. In this chapter we will concentrate on the extracranial anatomy and relations of the skull base. Ideally read this section using a skull alongside to gain a better understanding of the complex anatomy.

The skull base can be subdivided into three regions:
- the anterior,
- the middle, and
- the posterior.

Anterior skull base

Anterior skull base contains the orbits and the paranasal sinuses (Table 19.1).

Table 19.1 Orbit: anatomical relations

Boundaries	Structures
Posterior wall	
Foramen	Structures passing through
Optic canal	II and ophthalmic artery
Superior Orbital Fissure	III, IV, VI, V1, and ophtahlmic veins
Inferior Orbital Fissure	V2 and infraorbital vessels
Medial wall	Frontal process of maxilla, lacrimal, ethmoid and sphenoid
Foramen	Structures passing through
Anterior ethmoidal foramen	Anterior ethmoidal artery
Posterior ethmoidal foramen	Posterior ethmoidal artery

The anterior ethmoidal artery lies approximately at 24mm from the lacrimal crest of the maxillary bone, the posterior ethmoid artery lies 12mm posterior to it, and the optic nerve a further 6mm posteriorly. These relationships are important to remember when considering surgery for epistaxis.

Lateral wall	Greater wing of sphenoid and zygoma
Floor	Maxilla, zygomatic, orbital process of palatine
Roof	Orbital part of frontal and lesser wing of sphenoid

Ethmoid and frontal sinuses

- The ethmoid sinuses are inferior to the anterior cranial fossa and medial to the orbits.
- The frontal sinuses are in front and above of the ethmoid cells, and have a thick anterior and thinner posterior wall.
- Intracranial contents of anterior skull base;
  - Frontal lobes, olfactory bulb and tract.

Middle skull base

The middle skull base can be further subdivided into one central and two lateral compartments by a line that joins the medial pterygoid plate with the occipital condyle in each side.

Table 19.2 Middle skull base: Anatomical relations

Boundaries	Structures
Anterior	Postero-lateral wall of maxillary sinus
Posterior	Petro-occipital suture
Roof	Greater wing of sphenoid and temporal bone
Central compartment	Body of sphenoid and nasopharynx
Intracranial contents: the pituitary fossa, the optic nerves and chiasma, the cavernous sinus [ICA superomedially, VI superolaterally, and from superior to inferior along the lateral wall: III (superior and inferior divisions), IV, and V1, and V2], the anterior communicating artery and the trigeminal ganglion (in Meckel's cave).	
Lateral compartment = Infra-temporal fossa	
Anterior	Posterior wall maxillary sinus
Posterior	Tympanic and mastoid portions of temporal bone
Medial	Lateral pterygoid and sphenoid sinus
Lateral	Zygomatic arch, ramus, and condyle of mandible

Contains the muscles of mastication (temporalis, masseter, and medial and lateral pterygoid muscles), the internal maxillary artery, and further medially the Eustachian tube, and tensor and levator veli palatini muscles.

Also laterally contains the deep lobe of the parotid gland and the facial nerve.

Anteriorly lies the pterygomaxillary fossa, this connects with the infratemporal fossa via the pterygomaxillary fissure, which transmits the maxillary artery. Also the vidian nerve enters the fossa via the vidian or pterygoid canal to join the pterygopalatine ganglion.

Intracranial contents: the temporal lobe and the greater superficial petrosal nerve.

Also the arcuate eminence, which is an important landmark in middle cranial fossa approach to IAM.

Foramina of the middle skull base/infratemporal fossa are given in Table 19.3.

Table 19.3 Middle skull base: Foramina

Foramen	Structures passing through	
Rotundum	V2 into pterygoplatine fossa	
Ovale	V3, accesory meningeal artery and superficial petrosal nerve	
Spinosum	Middle meningeal artery and meningeal branch of VII	
Carotid canal	Internal carotid artery	
Lacerum		
Jugular	Anterior compartment	Inferior petrosal sinus and IX
	Posterior compartment	X, XI and internal jugular vein
Stylomastoid	VII	

Posterior skull base

Table 19.4 Posterior skull base: Anatomical relations

Boundaries	Structures
Anterior	Clivus
Lateral	Petrous temporal bone
Posterior	Occipital bone
Foramen	**Structures passing through**
Porus acousticus	VII, VIII, nervus intermedius and AICA
Vestibular aqueduct	Endolymphatic duct
Hypoglossal foramen	XII, a meningeal branch of the ascending pharyngeal artery and a venous plexus
Foramen magnum	Medulla oblongata, spinal accessory nerve and vertebral and posterior spinal arteries

Contents are muscles (sternomastoid, posterior digastric muscle, trapezius, splenius capitis and cervicis muscles, and semispinalis capitis muscle).

Also contains the occipital artery, vertebral artery, veins, the greater occipital nerve, and the C-1 nerve.

Intracranially the posterior fossa contains the cerebellar hemispheres, midbrain, pons, medulla oblongata and VIIth to XIIth cranial nerves.

Tumours of the cerebello-pontine angle

CPA tumours account for 10% of all the intracranial tumours. Of these, 80% are acoustic neuromas (Fig. 19.1).

Acoustic neuroma

- More accurately a vestibular schwannoma.
- It is a benign, slow-growing tumour originating commonly from the superior vestibular nerve.
- Incidence: 1 per 100 000 per year, but post-mortem studies suggest that this tumour is under-diagnosed.
- Acoustic neuromas occur in two forms:
  - Sporadic presentation (95%).
  - Genetic (5%): neurofibromatosis type 2 (chromosome 22 abnormality), presenting with bilateral acoustic neuromas, meningiomas, facial-nerve neuromas, gliomas, spinal neurofibromas, and cataracts.

Signs and symptoms

- Unilateral sensori-neural hearing loss.
- Unilateral tinnitus.
- Sudden (acute onset) sensori-neural hearing loss in 10% of cases.
- Reduced corneal reflex, facial weakness, and Hitselberger's sign (anesthesia of the posterior external auditory meatus) are signs of trigeminal and facial nerve compression.
- Dysequilibrium occurs less commonly than one would expect, due to its slow growth that allows central compensation to occur.
- Signs and symptoms of raised intracranial pressure such as headache or visual disturbance.
- Ataxia and dysdiadochokinesis will be present in large tumours with brainstem compression.

Diagnosis

- Unilateral SNHL on PTA.
- MRI of IAM (± gadolinium contrast) is the diagnostic imaging of choice and has superseded ...
- ABR, whose typical finding is an inter-aural latency of V wave = 0.2–0.4ms in 80% of cases, however this technique may not detect small tumours.

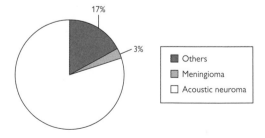

Fig. 19.1 Classification and incidence of CPA tumours.

Management

Options depend on the status of the hearing and facial nerve, size and position of the tumour, surgical morbidity, and patient preference:
- **Watchful waiting**: monitoring with serial MRI scans at yearly intervals. 50% tumours will have no or little growth (<0.2mm per year) for several years. A small percentage show tumour regression.
- **Surgical excision**: via translabyrinthine, retrosigmoid or middle fossa approach.

Translabyrinthine approach
- In this approach the hearing will be completely lost.
- It is used for tumours up to 3cm or for poor residual hearing.
- The facial nerve can be preserved.

Consists of a complete mastoidectomy and Labyrinthectomy, extending laterally to expose 270 degrees around the IAC (Internal auditory canal) until 'Bill's bar' is identified (vertical bony ridge in the IAC that separates the facial from the superior vestibular nerve). Then dura is incised and the tumour can then be removed with the help of an ultrasonic device (CUSA- Cavitational Ultrasonic Surgical Aspirator). The middle ear and Eustachian tube are obliterated with muscle and fat and the ear canal closed.

Retrosigmoid approach
- In this approach hearing and facial nerve can be monitored during the dissection and with care, preserved.
- Used for larger tumours (>3cm).

A complete mastoidectomy is performed to expose both in front and behind the sigmoid sinus which is compressed to improve access. The posterior fossa dura is incised. The cerebellum is retracted posteriorly and the bone of the posterior IAC is removed. AICA must be identified and preserved. Facial nerve and cochlear can be identified and preserved, the tumour then is dissected. The dura is closed and the mastoid obliterated with fat.

Middle fossa approach
- This approach is especially suitable for small intracanalicular tumours (<1cm).
- In this approach hearing and facial nerve can also be preserved.

A craniotomy is performed, creating a window in the squamous portion of the temporal bone just above the floor of the middle cranial fossa. Dura is elevated and landmarks identified: the greater superficial nerve and middle meningeal artery anteriorly, and the arcuate eminence posteriorly. The fundus of the IAC is exposed by drilling the bone in the area of the bisection of the angle formed by the greater superficial nerve and the arcuate eminence. The tumour is removed with care to preserve both facial and cochlear nerves. Fascia and fat are used to close the bony defect.

Stereotactic radiosurgery (gamma-knife)
- This is a multiplanar method of delivering radiotherapy to a very localized area with less risk of damaging neighbouring structures.
- It is used for tumours of <3cm in size.
- There is a low risk of facial-nerve damage and hearing loss.

Complications
The complications of surgery are:
- Facial-nerve injury.
- Hearing loss (inevitable in translabyrinthine approach).
- Intracranial haemorrhage/haematoma.
- Meningitis.
- Death (1%).

Following middle cranial fossa approach the patient will need prophylactic anticonvulsant therapy for 12 months and will be unable to drive during this time.

Glomus tumours

- Also known as paraganglioma or chemodectoma. They arise from the chemoreceptor tissue along the parasympathetic nerves in skull base, neck and thorax.
- Most common benign tumour in the temporal bone.
- Familial distribution in 10% of cases (MEN syndrome).
- Secrete catecholamines in approximately 10% of cases.
- 10% have multiple tumours, and similar figure will show malignant transformation with rapid bony erosion, metastases and short survival.

Classification

- Glomus tympanicum, the tumour is confined to the middle ear space.
- Glomus jugulare, arises in the jugular foramen may extend upwards to fill the middle ear.
- Glomus vagale, arises in the neck extending to the jugular foramen.
- Carotid body tumour, splays the carotid bifurcation.

Signs and symptoms

- Pulsatile tinnitus is key.
- Conductive hearing loss.
- Large tumours can expand laterally to the tympanic membrane causing otalgia and otorrhoea (blood and/or suppuration), or medially invading the labyrinth (sensori-neural hearing loss and vertigo) and involving cranial nerves VII, IX, X, XI, XII, and VI.
- Otoscopic examination reveals a red-blue mass behind the tympanic membrane. Glomus jugulare, will errode the floor of the middle ear giving the typical 'rising sun' appearance on otoscopy.
- The mass blanches when compressed using the pneumatic Siegle's speculum.

Diagnosis

- History and clinical examination.
- Special investigations.
- PTA, tympanogram and tuning-fork testing.
- CT scan to assess size tumour and bone erosion.
- MRI scan to assess intracranial extent and exclude multiple tumours. Typical 'salt and pepper' appearance due to areas of slow and fast blood flow within the tumour.
- Angiography for diagnostic purposes and pre-operative embolization. A carotid balloon occlusion test can be performed during the angiography to assess collateral circulation.
- Urine catecholamines (adrenaline, noradrenaline) and their metabolites (vanillylmandelic acid, VMA) in a 24h urine collection.
- If the tumour is secreting, it is necessary to exclude an associated phaeocromocytoma (MEN syndrome) with an MRI of the adrenal glands.
- Patients with secreting tumours need to have alpha- and beta-blockade prior to surgical treatment and intra-operative magnesium infusion to protect against the potentially devastating cardiovascular effects of any catecholamines released during handling of the tumour.

> **Box 19.1 Fisch classification of middle ear glomus tumours**
>
> - Type A: tumour localized to the middle-ear cleft.
> - Type B: tumour in the middle ear and mastoid with no destruction of bone in the infra-labyrinthine compartment.
> - Type C: tumour invading the bone in the infra-labyrinthine compartment of the temporal bone.
> - Type D: tumour with intracranial extension.

Treatment

- Depending on tumour and patient factors, the treatment intent can be curative or palliative, and may involve surgery, radiotherapy, or chemotherapy.
- Mainsaty of treatment is surgery with radiotherapy reserved for frail patients and recurrent/residual disease.
- Glomus tympanicum tumours (or Fisch type A) can be excised via a transcanal approach, using laser or diathermy for heamostasis.
- Type B glomus tumours need a post-auricular approach, as in mastoid exploration, with extended facial-recess dissection to allow exposure of the jugular bulb area.
- Larger glomus jugulare tumours (types C and D) are usually embolized pre-operatively, the major vessels must be controlled in the neck and neurosurgical input may be necessary to deal with any intracranial component.
- The transtemporal skull-base or infratemporal approaches are used.
- Surgical steps include:
  - Dissection of the neck to control vessels.
  - Identification of the facial nerve in parotid.
  - Blind sac closure of the external auditory canal (infratemporal approach only).
  - Extensive cortical mastoidectomy.
  - Subtotal petrosectomy (infratemporal approach only).
  - Anterior transposition of the facial nerve (infratemporal approach only).
  - Ligation of the sigmoid sinus (infratemporal approach only).
  - Control of the distal internal carotid artery.
  - Obliteration of the Eustachian tube (infratemporal approach only).
  - Ligation of the internal jugular vein.
  - Dissection of the tumour.

Contraindications

- Carotid involvement with poor collateral cerebral circulation.
- Neurosurgically unresectable tumour.
- The tumour affects the only patent sigmoid sinus/internal jugular vein. In which case wait for the tumour to grow and collateral drainage pathways open.

Lateral temporal bone resection

Is a partial resection of the temporal bone, lateral to the facial nerve (tympanic membrane and middle ear included).

Indications

Malignant tumours of the temporal bone.

Consent

Special considerations as per mastoidectomy and parotidectomy operations (see 📖 p. 396, 126).

Technique

- The procedure is in itself an extended radical mastoidectomy, with preservation of stapes superstructure, facial nerve, labyrinth, temporo-mandibular joint, and external auditory meatus, if the latter two are not involved.
- May be combined with parotidectomy to clear disease that spreads directly either to the gland or to remove intraparotid lymph nodes.
- Approach is post-auricular, incision extending to allow exposure to perform a parotidectomy (Fig.19.2).
- Subplatysmal and subperiosteal flaps are elevated as for parotidectomy and mastoidectomy procedures.
- Parotidectomy performed with preservation of the facial nerve.
- Cortical mastoidectomy is performed with a large, posterior tympanotomy to allow resection of the facial recess. This will allow a plane to develop between the jugular bulb and the tympanic ring, extending anteriorly to the glenoid fossa.
- Incudostapedial joint is disarticulated and incus removed.
- Bone is removed above the tympanic ring without injury to the middle cranial fossa dura, until the anterior epitympanum is reached.
- Stylomastoid foramen is skeletonized and the mastoid tip removed.
- The specimen is then lifted *en block* with the help of an osteotome to free any remaining bony attachment (Fig.19.3).
- Frozen sections of the parotid margin may be taken and further excision perfomed, if necessary.
- Mobilise temperalis muscle onto mastoid cavity.
- Closure of ear canal and insert neck drain.

Complications

- Also as per mastoidectomy and parotidectomy.
- Oteoradionecrosis can complicate radiotherapy post-operatively. It may be treated with hyperbaric oxygen, debridement and regular aural toilet, or further excision of necrotic tissue ± free flap reconstruction.

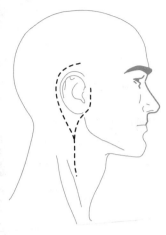

Fig. 19.2 Incision for temporal bone resection.

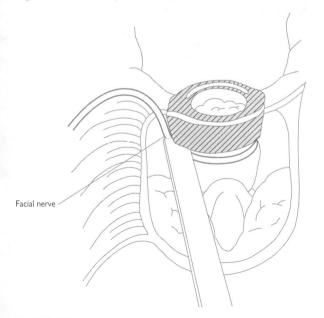

Facial nerve

Fig. 19.3 En block resection of ear canal and tympanic ring lateral to facial nerve (left ear).

Total petrosectomy

Indications

Advanced malignant tumours of the ear canal and temporal bone.

Consent

Special considerations as per mastoidectomy and parotidectomy operations.

Technique

- Preauricular incision as per parotidectomy with a superior extension.
- Subplatysmal flap and subperiosteal flaps are elevated.
- The upper neck is explored and major vessels (carotid and jugular) identified and controlled.
- The facial nerve may have to be divided and grafted (with greater auricular nerve cable graft).
- An osteotomy divides the zygomatic arch and ramus of mandible.
- Infratemporal fossa structures can then be excised (preserving the deep temporal artery).
- The Eustachain tube is divided and transfixed and the internal carotid artery exposed.
- Middle cranial fossa dura is retracted superiorly.
- Transverse and sigmoid sinuses exposed posteriorly.
- Temporal bone can be then removed.
- The internal carotid artery can be preserved or resected if patient has passed pre-op occlusion test.
- Free tissue transfer to fill the defect ± skin cover.
- Closure of the ear canal.

Complications

As in lateral temporal bone resection plus:
- CVA.
- CSF leak.
- Meningitis.
- Aspiration pneumonia due to lower cranial nerve palsies.

The nose and postnasal space

Anatomy

Embryology

By the end of the 4th week, three facial prominences from the 1st pharyngeal arch, are visible on the ventral surface of the embryo: the frontonasal prominence, most of the nose, and the upper part of the stomodeum. By the end of the 5th week, local thickenings on the surface ectoderm forms the nasal placode, which invaginates to form the nasal pits. In doing so, ridges of tissue surrounding each pit, form the medial and lateral nasal prominence, which eventually will form the columella, tip, and alae of the nose (Fig. 20.1a). The nasal pits deepen considerably and are initially separated from the primitive oral cavity by the bucconasal membrane, which will breakdown later to form the choanae.

External anatomy

Externally, the nose consists of the nasal bones superiorly, upper and lower lateral cartilages inferiorly, with the nasal septum supporting them in the midline. Laterally it is bounded by the ascending process of the maxilla. Fibro-fatty tissue containing sesamoid cartilages forms the lateral boundary of the nostril itself. The major supports for the nose are:
- the keystone area (where the upper lateral cartilages are attached to the undersurface of the nasal bones);
- the scroll area (where the lower lateral cartilages are attached to the undersurface of the upper lateral cartilages) (Fig. 20.1b); where the medial crura of the lower lateral cartilages are attached to the nasal septum.

All the cartilages and bone are covered with facial muscles (part of the SMAS layer) and skin, which contains many sebaceous glands. The skin is thicker at the nasal tip and nasion (the root of the nose) and thinner over the rhinion (the most prominent part of the dorsum). The skin extends into the vestibule of the nostrils for about 1cm and here is a variable crop of stiff hairs. The muco-cutaneous junction lies just beyond the hair-bearing area.

Aesthetically, the nose should be proportional to the rest of the face. The nose should also be set onto the face at the appropriate angle (Fig. 20.1c).

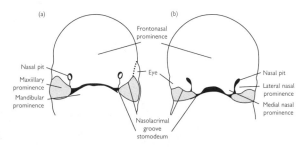

Fig. 20.1 a Embryology of the external nose.

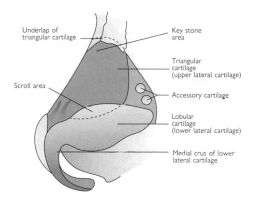

Fig. 20.1 b External nasal anatomy.

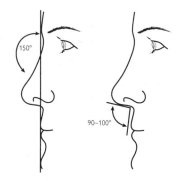

Fig. 20.1 c Nasofrontal and nasolabial angles.

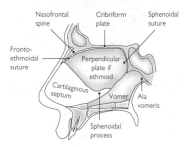

Fig. 20.1 d Anatomy of the nasal septum.

Internal anatomy

Septum, posterior choana and postnasal space (Fig. 20.1d)

The septum divides the nasal cavity into two parts. Superiorly the septum supports the nasal bones and lateral cartilages and inferiorly it rests on the maxillary crest. The anterior-third of the septum is formed by the quadrilateral cartilage, whilst posteriorly it is formed by the perpendicular plate of the ethmoid above and the vomer below. The anterior septum may be thickened by erectile tissue to form a septal tubercle or organ of Zuckerkandl. Posterior choana is the opening of the nasal cavity into the postnasal space. The postnasal space is a 4 x 4 x 2cm space and it usually contains lymphoid tissue. In children, distinct finger like projections of the adenoids are seen on the posterior superior wall. On the lateral wall of the postnasal space lies the opening of the Eustachian tube, with the fossa of Rosenmuller extending posterior to the medial crus of the tube for a variable distance. The fossa is difficult to inspect endoscopically and this the commonest site for nasopharyngeal carcinoma.

Lateral nasal wall (Fig. 20.1e)

● The lateral nasal wall contains the inferior, middle, and superior turbinates (or conchae) projecting down like scrolls. The space lateral to each turbinate is known as its meatus.

● The inferior turbinate is the longest turbinate and is lined by mucosa containing large vascular spaces. It can become engorged in response to infection or allergy causing nasal blockage. The inferior meatus receives the nasolacrimal duct about 2cm behind the nostrils.

● The middle turbinate is attached to the lateral nasal wall in three parts:
  ● a horizontal anterior attachment;
  ● a vertical attachment (also known as basal lamella); and
  ● a shorter posterior inferior horizontal attachment.

● Occasionally, the middle turbinate can be pneumatized when it is known as a 'concha bullosa'.

● All the anterior sinuses drain into the middle meatus. The ethmoid bulla (containing anterior ethmoid aircells) forms a convex bulge in the middle meatus. The hiatus semilunaris is a 2D slit-like area just anterior to the bulge of the bulla.

- Lateral to the hiatus is the infundibulum, which drains the frontal sinus via the frontal recess (Fig. 20.1f) and the maxillary sinus via its ostium. The bone anterior to the hiatus is the sickle-shaped uncinate process and this can have a variable superior attachment. This in turn will influence the final drainage pathway for the frontal sinus.
- In front of the uncinate process lies the nasolacrimal duct which is covered by thick maxillary bone.
- At the posterior end of the middle meatus, just below the basal lamella lies the sphenopalatine foramen.
- The superior turbinate is the smallest of the three turbinate bones. Laterally the superior meatus drains the posterior ethmoidal cells. Above the superior turbinate lies the sphenoethmoidal recess and the sphenoid ostium opening can often be seen here.

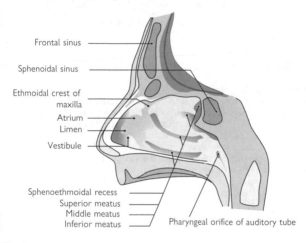

Frontal sinus

Sphenoidal sinus

Ethmoidal crest of maxilla

Atrium
Limen

Vestibule

Sphenoethmoidal recess
Superior meatus
Middle meatus
Inferior meatus

Pharyngeal orifice of auditory tube

Fig. 20.1 e Anatomy of the lateral nasal wall.

Epithelial lining

Most of the nasal cavity is lined by respiratory epithelium (pseudostratified, ciliated, columnar epithelium with goblet cells). Superior part of the nasal cavity, the superior turbinate, and part of the middle turbinate has olfactory epithelium. The vestibule is lined by skin.

Blood supply

External (Fig. 20.1g)

- Dorsal nasal artery (from the ophthalmic artery) supplies the base of the nose.
- The external nasal artery (from the anterior ethmoidal) supplies the area around the upper lateral cartilages, whilst the facial artery and its superior labial branch supplies the lower part of the nose.

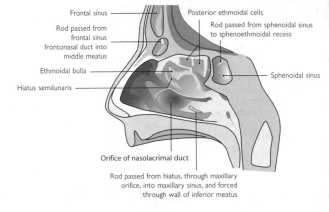

Frontal sinus

Rod passed from
frontal sinus
frontonasal duct into
middle meatus

Ethmoidal bulla

Hiatus semilunaris

Posterior ethmoidal cells

Rod passed from sphenoidal sinus
to sphenoethmoidal recess

Sphenoidal sinus

Orifice of nasolacrimal duct

Rod passed from hiatus, through maxillary
orifice, into maxillary sinus, and forced
through wall of inferior meatus

Fig. 20.1 f Anatomy of lateral nasal wall following removal of turbinate bones.

Internal (Fig. 20.1 g+h)
- The sphenopalatine artery enters the nasal cavity through the sphenopalatine foramen and supplies the posterior nasal cavity and runs anteriorly to end in Kiesselbach's plexus at Little's area.
- Anterior and posterior ethmoidal arteries run along the roof of the cavity and also anastomose with other vessels at Little's area.
- The superior labial artery supplies the vestibule and Little's area.
- Finally, the greater palatine artery runs along the hard palate and has an ascending branch entering the floor of the nasal cavity through the incisive foramen to terminate in Kiesselbach's plexus.

Nerve supply
Sensory
External
- The external nasal nerve (the terminal branch of the anterior ethmoidal nerve) notches the nasal bone and passes down on the upper and lower lateral cartilages to the tip of the nose. The area around the nostrils is also supplied by a medial branch of the infra-orbital nerve.
- The upper part of the nose is supplied by the supratrochlear and infratrochlear nerves from the frontal and nasociliary nerves, respectively.

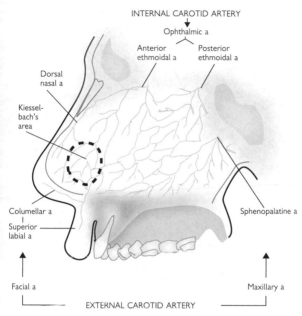

Fig. 20.1 g Blood supply of the nasal septum.

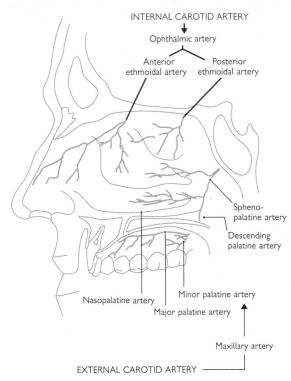

Fig. 20.1 h Blood supply of the lateral nasal wall.

Internal
- Nasopalatine nerve runs with the sphenopalatine artery to supply a similar area in the posterior nasal cavity.
- The anterior ethmoidal nerve runs with its artery to supply the anterior superior part of the nasal cavity.
- The olfactory nerve covers the superior turbinate, part of the middle turbinate, the roof of the nasal cavity, and corresponding septum.

Autonomic
- Parasympathetic innervation is by the superior salivatory ganglion, facial nerve, and greater superficial petrosal nerve synapsing in the pterygopalatine ganglion. Postsynaptic secretomotor neurones run with branches of maxillary nerve. Parasympathetic innervation causes vasodilation.
- Postsynaptic sympathetic fibres are from the superior cervical ganglion forming the deep petrosal nerve in the foramen lacerum joining with the greater superficial petrosal nerve to form the nerve of the pterygoid canal (Vidian nerve) in the pterygopalatine fossa. The sympathetic fibres are distributed with the branches of the maxillary nerve. Sympathetic innervation causes vasoconstriction.

Lymphatic drainage
External
The skin of the nose drains to the submandibular and upper deep cervical nodes. The area over the frontal sinus drains to the pre-auricular nodes and metastasis may present as a parotid swelling.

Internal
The front half of the nasal cavity drains to the submandibular nodes and the posterior part of the nose drains to the retropharyngeal and upper deep cervical nodes.

Nasal respiration
Most important sites of airway resistance are:
- the external nasal valve (caudal end of lower lateral alar cartilage, columella, and nostril sill); and
- the internal nasal valve (caudal end of upper lateral cartilages, corresponding parts of septum and inferior turbinate).

Any change in this area will have major effects on cross-sectional area and alter flow by up to four times.

Inspired air travels by laminar flow throughout the nasal cavity. Odourants depolarize the olfactory fibres in the roof of the nose. Nasal obstruction produces noisy, turbulent airflow in the nose. The nasal cavity filters particles >2µm and prevent them from reaching the lungs. House-dust mite faeces (approx 20µm) ∴ are trapped in the nose and can cause allergic rhinitis.

Most normal subjects demonstrate a nasal cycle with alternating periods of nasal mucosal congestion and vasoconstriction lasting 20min to 3h primarily affecting the inferior turbinates. This is absent in laryngectomees.

Trauma to mid-third of face

Definition
- Fractures involving the area between the supraorbital ridge and upper teeth.
- Central fractures involve the nasomaxillary complex and are usually classified as Le Fort I, II, or III (Fig 20.2). Le Fort fractures were originally described after studying the effects of dropping cannon balls on the faces of dead soldiers. This is unlikely to get ethical approval nowadays!
- Lateral fractures involve the malar-maxillary complex.

Aetiology
- Central fractures usually involve antero-posterior forces, e.g. head on crashes.
- Lateral fractures involve blows from the side.

Clinical features
As well as assessing the facial skeleton, it must be remembered that the patient has had serious head trauma and any injury to the brain and cervical spine will take priority over management of facial fractures.
   Midfacial trauma can damage the following areas:
- Nasal structures: often the nasal bones, ethmoids, ascending process of maxilla, and septum are fractured causing epistaxis and/or CSF rhinorrhoea. Skull-base fractures can cause anosmia. The central-third of the face can collapse to produce a 'dish-face' deformity.
- Orbit: check for proptosis or diplopia. The inferior rectus muscle can be trapped in an orbital floor fracture so the globe cannot be rotated superiorly.
- Nasolacrimal apparatus causing epiphora.
- The bite causing malocclusion, especially with Le Fort fractures.
- Infra-orbital nerve: causing anaesthesia of the cheek.
- There may also be a step deformity around the orbital rim, flattening of the malar eminence or trismus due the involvement of the TMJ or coronoid process.

Investigations
- Facial views on skull Xray may show the fracture or an opaque antrum.
- CT scan of midface.

Treatment
Where possible, patients are best managed jointly with the maxillo-facial team. Displaced fractures need reduction and splinting or fixation especially if there is malocclusion. Open reduction is required for severe displacement and Le Fort II and III fractures. Le Fort I fractures can usually be treated by inter-dental elastic fixation, with firm fibrous union achieved by 4 weeks. Lateral fractures can be reduced by external or internal (incision in buccal sulcus) open fixation with wires or plating. Orbital-floor support may by achieved by performing a Caldwell Luc procedure and a large antrostomy and packing the antrum with gauze or by supporting with a balloon.

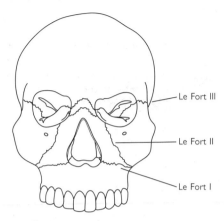

Fig. 20.2 Le Fort classification of central fractures of midface.

Epistaxis

Definition

Derived from Greek term, *epistazein* 'to bleed/drip from the nose'.

Anatomy

Branches of the external and internal carotid arteries meet over Little's area (Kiesselbach's plexus), over the anterior-inferior part of the septum, and this is the commonest site of bleeding (Fig 20.1g).

Aetiology

- Idiopathic (85%).
- Coagulopathy, e.g. ITP, DIC.
- Rhinitis: viral, allergic, drug-induced.
- Traumatic: nose picking, iatrogenic, e.g. septoplasty, FESS.
- Drugs: aspirin, clopidogrel, warfarin.
- Chronic granulomatous disease: Wegener's, sarcoidosis.
- Neoplastic: SCC, adenocarcinoma, inverted papilloma, juvenile angiofibroma.
- Heriditary: Osler Weber Rendu syndrome, haemophilia, von Willebrand's disease.

▶ Hypertension tends to prolong epistaxis rather than cause it.

Investigations

Minimal investigations for admitted patients include FBC, clotting ± group + save.

Stepwise treatment for epistaxis

1. Correct first aid: lean forward, pinch soft cartilaginous part of nose over lower lateral cartilages to exert pressure internally on little's area, ice on forehead or nape of neck.
2. Resuscitation, if necessary: assess blood loss, obtain IV access, start IV fluids or blood as necessary.
3. Cauterization.
4. Anterior packing.
5. Anterior and posterior packing.
6. Surgery.

Principles: closer to source of bleeding, more effective the procedure:

- EUA nose: electrocautery including suction bipolar diathermy, packing ± septoplasty.
- Arterial ligation:
    - Anterior and posterior ethmoid artery ligation.
    - Sphenopalatine artery ligation.
    - Maxillary artery ligation via transantral approach.
    - External carotid artery.

7. Embolization.

Cauterization

- Cauterization is performed with silver nitrate sticks, hot wire, or electrocautery.
- Silver nitrate breaks down when in contact with a wet surface to form nitric acid, which causes a chemical burn.
- Cautery is more effective if the bleeding can be slowed or stopped with local pressure or with adrenaline to reveal the precise bleeding point.

Technique

- Equipment: headlight, thudichum nasal speculum, suction, endoscopes, cautery.
- Suck out any large clots from the nasal cavity.
- Use a topical local anaesthetic/phenylephedrine spray, e.g. co-phenylcaine to anaesthetize the nasal cavity. Additional pledgets moistened with vasoconstriction spray may be placed over the bleeding areas to try and slow the bleeding further.
- Begin by cauterizing the exact bleeding point and lightly cauterize the surrounding area to reduce blood flow to bleeding point. Some surgeons will cauterize the surrounding area first, moving centrally to the source of the bleeding.
- If the bleeding continues, you may have to place pledgets moistened with vasoconstrictor over the area for a few minutes and then repeat the cautery as above. This may need to be repeated up to three times.
- Apply Naseptrin® cream into the nostril and ask the patient to gently sniff it deep into the nasal cavity. The cream should be used three times a day for a week.

▶ Avoid heavily cauterizing a particular spot too often because of the risk of causing a septal perforation. Do not apply cautery to the same spot for more than 2min. Remember bilateral cautery, especially over Little's area, can also cause septal necrosis and perforation. Protect the upper lip with petroleum jelly to avoid a chemical burn from silver nitrate 'leak'.

Anterior nasal packing

- This is performed with ribbon gauze or dehydrated sponges, e.g. Merocel® packs.
- Nasal packing is performed if cautery fails or bleeding point not easily identified.
- Antibiotics not routinely used, unless medically indicated, e.g. prosthetic valve or if packs left in for >48h.

Merocel® pack insertion

Easy to insert and provides light packing for the nasal cavity.

Technique

- Suck out any large clots from the nasal cavity.
- Use a topical local anaesthetic/decongestant spray, e.g. co-phenylcaine to anaesthetize the nasal cavity.
- Lubricate the pack with KY jelly or naseptrin cream.

- Staying close to the nasal septum and the floor of the nasal cavity, the Merocel® pack is inserted horizontally into the nose aiming for the occiput, i.e. not cranially towards the vertex. The pack should be fully pushed in for about 5–8cm.
- Hydrate the packs with 5–8ml of water.
- To remove the packs, place ice on the nasal bridge first. Moisten packs with 5–8ml of water and gently slide out. Keep ice on nose for 5min after pack removal.

BIPP packing (Fig. 20.3a)
- Bismuth iodoform paraffin packing provides better tamponade of bleeding but is not as easy to insert as Merocel®.

Technique
- Suck out any large clots from the nasal cavity.
- Use a topical local anaesthetic/phenylephedrine spray, e.g. co-phenylcaine to anaesthetize the nasal cavity.
- Using a thudichum nasal speculum and nasal-packing forceps, BIPP ribbon is gradually introduced into the nasal cavity, packing from the floor of the nose towards the roof, i.e. from near the inferior turbinate to the superior turbinate.
- After every loop of BIPP ribbon has been introduced, the pack is compressed down to create room for the next loop of ribbon.
- If more than one ribbon is needed, the end of the first pack is tied to the beginning of the second pack to facilitate later removal of the packs.
- Prior to removal, place ice on the nasal bridge and then gradually remove the ribbon, removing the pack from the superior part of the cavity first. Keep ice on nose for 5min after pack removal.

▶ Placing ice on the nose prior to pack removal is said to cause local vasoconstriction helping to minimize the chances of rebleeding. It may also help reduce the discomfort of pack removal.

Posterior nasal packing
Used for posterior bleeds. It is usually inserted in combination with an anterior nasal pack and can be left *in situ* for up to 48h.
Types:
- Inflatable posterior nasal pack, e.g. Foley catheter or Brighton balloon.
- Pre-made cotton nasopharyngeal packs: usually inserted in theatre and used to control post-adenoidectomy bleeds (Fig. 20.3b).

Inflatable posterior packs
Standard male or female 12–16F Foley urinary catheter (single balloon) or custom-made Brighton epistaxis double-balloon catheter used.

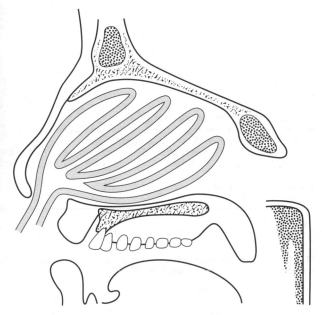

Fig. 20.3 a Nasal packing (anterior)

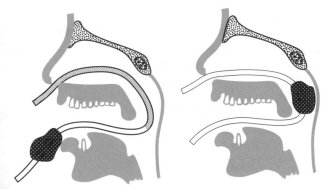

Fig. 20.3 b Inserting a posterior nasal pack.

Technique
- Suck out any large clots from the nasal cavity.
- Use a topical local anaesthetic/phenylephrine spray,
  e.g. co-phenylcaine to anaesthetize the nasal cavity.
- The catheter is introduced into the floor of the nasal cavity and gently advanced until the tip of the catheter is just visible per orally behind the soft palate.
- The catheter is gradually inflated with 7–10ml of air or water (danger of aspiration if balloon burst) and then gently pulled anteriorly to occlude the ipsilateral posterior choana
- If necessary, a posterior pack is inserted in the contra-lateral nasal cavity to occlude the contra-lateral posterior choana.
- Anterior nasal cavity is packed above the catheter with either BIPP or Merocel® (see above). If a Brighton balloon has been used, the anterior balloon can be inflated.
- Whilst maintaining anterior traction on the catheter, it is secured with a gate clamp or an umbilical clamp.
- To remove the posterior pack, the clamp is released and the balloon deflated fully but left *in situ*.
- If there is bleeding, the balloon is re-inflated. Otherwise, the catheter is removed as is the anterior pack.

❶ It is imperative that heavy gauze padding is applied around the base of the clamp to prevent pressure necrosis of the alar rim.

Pre-made cotton postnasal packs
Available in three sizes: small (for children), medium (standard for adults), and large. Usually used for post-adenoidectomy bleeds. Can be made by sewing together gauze swabs and attaching three pieces of ½-in ribbon gauze: 1 near the middle of the pack, and 1 each laterally from side of the pack.

Technique (Fig. 20.3b)
- Pre-made posterior packs are usually inserted in theatre under a general anaesthetic.
- Suck out any large clots from the nasal cavity.
- A suction or Foley catheter is inserted down each nostril.
- A Boyle–Davis gag is inserted into the oral cavity and opened.
- The suction or Foley catheter is retrieved per orally from behind the soft palate and the tip is brought out through the mouth.
- The lateral ribbons on the posterior pack are sutured to the tips of the catheter.
- The catheters are gently retracted from the nostrils and, at the same time, the posterior pack is delivered into the mouth and then behind the soft palate to snugly occlude both posterior choanae.
- Anterior nasal cavity is packed above the catheter with either BIPP or Merocel® (see above).
- The ribbon from each nostril is tied over the columella anteriorly ensuring adequate padding to protect alar rim and the third remaining ribbon coming out the mouth is taped to the cheek.
- To remove the posterior pack, first the anterior pack is removed.

- The columella ribbons are cut, and then the third oral ribbon is gently pulled to release the posterior pack from the postnasal space into the oral cavity. The pack is removed from the mouth.

❶ Heavy gauze padding must be applied around the columella ribbons to avoid pressure necrosis of this area. Young children do not tolerate posterior packing and often they need to be ventilated on PICU. These patients often need to go back to theatre to have their pack removed.

Embolization

- Considered in resistant cases of epistaxis or if surgery is contraindicated on medical grounds. Only branches of the external carotid artery (maxillary artery branches) can be embolized. Effectiveness of embolization is largely dictated by expertise of interventional radiologist and available local facilities. Vessels as small as 2mm can be occluded. If the patient is actively bleeding or oozing through the pack, it is easier to identify the offending branch.
- Particles used: latex, metal coils, gelatin sponge.
- Technique: performed under local anaesthesia ± sedation. Angiocatheter is introduced via the femoral artery, aorta and then into the carotid system under image guidance.
- Risks: reflux of particles up internal carotid artery with subsequent cerebrovascular accident, dissection of aorta or carotid arteries, blindness, facial pain.
- Contraindications: high risk of cerebrovascular accident, e.g. carotid artery stenosis, clotting problems, allergy to contrast or embolization particles.
- Minimal pre-operative investigations: FBC and clotting, group and save.

Surgery for epistaxis

EUA nose, electrocautery, ± septoplasty, ± packing

- The nasal cavity is examined under a hypotensive general anaesthetic with throat pack.
- The nose is often prepared with Moffat's solution (1ml of 1 : 1000 adrenaline, 2ml of 10% cocaine, and 2ml of 8.4% sodium bicarbonate), either sprayed in the nasal cavity or applied on pledgets. Avoid Moffat's solution if there is a known history of cocaine allergy, severe ischaemic heart disease, or arrhythmias.
- If the bleeding point is seen, it is cauterized either with the monopolar Abbe needle or with suitable bipolar forceps.
- If there is a septal deviation obscuring the site of bleeding, a septoplasty is performed to facilitate access, improve visualization and also for more effective packing if necessary.

Arterial ligation

Anterior and posterior ethmoidal arteries

The arteries are usually approached externally for the treatment of high anterior epistaxis. The arteries are indirectly derived from the internal carotid artery via the ophthalmic artery. The anterior ethmoidal artery is found approximately 24mm posterior to the anterior lacrimal crest and the posterior ethmoidal artery is found 12mm behind this. The optic nerve is approximately 6mm behind the posterior ethmoidal artery. Furthermore, the position of the posterior ethmoidal artery is rather variable and it is occasional absent.

Steps

- The procedure is performed under a general anaesthetic and it is often combined with surgery to the sphenopalatine artery.
- The patient is positioned supine on a head ring with a slight head-up tilt.
- The eye is protected with a temporary tarsorrhaphy.
- The skin is infiltrated with 2.2ml of xylocaine 2%/adrenaline 1 : 80 000 and a curved incision is made down to the nasal bones midway between the medial canthus and the dorsum (Fig. 20.4a) often with a 'z' or 'w' in the middle of the incision to reduce the chances of post-operative webbing of the scar.
- A Freer elevator is used to elevate the tissues in a subperiosteal plane to identify the anterior lacrimal crest.
- The lacrimal sac is lifted out laterally and the subperiosteal elevation is continued deep to it to identify the anterior ethmoidal artery, which is most often noted as tethering of the periosteum to the ethmoidal foramen. A malleable copper retractor or a Ferris-Smith retractor will aid visualization.
- Two metal clips are placed on the anterior artery and, if the posterior ethmoidal artery is to be approached, the anterior ethmoidal artery is divided between the clips to allow the subperiosteal elevation to continue.

- Care must be taken to correctly identify the posterior ethmoidal artery from the optic nerve, given their close relation and the variable anatomy in this area.
- The incision is closed carefully to avoid webbing near the inner canthus.

Endoscopic sphenopalatine artery ligation

This large artery is usually responsible for posterior epistaxis. It is the main branch of the maxillary artery, the terminal branch of the external carotid artery.

Steps

- The procedure is performed with a hypotensive general anaesthetic with throat pack.
- The patient is positioned supine on a head ring with a slight head-up tilt.
- The nasal cavity mucosa is vasoconstricted with Moffatt's solution (1ml of 1 : 1000 adrenaline, 2ml of 10% cocaine and 2 ml of 8.4% sodium bicarbonate) either sprayed in the nasal cavity or applied on pledgets.
- Using a FESS setup in theatre, an endoscopic uncinectomy is performed removing all the inferior part of the uncinate process.
- The natural maxillary sinus ostium should now be visible and a wide, middle-meatal antrostomy is performed extending it as posteriorly as possible, so that the posterior wall of the antrum is clearly visible. The ethmoid bulla is not usually opened unless it impedes the antrostomy formation. The antrum is usually full of old blood that should be sucked out.
- A lateral nasal-wall mucoperiosteal flap is raised from the posterior edge of the antrostomy with a Freer elevator. Two horizontal incisions at the upper and lower end of the flap will make it easier to continue raising the flap posteriorly.
- The artery is usually seen as tethering of the mucoperiosteal flap just behind the posterior end of the middle turbinate. It lies approximately at the same depth as the posterior wall of the antrum, which should be easily visible through the wide, middle-meatal antrostomy.
- The sphenopalatine foramen has a superior bony crest that often needs to be removed with a curette or diamond burr if the artery needs to be exposed further.
- The artery is diathermied with suitable bipolar forceps or ligaclips are applied.
- The mucoperiosteal flap is replaced back over the lateral nasal wall and the middle meatus is packed with a small Merocel® pack, if needed.

❶ Avoid using monopolar diathermy near sphenopalatine foramen because of the risk of arcing with optic nerve damage (it is less than 13mm away).

Maxillary artery ligation (Fig. 20.4b)

This procedure has largely been replaced by endoscopic sphenopalatine artery ligation but it is still useful when there is active per-operative bleeding into the nasal cavity, when the sphenopalatine artery can be difficult to identify. In this situation, the maxillary artery is easier to ligate via a Caldwell Luc antrostomy, as there is a relatively bloodless field in the antrum.

Steps

- The operation is performed under a hypotensive general anaesthesia with the head on a head ring, with the bed on a 30-degree head-up tilt.
- The canine fossa is infiltrated and a Caldwell Luc antrostomy is performed to create a large anterior antral window.
- A 300mm focal length microscope is used and the mucosa over the posterior wall of the antrum is removed.
- The bone of the posterior wall is then removed. If it is thin, it can be fractured with a Freer elevator and then gently lifted off to expose the periosteum. If it is thick, it is thinned with a burr.
- Any veins under the periosteum are coagulated and the periosteum is opened.
- The main trunk of the maxillary artery is identified in the fat of the pterygopalatine fossa. It always lies superficial to the maxillary nerve. It is lifted up with a blunt nerve hook to allow cleaning of the artery and enable identification of the other branches.
- The main trunk and branches are ligated with surgical clips.
- The canine fossa incision is closed with vicryl.

External carotid artery ligation

This is generally not as successful as the above procedures, as the external carotid artery is relatively far from the point of bleeding, with collaterals opening up quickly. The closer you are to the source of bleeding, the more effective the procedure. Often used as a last resort. The procedure is however quick and easy to perform and ∴ suitable for most elderly patients with multiple co-morbidities. Rarely, external carotid artery ligation is required to control post tonsillectomy haemorrhage.

Steps

- The procedure is performed under local or general anaesthesia.
- The patient is positioned supine with a shoulder bag and small head ring, and the neck is slightly turned to the opposite side.
- A horizontal incision is planned at the level of the greater cornu of the hyoid bone (Fig. 20.4c). The area is infiltrated with 2.2ml of xylocaine 2%/adrenaline 1 : 80 000 prior to making the incision.
- Subplatysmal flaps are raised, clearly identifying the anterior border of sternomastoid muscle and the deep cervical fascia. The greater auricular nerve should be preserved, if possible. The facial vein is ligated and divided.
- The carotid sheath is found deep to the anterior edge of the sternomastoid muscle. The internal jugular vein is first identified and carefully retracted to expose the carotid arteries. The external carotid artery has multiple branches whilst the internal carotid artery has none (Fig. 20.4d).
- The vagus nerve is identified in the carotid sheath. The hypoglossal nerve may be identified crossing the lingual artery. All nerves should be preserved.
- The external carotid artery should be doubly tied above the lingual artery having clearly identified the external carotid by seeing more than one branch.
- A drain is inserted and the incision is closed in two layers, one to platysma and the second for skin.

(a)

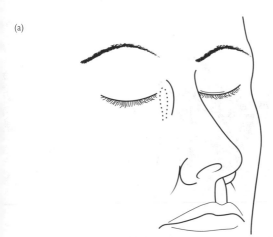

Fig. 20.4 a Ethmodal arteries ligation: skin incision.

(b)

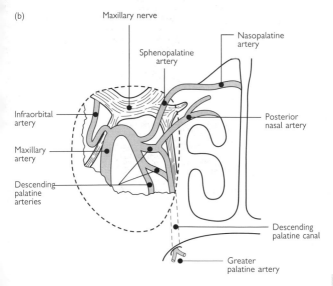

Fig. 20.4 b View at transantral maxillary artery ligation.

(c)

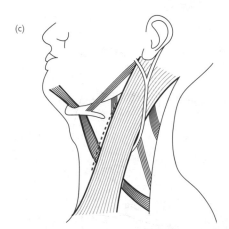

Fig. 20.4 c External carotid artery ligation: skin incision.

(d)

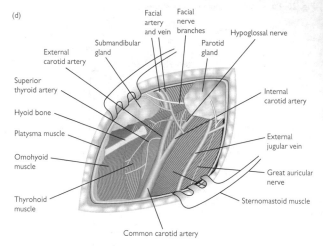

Fig. 20.4 d Relations of the external carotid artery.

Reduction of fractured nasal bones

Nasal fractures are the most common facial fracture and reduction is usually carried out 10–14 days after injury.

Indications

Main indication is displacement of the nasal bones causing unacceptable cosmetic deformity for the patient. The best time for review is within 1h of injury or between 7–10 days after the incident, as local oedema during the intervening period will make assessment difficult. Severe facial trauma causes more complex injuries involving multiple bones of the facial skeleton and can cause neuro-opthalmological problems; these take precedence over the treatment of simple nasal bone fractures, as do associated cervical spine fractures. Central fractures usually involve antero-posterior forces, e.g. head-on crashes.

Classification

- Type 1: frontal blows cause a depressed or displaced distal portion of nasal bone. Associated with a vertical fracture of the septum (Chevallet).
- Type 2: due to lateral trauma causing lateral deviation of the nasal bone and associated with a horizontal (Jarjavay) or a C-shaped fracture of the septum.
- Type 3: severe trauma causing a fracture of ethmoids and nasal bone. The perpendicular plate of the ethmoids rotates backwards as the septum collapses into the face, turning up the tip of the nose and revealing the nostrils. There is apparent widening of the space between the eyes (telecanthus).

Pre-operative assessment

History

The nature and direction of injury are noted as are details of previous injury or surgery to the nose. Was the nose perfectly straight before the current injury? MUA fractured nasal bones are unlikely to straighten a previously bent nose! Clear rhinorrhoea may indicate a CSF leak.

Examination

- Nasal pyramid: attention is focused on the nasal bones forming the upper-third of the nasal pyramid. This is best assessed from above and from below rather than face on.
- Nasal septum: the septum is assessed for significant deviation and for the presence of septal haematoma. Haematoma will require immediate surgical drainage.
- Surrounding structures: eye movements are assessed, any ridges on the infra-orbital rim and any impairment of infra-orbital sensation are noted, and may indicate a more extensive fracture.

Investigations

A simple fracture of the nasal bones is a clinical diagnosis and there is no role for an X-ray of the nasal bones in this situation. However, facial X-rays and CT scans may be helpful if more complex injuries are suspected clinically.

Surgical technique
Preparation
The procedure can be performed under local or general anaesthesia, although the latter is more favourable for most surgeons and patients. Local anaesthesia involves external infiltration of the infra-trochlear nerve, external nasal nerve, and the infra-orbital nerve (Fig. 20.5) and internal topical anaesthesia, with pledgets of cocaine, in the region of the sphenopalatine nerve behind the middle turbinate and the anterior ethmoidal nerve, high in the middle meatus. However, general anaesthesia with intubation or laryngeal mask is the preferred option in most cases. Topical vasoconstricting anaesthesia is often sprayed into the nose, e.g. lignocaine 5% with phenylephrine 0.5%. The patient is placed 30 degrees head-up on a head ring.

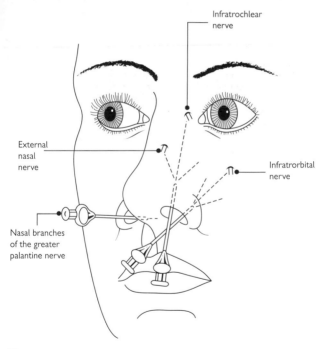

Fig. 20.5 Reduction of fractural nasal bones: local anaesthesia.

Procedure
- A Hill's elevator or Walsham's forcep is introduced via the nasal cavity and placed on the under-surface of the nasal bone. The nasal bones are then rotated laterally to out-fracture them.
- The nasal bones are then infractured by using external pressure from one's thumb to narrow and shape the nasal bones.
- BIPP packing is used if the nasal bones need further support or if there is heavy bleeding.
- Some surgeons attempt to manipulate septal fractures using Asch forceps. Some will even perform a conservative septoplasty to reduce acute septal fractures. Most will leave the septum alone at this stage and reassess it in 6 weeks and perform an elective septoplasty if required.
- If the nasal fracture is stable, nasal tape is used to reduce oedema over the dorsum. If the nasal bones are unstable and mobile, a thermoplastic splint or plaster-of-Paris cast is used. Occasionally, a small nasal pack is needed to support a nasal bone which has a tendency to fall in.
- The tape, splint, or cast is removed after 5–7 days.

Post-operative management
Most patients are managed as day-cases. If nasal packs are inserted for epistaxis, the patient usually stays in overnight. Packs inserted to support the nasal bones are removed after 5–7 days. Antibiotics are only given if packs are inserted for more than 24h.

Complications
Haemorrhage is managed by nasal packing. Imperfect result may require an elective septorhinoplasty.

Rhinitis

Definition

Inflammation of the nasal mucosa. May be acute or chronic.

Aetiology

Commonest causes are allergic and infective. See Table 20.1 for a simple classification system. Nearly all smokers will have a degree of rhinitis.

Clinical features

Rhinitis can be diagnosed if 2 out of 3 of the following are present for more than 1h every day for more than 2 weeks:
- Nasal congestion.
- Rhinorrhoea (anterior or posterior).
- Sneezing.
- Patients may also complain of itching of the nasal cavity, mild facial pain, and hyposmia.

Investigations

- Anterior rhinoscopy: this will reveal inflamed nasal mucosa, often with fine or occasionally thick mucus traversing the nasal cavity. The inferior turbinate is often engorged, although occasionally it can be pale and wet—especially in allergic rhinitis.
- Posterior rhinoscopy: to look for associated sinus disease (oedema, mucus or pus in the middle meatus) or septal deflections.
- Skin-prick tests (SPT) or RAST: identifies any sensitivity to common aeroallergens, e.g. grass, pollen, house-dust mite, cat and dog dander, feathers, and fungal spores.
- Blood tests: if a systemic cause is suspected, e.g. immunoglobulin levels, ACE levels, ANCA levels (see Table 20.1)
- CT scan of sinuses: if co-existing sinus disease is suspected.
- Saccharin clearance test: a small tablet of saccharin is placed on the anterior end of the inferior turbinate. Patient should taste it 5–15min. Delay of >20min raises the possibility of mucociliary dyskinesia.
- Nasal biopsy: electromicroscopy may show evidence of ciliary abnormalities.

Table 20.1 Classification of rhinitis

Common Allergic	Infective	Part of systemic disease	Rare Other
Seasonal	Acute	Primary mucus defect:	Idiopathic
Perennial	Chronic	Cystic fibrosis	NARES (non-allergic rhinitis with eosino-philia)
Occupational		Young's disease	
		Primary ciliary dyskinesis:	Drug-induced
		Kartagener's syndrome	β-blockers
		Immunological:	Oral contra-ceptives
		SLE	Aspirin
		Rheumatoid arthritis	NSAIDS
		AIDS	Local decon-gestants
		Antibody deficiency	
		Granulomatous disease:	Autonomic
		Wegener's/sarcoidosis	Atrophic
		Hormonal:	Neoplastic
		Hypothyroidism	
		Pregnancy	

Medical treatment of rhinitis

Nearly all patients are controlled with medical treatment.

Allergen avoidance
- If an allergen can be identified either via the history or clinically with SPT or RAST, then avoidance can be practised.
- The patient can also be advised on how to limit exposure, e.g. hot-washing bedsheets or using anti-allergy covers in house-dust mite allergy.
- SPT also provide a good visual feedback and understanding for the patient: the reaction occurring on the forearm is similar to the reaction in their nose on exposure to antigen.

Pharmacological measures
Choice of drug depends on severity of symptoms, seasonal nature, and nature of symptom (see Table 20.2).

Steroids
- Reduces the inflammation in the nasal cavity. Sprays, e.g. beclomethasone, fluticasone and mometasone are safest as they have lowest dose of steroid but consequently may take up to 6 weeks to take effect. The sprays should be directed laterally in the nasal cavity onto the inferior turbinate rather than onto the septum, to reduce the risk of aerosol-associated epistaxis and septal ulceration.
- Drops are much more potent and work within a week but may cause systemic side-effects if used continuously for more than 6 weeks. The drops should be applied in a head-down position to maximize delivery to the nasal cavity and sinuses (if the drops are applied simply with the head back, then the drops are swallowed quickly and do not have time to work topically and are thus less effective) (Fig. 20.6).
- Oral steroids are extremely effective and are occasionally used in the treatment of severe rhinitis unresponsive to other treatment. They should not be used more than a week.
- Typical regime for treatment of severe rhinitis is 1-month course of steroid drops, e.g. fluticasone nasules or betamethasone drops, to be followed by long-term nasal steroid sprays. All steroids are contraindicated in pregnancy, breast-feeding, glaucoma, and in the presence of active infection.

Antihistamines
- Reduces the systemic allergic response. These are used for treatment of mild allergic rhinitis. Also available in topical form, e.g. azelastine. They work very quickly and are safer then steroids. They are ideal for the treatment of seasonal allergy, e.g. hayfever.
- Second-generation antihistamines, e.g. terfenidine.are non-sedating and third-generation antihistamines, e.g. desloratidine, also have a mild anti-inflammatory action.

Table 20.2 Medications and their symptom control

	Sneezing	Discharge	Blockage	Anosmia
Cromoglycate	++	+	+	–
Decongestant	–	–	+++	–
Antihistamine	+++	++	±	–
Ipratropium	–	++	–	–
Topical steroids	+++	++	++	+
Oral steroids	++	++	+++	++

▶ Degree of benefit where +++ is maximum and – is minimum.

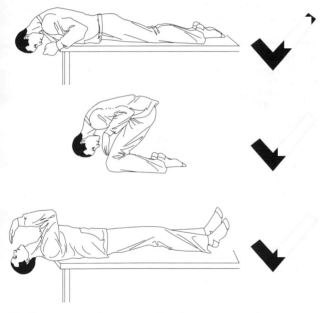

Fig. 20.6 Correct head position to instill nasal drops into the middle meatus.

Montelukast
- Mast-cell stabilizer and reduces the inflammatory response. Well tolerated. Mainly used for patients who have rhinitis and asthma, and also patients with Samter's triad (aspirin intolerance, nasal polyps, and asthma caused by a genetic defect in leukotriene metabolism).

Saline douche
- Extremely safe irrigation solution for the nasal cavity and very effective at clearing postnasal discharge. Can be used on snuffly infants, who are obligate nasal breathers, to aid sucking.

Ipratropium bromide
- An anticholinergic drug useful for drying the 'dew drop nose' of old-age rhinitis.

Sodium chromoglycate
- Mast-cell stabilizer that is effective in children with seasonal allergic rhinitis but limited somewhat because it needs to be used up to 6 times a day.

Nasal decongestants, e.g. ephedrine or xylometazoline
- Used mainly for viral rhinitis for maximum duration of a week.
- Produces rapid vasoconstriction of nasal mucosa and inferior turbinate to improve breathing.
- Can be combined with nasal steroid sprays to allow better delivery of medication in a congested nasal cavity.
- Long-term use of nasal decongestants will produce rebound congestion (rhinitis medicantosa) characterized by thick, boggy nasal mucosa, which is unresponsive to further decongestant treatment.

Desensitization
- This may be effective in patients allergic to one or two aeroallergens.
- Increasing doses of the purified allergen is injected hoping to produce blocking IgG antibodies.
- The length of treatment may be as long as 3 years.
- It is not widely practised in the UK because of the small risk of anaphylaxis.
- More recently, sublingual immunotherapy has been available for grass-pollen allergy and has been shown to provide long-term relief of hayfever symptoms.

Surgical treatment of rhinitis

Surgery may produce limited improvements of some of the symptoms of rhinitis especially nasal congestion. Surgical procedures are directed at the effects of rhinitis, e.g. enlarged turbinate, rather than the underlying cause. Consequently, the effects of surgical treatment of rhinitis are short lived and last about 12–18 months. However, improving the nasal airway will improve delivery of topical medication so that medical treatment of rhinitis is more effective.

Inferior turbinate surgery

- Linear cautery of inferior turbinate: surface electrocautery along the full length of the inferior turbinate using a monopolar Abbe needle and insulated thudichum speculum. Preferable in children as it carries the least risk of bleeding compared to the other methods of turbinate surgery.
- Submucous diathermy of inferior turbinate (Fig. 20.7a). The anterior end of the inferior turbinate is pierced with the monopolar Abbe needle, which is passed under the mucosal surface to the posterior part of the turbinate. As the needle is withdrawn, the mucosa is electrocauterized and care is taken not to damage the skin of the anterior nares. Maximum of three passes per turbinate bone because of the risk of osteonecrosis.
- Multiple outfracture of the inferior turbinate: the turbinate is pushed laterally with a Hill's elevator.
- Turbinoplasty (Fig. 20.7b–d): whereby the mucosa is elevated of the underlying bone at the anterior end of the inferior turbinate. The exposed anterior bone is then resected and the previously elevated mucosa is then folded back onto the remaining bare bone. Technically difficult but less risk of bleeding and atrophic rhinitis, compared to trimming the whole turbinate.
- Trimming of inferior turbinate (Fig. 20.7e): The inferior turbinate is fractured inwards with a Hill's elevator. The pedicle of the turbinate is then crushed with a straight clip for 1min. The clip is then removed and the crushed pedicle is cut with turbinectomy scissors. The detached turbinate is removed. Sometimes the severed turbinate needs to be pushed back into the postnasal space to free it from its remaining attachments before it is pulled out through nostril. The bleeding stump is often cauterized with an Abbe needle. There is a significant risk of bleeding with this procedure—especially from the remaining posterior stump of inferior turbinate, which is supplied by a branch of the sphenopalatine artery. Better visualization with rigid endoscopes and using diathermy reduces this risk. Trimming is also a more effective method of turbinate reduction than the other techniques.

(a)

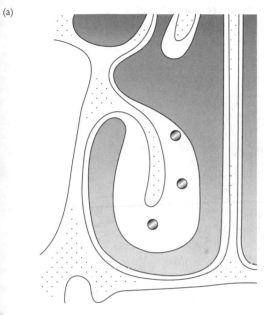

Fig. 20.7 a Submucous diathermy of inferior turbinate.

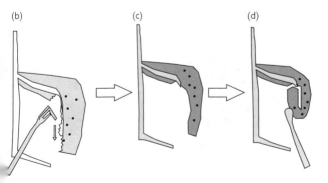

Fig. 20.7 b–d Turbinoplasty.

Treat any associated septal deviation
See 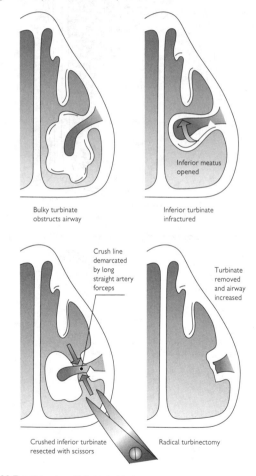 p. 548.

Treat any associate sinus disease
- E.g. polyps (see p. 580).
- Mild sinus disease often coexists with chronic rhinitis and it should be regarded as part of the same spectrum of disease.

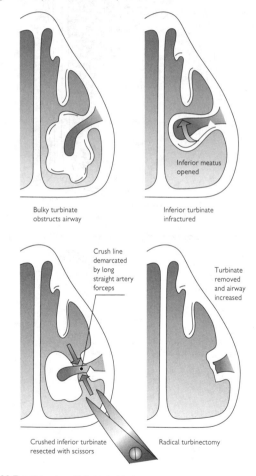

Bulky turbinate
obstructs airway

Inferior meatus
opened

Inferior turbinate
infractured

Crush line
demarcated
by long
straight artery
forceps

Turbinate
removed
and airway
increased

Crushed inferior turbinate
resected with scissors

Radical turbinectomy

Fig. 20.7 e Trimming of inferior turbinate.

Septoplasty and submucous resection of septum

Aims
- The goal of septoplasty is to reposition the misplaced septum by freeing the quadrilateral cartilage from its inferior and posterior attachments, so the anterior septum is hinging from the dorsum only ('swinging door' technique).
- The aim of submucous resection is to remove the misplaced quadrilateral cartilage, except for a 1cm dorsal strut and 1cm columella strip, which are left to prevent saddling and columellar retraction, respectively.

Indications
- Septal deformity, especially in the internal nasal valve area, producing nasal obstruction.
- As part of another procedure, e.g. septorhinoplasty, to correct an external deviation of the nose especially the cartilaginous dorsum.
- As a donor procedure to obtain cartilage, e.g. augmentation of a saddle deformity.
- Repair of a septal perforation.

Pre-operative management
- Full nasal examination including anterior rhinoscopy and nasal endoscopy is performed.
- The presence of alar collapse on normal inspiration is noted.
- The position of the caudal end of the septum is also noted, as it may dictate the surgical approach.

Surgical technique
Preparation
- The nasal mucosa is anaesthetized with a topical vasoconstricting solution, e.g. Moffat's solution (see 🕮 p. 528), 10% cocaine paste or solution. It can be applied on ribbon gauze or sprayed in the nasal cavity in the anaesthetic room.
- The patient is usually intubated with a throat pack but the procedure can also be performed with a laryngeal mask. A hypotensive anaesthetic is preferable.
- The patient is placed 30 degree head-up with the head slightly rotated towards the surgeon.
- Septal mucoperichondrial flaps are raised by hydro-dissection by infiltrating with 4.4ml of xylocaine 2% with 1 : 80 000 adrenaline with a dental syringe.

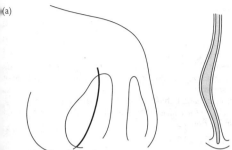

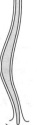

Fig. 20.8 a Submucous resection of septum: killian incision

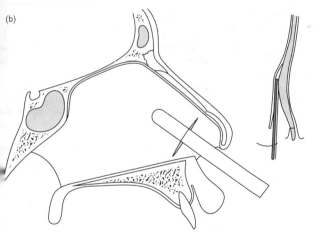

Fig. 20.8 b Submucous resection of septum: flap elevation.

Approaches

Killian incision (Fig. 20.8a and b)

- This is a mucosal incision about 15mm behind the caudal edge of the septal cartilage. It is relatively easy to get in the correct plane at this level and raise an intact mucoperichondrial flap over the underlying cartilage with the aid of a Freer elevator and Killian or Cottle speculum.
- The cartilage is seen as bluish-white and should have no vessels over it. Sharp dissection with a long-handled no.15 blade is often required over fracture sites and spurs.
- Because the incision is made behind the free edge of the septum, this approach is not suitable for addressing columellar dislocation or anterior nasal spine problems.

Hemitransfixion incision (Fig. 20.8c)

- This is a J-shaped vestibular incision over the caudal free edge of the cartilage extending over to the floor of the nasal cavity.
- The mucoperichondrium is tightly bound to the underlying cartilage for the first 8mm and it is not easy to enter a plane of dissection.
- For this initial part of the dissection, iris scissors or a no.15 blade are used with a Cottle speculum and toothed forceps.
- Eventually, further posteriorly, the mucoperichondrium strips easily with the aid of the Freer elevator.
- This approach is most suitable for addressing columellar dislocation or anterior nasal spine problems.

Flap elevation

- Once the correct relatively avascular plane is reached, the mucoperichondrium easily strips off the underlying bluish-white cartilage.
- The Freer elevator is used in an up and down motion, rather than a to and fro action.
- The flap can be difficult to raise at the septovomerine, septoethmoid junction, and at fracture sites, and sharp dissection is occasionally required.
- If a large spur is present, then a inferior tunnel should be created on the floor of the nasal cavity, which is connected with the mucoperichondrial flap above.
- Depending on the septal deformity, unilateral or bilateral mucoperichondrial elevation is performed but bilateral mucoperiosteal flap elevation is always performed.

(c)

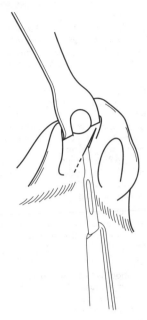

Fig. 20.8 c Septoplasty: right hemitransfixion incision.

(d)

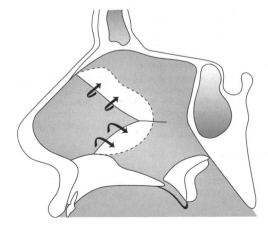

Fig. 20.8 d Septoplasty: resection at osteochondral junction.

Cartilage/bone/spur resection
- Any tissue to be resected must be clearly visible and free from its overlying mucoperichondrium or mucoperiosteum.
- The basic technique is described below but additional resection of deviated posterior bony septum and prominent spurs may be required if it is deemed symptomatic.

Septoplasty resection (Fig. 20.8d)
- After full exposure, a no.15 blade is used to remove a wedge shaped piece of cartilage inferiorly.
- A posterior chondrotomy is performed and cartilage and bone are removed posteriorly with Tilley–Hinchel forceps to free the quadrilateral cartilage from the ethmoid and vomer.
- Once the quadrilateral cartilage has been freed from its inferior and posterior attachments, it can be positioned in the required position.
- If the cartilage is still bent, the concave surface is scored to break the tension within the cartilage and lengthen it.

Submucous resection of septum
- After full exposure, the quadrilateral cartilage is resected preserving 1cm columellar and 1cm dorsal struts using a no.15 blade or a Ballenger swivel knife.

Closure and packing
- The hemitransfixion incision is closed with Vicryl. Some surgeons may elect not to close a Killian incision.
- The remaining flaps are approximated together with a quilting suture to eliminate dead space and reduce the chances of post-operative bleeding and haematoma.
- Any flap tears are repaired, if possible.
- If there are bilateral flap tears, resected straight septal cartilage is replaced between the torn flaps and they are approximated to reduce the chances of post-operative septal perforation.
- If there is excessive bleeding following closure, a non-adherent dressing, e.g. telfa or Merocel® is inserted for 24–48h.

Post-operative management
- Nasal packing is removed after 24–48h and the patient discharged.
- There will be sero-sanginous nasal discharge for up to 2 weeks post-operative. Nasal saline douche or Oxymetazoline drops are often prescribed after surgery to help clear the nasal cavity.
- The patient is advised to remain off work for 2 weeks and to avoid contact with individuals with URTIs.

Complications
Bleeding, infection, septal haematoma and abscess requiring prompt intervention, septal perforation, saddling of dorsum, columellar retraction are all recognised complications of septal surgery.

Septal perforations

Definition

Full-thickness defect in the cartilaginous and/or bony septum allowing one side of the nasal cavity to communicate with the other.

Aetiology

- Trauma, e.g. nose picking, after septal haematoma and abscess.
- Iatrogenic, e.g. following aggressive septal cautery, septal surgery especially SMR.
- Granulomatous disease, e.g. Wegener's disease, sarcoidosis, TB, syphilis (usually affects posterior bony septum).
- Drugs, e.g. cocaine sniffing, snuff, chrome workers.
- Neoplasia, e.g. SCC, BCC, T-cell lymphoma.
- Idiopathic.

Clinical features

Most are asymptomatic. Small anterior septal perforations can cause whistling. Others can present as epistaxis, excessive crusting and they can even cause nasal obstruction due to loss of laminar airflow within the nasal cavity.

Investigations

- Unless there is an obvious cause, most patients should have baseline investigations.
- Blood tests: FBC, ESR, ANCA, ACE levels, ?VDRL.
- Consider urinalysis and CXR.
- Consider biopsy, especially if there is a prominent granular area.

Treatment

Most asymptomatic septal perforations require no treatment.

Medical treatment for symptomatic perforations

- Reduce crusting with nasal saline douche, 25% glucose in glycerine solution or naseptrin.
- Granular areas causing epistaxis can be lightly cauterized.

Surgical treatment following failure of medical treatment

- Silastic septal button: if large, anterior perforation, especially if there is an inferior ridge of septum below the perforation to support the button.
- Surgery can be considered for small- to medium-size perforations (<2cm) but the results of surgical treatment to close the perforation is variable, even in experienced hands.
- Exposure to the anterior septum is by an open septoplasty or lateral rhinotomy approach.
- Sliding mucoperichondrial flaps, tunnelled buccal mucosal flaps, and composite grafts utilizing cartilage from the conchal bowl or posterior septum have been described for small- to medium-sized perforations. Success relies upon closure with multiple layers and having good vasculature to the repositioned tissue.

Granulomatous diseases of the nose

Definition
An uncommon group of conditions causing chronic inflammation in the nasal cavity and paranasal sinuses characterized histologically by granuloma formation.

Aetiology
- Autoimmune: Wegener's, Polyarteritis nodosa, SLE.
- Chronic infection: TB or syphilis.
- Unknown: sarcoidosis.

Clinical features
- Sinonasal symptoms and signs including crusting, granulation, ulceration, and septal perforation. Granulomatous disease tends to be more aggressive and destructive than 'normal' chronic rhinosinusitis.
- Systemic symptoms and signs, e.g. cough, urinary symptoms, eye problems, weight loss, skin nodules.

Investigations
- Blood tests: FBC, ESR, U+Es, ANCA, ACE levels, TPA/VDRL.
- CT of paranasal sinuses looking for extensive sinusitis with bone destruction.
- Urinalysis ± renal biopsy.
- Chest X-ray/CT chest scan.
- Biopsy of granular areas in nasal cavity.

Treatment
Medical

Patients often require long-term steroids and other immunosuppressants, e.g. methotrexate or azathioprine. Low-dose septrin can be used to prevent relapse in Wegener's disease. Patients are best managed in conjunction with a clinical immunologist or chest or renal physician.

Surgical

If the patient has chronic sinusitis unresponsive to medical treatment, then endoscopic surgery can be considered. However, these patients often have higher risk of intra-operative bleeding, post-operative complications, e.g. infection, and recurrent problems. Septal perforations are best managed conservatively or with a silastic button.

Nasopharyngeal carcinoma

Aetiology

- Genetic: certain HLA types, e.g. HLA-A2 and A5 in Singaporeans and Southern Chinese people predispose them to NPC.
- EBV infection is related to undifferentiated or poorly differentiated NPC. Antibodies to viral capsid antigen and early antigen detected in affected individuals or can be used to screen high risk (Chinese) population.
- Dietary habit: salted fish, commonly eaten by Chinese population, are high in nitrosamines, which are potent carcinogens.

Pathology (WHO histologic classification for NPC)

- Keratinizing squamous cell carcinoma (25%): above factors not involved. These tumours tend to occur in elderly smokers.
- Non-keratinizing squamous cell carcinoma (12%).
- Undifferentiated carcinoma of nasopharynx (63%): tend to occur in young patients with above risk factors.

Clinical features

- Lymph node metastases (70%): retropharyngeal nodes are involved early and occasionally seen as a bulge in the posterior pharyngeal wall. Palpable cervical metastases, usually level II or V, may be unilateral or bilateral.
- Symptoms of local invasion (Trotter's triad): glue ear due to Eustachian-tube involvement, reduced mobility of ipsilateral soft palate due to direct infiltration, and trigeminal pain due to irritation of V nerve.
- Other symptoms of invasion: involvement of cranial nerves II, III, IV, and VI due to involvement of orbital apex or cavernous sinus. Jugular foramen syndrome with paresis of cranial nerves IX, X, XI. Horner's syndrome, if cervical sympathetic chain involved.
- Nasal obstruction in proliferative lesions.
- Serosanginous discharge or epistaxis, especially in ulcerating lesions.
- Many tumours are submucosal and difficult to see, even with an endoscope. Contact bleeding or irregular mucosa may be the only tell-tale signs. The fossae of Rosenmuller, posterior to the medial crus of the Eustachian tube must be inspected thoroughly.

Investigations

- Routine blood tests, especially if recurrent epistaxis is a problem or distant metastasis are suspected.
- Audiometry, including tympanometry, if there are any otological symptoms.
- CT/MRI scan from head to abdominal cavity to delineate the extent of the primary lesion, including intracranial extension, any associated neck disease, and the presence of distant metastasis.

- Biopsy of nasopharyngeal mass. If a NPC is suspected but the postnasal space looks normal, the area should be curetted and tissue submitted for histology or a blind biopsy of fossae of Rosenmuller should be performed. Some care should be taken as the fossa can be up to 25mm deep and the internal carotid artery lies in its depths!
- FNA of any palpable neck masses.

Differential diagnosis of a irregular nasopharyngeal mass

- Nasopharyngeal carcinoma.
- Non-epithelial tumours, e.g. lymphoma, rhabdomyosarcoma.
- Other epithelial tumours, e.g. adenocarcinoma, adenoid cystic carcinoma, malignant melanoma.
- 'Normal' adenoid tissue.

Box 20.1 Staging (TNM system)

T0 No evidence of tumour.
T1 Tumour confined to nasopharynx.
T2 Tumour extends to soft tissues of oropharynx and/or nasal fossa.
T3 Tumour invades bony structures and/or paranasal sinuses.
T4 Tumour with involvement of cranial nerves or extension to cranial cavity, infratemporal fossa, hypopharynx or orbit.
N0 No regional lymph node metastasis.
N1 Unilateral lymph node metastasis, <6cm, above supraclavicular fossa.
N2 Bilateral lymph node metastasis, <6cm, above supraclavicular fossa
N3 Lymph node metastasis, >6cm or in supraclavicular fossa.
M0 No distant metastasis.
M1 Distant metastasis.

▶ The 'N' classification for nasopharyngeal SCCs is different to other head and neck SCCs.

Treatment

- Any treatment decisions should be made in the context of a multidisciplinary team clinic.

Curative

- Radical radiotherapy to nasopharynx, retropharyngeal node, and bilateral neck, even if no nodes are present.
- Even bulky neck disease in NPC is highly sensitive to radiotherapy. Because of the wide field involved, patients get severe side-effects from the irradiation, especially anorexia and mucositis, sometimes requiring a gastrostomy.
- Often platinum-based chemotherapy may be given in conjunction with radiotherapy.
- Recurrent disease may be amenable for further external beam radiotherapy or brachytherapy.
- Surgery is reserved for recurrent disease in the neck and occasionally in the nasopharynx.
- If the nasopharynx is free of disease, recurrent/residual neck disease can be treated by radical neck dissection.

- Recurrent/residual disease in the nasopharynx generally carries a very poor prognosis.
- If it is limited with no bony involvement, laser excision has been described.
- In Hong Kong, maxillary swing procedures have been advocated for more advanced recurrences.

Palliative
- Offered if medically unfit, untreatable residual/recurrent disease or if distant metastasis are present.

Prognosis
- Primarily relates to the size of the primary and not to the presence of neck metastasis.
- T_1 and T_2 carries a 90% and 70% 5y survival, respectively.
- T_4 carries a 40% 5y survival.
- Undifferentiated carcinomas have a better prognosis than keratinizing SCCs.

Juvenile nasopharyngeal angiofibroma

Definition

A benign tumour, consisting of fibrous tissue with varying degrees of vascularity, arising from the base of the medial pterygoid plate and the region of the sphenopalatine foramen. It is the most common vascular neoplasm of the nasal cavity. Despite it being a benign tumour, it is locally recurrent if excision is incomplete and therefore potentially lethal.

Clinical features

It tends to affect adolescent males with peak incidence between the ages of 14 and 18. Symptoms include:
- progressive nasal obstruction,
- recurrent severe epistaxis,
- hyponasal speech ('rhinolalia clausa'),
- glue ear.

A smooth, lobulated rubbery tumour, which is reddish or grey in colour, may be seen in the nasopharynx.
   Advanced symptoms are due to extension to:
- Ethmoidal region: causing bowing of the medial orbital wall with hypertelorism and 'frog-face' deformity, diplopia, and even blindness.
- Pterygoid and pterygomaxillary fossae: and winding around the outside of the maxilla causing cheek swelling.
- Intracranial extension.

Investigations

- CT/MRI scan of postnasal space will delineate extent of lesion and extension into surrounding areas. Anterior bowing of the posterior maxillary wall with posterior bowing of the pterygoid plate is said to be diagnostic.
- Angiography is also diagnostic and is essential if pre-operative embolization 24–48h prior to surgery is planned. Blood supply is usually from the ascending pharyngeal artery and sphenopalatine artery.
- Biopsy should be avoided because of the risk of uncontrollable bleeding.

Treatment

Surgery

Surgical approaches to the nasopharyngeal area include:
- Combined lateral rhinotomy with transnasal approach.
- Mid-facial degloving, sometimes combined with Le Fort type I osteotomies.
- Transpalatal route through the junction of the hard and soft palate.
- Endoscopic transnasal approach for small tumours.
- Transantral route via Caldwell–Luc approach.
- Maxillary swing popularized by Professor Wei, Hong Kong, whereby the maxilla is retracted out of the way by leaving its lateral attachments which act as a hinge.
- Craniofacial resection, if cribriform plate is involved.

Haemorrhage is reduced by pre-operative embolization and by dissection in a subperiosteal plane. Recurrence is reduced by drilling out the basi-sphenoid.

Radiotherapy

Given for inoperable or recurrent disease. Radiotherapy will affect growth of mid-face in the adolescent and has a 4% lifelong malignant transformation rate.

Watchful waiting

Not an option if lesion is growing or causing significant bleeding.

Mid-facial degloving procedure

The skin over the mid-third of the face is elevated to allow access to the facial bones and the sinonasal cavity. It is feasible to perform a complete bilateral maxillectomy preserving the external nasal osseocartilaginous skeleton with this approach. The limits of the dissection are the ethmoids and cribriform plate superiorly, the posterior wall of the sphenoid, pterygoid muscles and plates posteriorly, and the coronoid process of the mandible laterally.

Indications
- Resection of benign sinonasal disease, e.g. inverted papillomas, angiofibromas.
- Repair of large septal perforations.
- Repair of mid-facial fractures.
- Resection of selected malignant tumours.

Surgery
Preparation
- The procedure is usually performed with a hypotensive general anaesthesia with an endotracheal tube and throat pack.
- The patient is placed supine on a head ring in the reverse Trendelenburg position.
- The nasal cavity mucosa is vasoconstricted with Moffatt's solution (1ml of 1 : 1000 adrenaline, 2ml of 10% cocaine, and 2ml of 8.4% sodium bicarbonate) either sprayed in the nasal cavity or applied on pledgets.
- The skin is cleaned with aqueous chlorhexidine, head draped, and a temporary bilateral tarsorrhaphy performed.
- Prophylactic broad-spectrum antibiotics, e.g. IV Augmentin® 1.2g are given.

Incision
- A bilateral sublabial incision is made down to bone from one maxillary tuberosity to the other (Fig. 20.9a).
- In the nasal cavity, intercartilaginous incisions are continued into a transfixion incision separating the medial crus of the lower lateral cartilage from the septum.
- The transfixion incision is extended to the anterior nasal spine and along the floor (Fig. 20.9b).
- The sublabial and nasal incisions are joined, staying on bone and defining the pyriform aperture.

Surgical technique
- The periosteum and soft tissues of the cheeks are elevated up to the infra-orbital nerves and as lateral as possible to facilitate flap retraction (Fig. 20.9c).

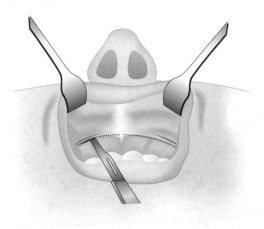

Fig. 20.9 a Midfacial degloving: bilateral sublabial incision.

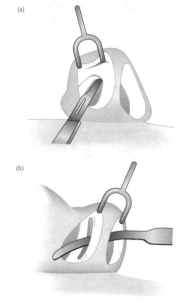

Fig. 20.9 b Midfacial degloving: intercartilaginous incision and full transfixion incision.

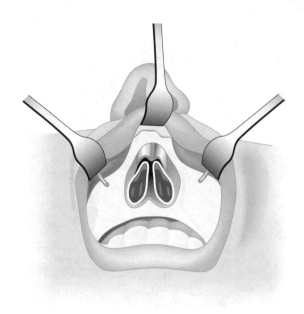

Fig. 20.9 c Midfacial degloving: final exposure.

- Through the intercartiliginous incisions, the soft tissues of the dorsum are elevated up to the root of the nose. It is joined laterally with the cheek dissection. The pyriform aperture with the attached upper lateral cartilages and both infra-orbital nerves should clearly be visible.
- With this access, a total or medial maxillectomy may be performed. Branches of the internal maxillary artery should be identified either posteriorly or laterally in the infratemporal fossa and ligated. The ethmoids can be cleared up to the cribriform plate and the sphenoid can also be explored if required.

Closure
- Haemostasis is achieved by bipolar diathermy or surgical clips. The resulting cavity is packed with Whitehead varnish pack.
- The intercartilaginous and sublabial incision is closed precisely with vicryl. The frenulum is correctly repositioned in the midline.
- Taping of the nose and application of a nasal plaster of Paris cast will help reduced facial oedema.

Post-operative management
- The patient is nursed 45 degrees head-up to reduce facial swelling due to venous congestion.
- The nasal packs are removed after 1–3 weeks, usually under a short GA, and the antibiotics are continued until this time.
- Saline douches are prescribed after the pack removal to reduce crusting and infection in the maxillectomy cavity.

Complications
- Vestibular stenosis, avoided by accurate suturing of the intercartilaginous incision.
- Paraesthesia over the infra-orbital nerve distribution preventable by avoiding enthusiastic retraction of the cheek flap.
- Oroantral fistula.
- Epiphora.
- Upward rotation of the nasal tip.

The sinuses

Anatomy of the paranasal sinuses

All the sinuses are considered as invaginations of the nasal cavity extending into bone and as such drain into the nasal cavity through their natural ostia. Their function is not known but they are responsible for mid-facial growth in childhood. They help in resonating the voice and lighten the weight of the skull. The paranasal sinuses also protect the brain from 'thermal' injury and facial trauma. The frontal sinus appears at the age of 2y and the other sinuses are only rudimentary air cells at birth.

Maxillary sinus

This sinus is roughly pyramidal is shape with the base towards the lateral nasal wall and its apex pointing into the zygomatic process of the maxilla. The roof of the sinus is the floor of the orbit and the floor of the sinus is the alveolar (tooth bearing area) part of the maxilla. The infra-orbital nerve runs in the roof of the sinus and often forms a ridge within the sinus at the junction of the roof and anterior wall. The size of the sinus varies. The roots of the three molar teeth (and occasionally the premolars) are separated from the floor of the antrum by a thin layer of compact bone. Tooth extraction can leave a oro-antral fistula. The natural ostium lies high up on the medial wall opening in the middle meatus of the lateral nasal wall, hidden behind the lower free end of the uncinate process. Occasionally a smaller accessory ostium is found more posteriorly and this may be visible by nasal endoscopy.

Ethmoidal sinus (Fig. 21.1a and b)

This sinus is not a single cavity but 3–18 cells lying within the ethmoidal labyrinth (lateral part of the ethmoid bone). The anterior cells are small and numerous, and correspond to the ethmoidal bulla draining into the middle meatus. The posterior cells are larger, fewer in number, and drain into the superior meatus.

An unusually large posterior ethmoidal cell that extends posterio-laterally around the sphenoid sinus to embrace the optic nerve is called an Onodi cell. A large infra-orbital ethmoidal cell near the maxillary sinus ostium is termed a Haller cell. An agger nasi cell is part of the anterior ethmoidal cell complex in the frontal process of the maxilla, anterior to the uncinate process but posterio-medial to the frontal recess.

The lateral wall of the ethmoid sinuses is the paper-thin lamina papyracea separating the sinus from the orbit and the roof is the cribriform plate separating it from the anterior cranial fossa. Disease can further thin the ethmoidal bone causing orbital and intracranial complications. The anterior, and occasionally the posterior, ethmoidal vessels can be seen in its roof.

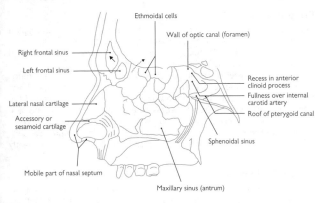

Fig. 21.1 a Parasagittal section through paranasal sinuses.

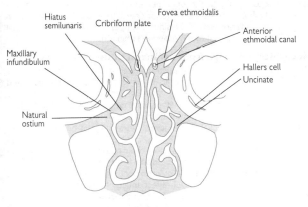

Fig. 21.1 b Coronal section through paranasai sinuses.

Frontal sinus (Fig. 21.1a)

These develop during the 2nd year of life as excavations into the diploe of the frontal bone and are really anterior ethmoidal air cells that have migrated upwards. Both frontal sinuses are variable in size and are separated from each other by a midline inter-sinus septum.

Immediately posterior to the posterior table of the sinus is the anterior cranial fossa. The floor of the sinus is related to the orbit. The sinus drains through its ostium at its lower medial corner into the anterior end of the semilunar hiatus via the frontal recess (previously called the frontonasal duct). The frontal recess has an hourglass shape and its volume may be further reduced by surrounding structures, e.g. prominent ethmoidal bulla or agger nasi cells. The frontal bone contains marrow and is consequently susceptible to osteomyelitis.

Sphenoid sinus (Fig. 21.1a)

These sinuses are located in the body of the sphenoid. The two sinuses are again variable in size and are separated from each other by an inter-sinus septum, which is usually not in the midline. The roof of the sinus is related to the pituitary fossa and the middle cranial fossa. Laterally lies the cavernous sinus with the optic nerve above and the internal carotid artery below. Posteriorly is the posterior cranial fossa and pons. The ostium is high on the anterior wall of the sinus and opens in the sphenoethmoidal recess (behind and medial to the superior turbinate).

Mucociliary drainage from paranasal sinuses (Fig. 21.1c)

The sinuses are lined with ciliated stratified or pseudostratified columnar epithelium. Mucous and serous glands lie beneath this epithelium and their secretions provide a biphasic mucous blanket with a thick 'gel' and thinner 'sol' layer. The gel layer traps inspired particles as small as 3µm and this tenacious layer is continually turned over by the wafting action of the cilia in the thin watery sol layer. On average, a healthy maxillary sinus renews its gel layer every 20–30min. The cilia of the ethmoid, maxillary and sphenoid sinuses beat towards their natural ostia but the cilia in the frontal sinuses can waft mucus away from the frontal recess. Cilia function better in a warm, humid environment. Severe infections, blocked ostia, and metabolic poisons will affect mucus production, consistency, and its transport in the sinuses. Decreased ciliary activity may make it easier for viruses and bacteria to penetrate the mucosa.

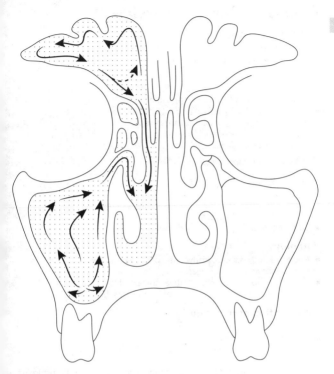

Fig. 21.1 c Mucociliary drainage pathways of paranasal sinus.

Rhinosinusitis: an overview

Definition (AAO-HNS)

An inflammatory response involving the:
- Mucous membrane of the nose and paranasal sinuses.
- Fluid within the cavities.
- And/or underlying bone.

With one or more of the following symptoms:
- Nasal obstruction/nasal congestion.
- Nasal discharge or purulent postnasal drip.
- Facial pain and pressure.
- Altered sense of smell.

Can be acute or chronic.

Aetiology

Multifactorial:
- Host: genetic, allergic, immune, anatomic, systemic.
- Enviromental: infectious, trauma, iatrogenic.
- Often preceded by acute viral illness.

Pathology

- Acute rhinosinusitis: exudative, necrotic, haemorrhagic process with neutrophils and macrophages.
- Chronic rhinosinusitis: proliferative, fibrosis of lamina propria with plasma cells, lymphocytes, eosinophils ± polyps, bacteria or fungi.

Classification of rhinosinusitis

- Acute: ≤4 weeks.
- Subacute: 4–12 weeks.
- Recurrent acute: ≥4 episodes/year.
- Chronic: ≥12 weeks.
- Acute on chronic: sudden worsening of chronic rhinosinusitis, returning to baseline after treatment.

Acute rhinosinusitis

Definition

Acute inflammation of the nasal and sinus lining lasting for up to 1 month. It is usually initially due to a viral upper respiratory-tract infection followed by a secondary bacterial infection. Occasionally it is due to dental sepsis or trauma.

Pathogens

- Viral: *rhinovirus, influenza*, RSV, *parainfluenza*.
- Bacterial: *Pneumococcus*, other streptococci, *Haemophilus influenza, Klebseilla, Escherischia coli*.

Clinical features

- Preceding URTI.
- Nasal congestion.
- Mucopurulent anterior and/or posterior rhinorrhoea.
- Facial pains especially over maxillary or frontal sinuses and the pain is characteristically worse on bending forward. Facial swelling is rare with uncomplicated acute sinusitis.
- Anterior rhinoscopy shows inflamed nasal mucosa ± mucopus in nasal cavity or oropharynx.
- Rigid nasal endoscopy shows oedematous middle meatus ± mucopus streaming back into the postnasal space.

Investigations

- Rarely necessary unless complications of acute sinusitis are suspected.
- Plain sinus X-ray are largely obsolete but may show air–fluid levels in frontal or maxillary sinuses.
- CT sinuses will show air–fluid levels in sinuses and thickened sinus mucosa.

Treatment

Most patients are treated effectively in the community with 2 weeks of full medical treatment consisting of:
- Broad-spectrum antibiotics, e.g. Augmentin® 625mg tds.
- Betnesol nose drops, 2 drops bd both nostrils.
- Steam inhalations often with added eucalyptus or menthol oils tds.
- Xylometazoline 0.5% 2 drops tds for a week.

In resistant cases, a pledget soaked in cocaine 10% solution placed in the middle meatus can produce rapid vasoconstriction to relieve obstruction of the osteomeatal unit and allow effective drainage of the sinuses. Other resistant cases may require an antral washout or urgent functional endoscopic sinus surgery (FESS), especially if complications of acute sinusitis are suspected (see p. 589).

Maxillary sinus lavage

Indications
- Diagnostic: proof puncture to obtain fluid for microbiology.
- Therapeutic: To remove secretions in acute infections.

Surgical technique

Preparation
- The procedure can be performed under local or general anaesthesia.
- Local anaesthesia can be administered by spraying lidocaine 5% with phenylephrine 0.5% into the nasal cavity. Additional topical anaesthesia can be applied to the inferior meatus by inserting a cottonwool-tipped probe dipped in cocaine paste under the inferior turbinate. The patient is seated, leaning forward slightly, holding a bowl under his mouth.
- General anaesthesia can be administered with an endotracheal tube with throat pack or via a laryngeal mask. The patient is placed in the head up position with the head on a head ring.

Procedure
- Using a thudichum nasal speculum to visualize the inferior turbinate, a Tilley–Lichwitz trocar is introduced into the inferior meatus (Fig. 21.2a).
- The tip of the trocar is gently passed near the roof of the inferior meatus, at the apex of attachment of the inferior turbinate, about 3.5cm posterior to the lateral edge of the vestibule in an adult. This is the thinnest part of the inferior meatal wall (Fig. 21.2b).
- The tip is directed towards the tragus of the ipsilateral ear and with moderate pressure and a gentle boring movement, the trocar pierces the bony wall of the meatus to enter the antrum. The handle of the trocar is placed in the palm of the hand and the index finger is extended along the shaft to prevent deeper penetration of the antrum.
- The trocar is removed and the cannula is advanced until it is judged to be in the middle of the antrum. If necessary, the cannula can be pushed against the lateral wall of the antrum and then withdrawn slightly.
- The antrum is aspirated and any pus sent for microbiology. Aspiration of air or fluid confirms that the cannula is in the maxillary sinus.
- A 20ml syringe containing sterile saline at 37°C is used to irrigate the antrum. Air must not be introduced because of the risk of air embolism. The eye is observed as the sinus is irrigated for periorbital swelling indicating misplacement of the cannula. The patency of the natural ostia is noted.
- If performed under LA, the patient is instructed to breathe through their mouth whilst the sinus is washed. As the patient leans forward, fluid flows out from the anterior nares.
- If performed under GA, a Belluci sucker removes irrigation fluid from the nasopharynx as the sinus is washed.
- Prior to removing the cannula, the antrum is aspirated to dryness.

▶ The maxillary sinus in a child is small and may contain unerupted dentition. Occasionally, adults may have hypoplastic antra.

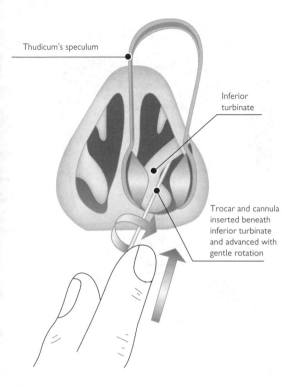

Fig. 21.2 a Maxillary sinus lavage: placement of trocar.

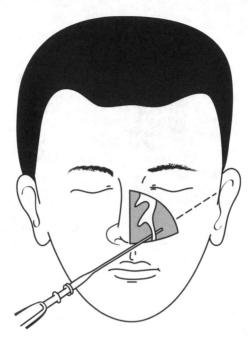

Fig. 21.2 b Maxillary sinus lavage: entering the antrum.

Complications

- Bleeding: there is usually minimal ooze following the procedure. If the antrostomy is made too posteriorly, a branch of the sphenopalatine artery may be damaged causing significant haemorrhage requiring nasal packing.
- Misplacement of the cannula into the soft tissue of the cheek or even the orbit. This will caused periorbital swelling and proptosis (and pain if the procedure is done under LA) as saline is introduced. The procedure should be abandoned immediately, antibiotics started and, if necessary, an urgent ophthalmology consultation sought.
- Epiphora, if the nasolacrimal duct is damaged by performing the antrostomy too anterior.
- Numbness of the incisors due to damage to the anterior superior alveolar nerve.
- Air embolism.

Chronic rhinosinusitis

Definition
Chronic inflammation of the nasal and sinus lining for over 3 months. It may be preceded by an acute episode.

Pathogens
Usually bacterial, e.g. *Streptococcus* incl. pneumococcus, anaerobes, *Pseudomonas*, *E. coli*.

Clinical features
Similar to acute sinusitis but less severe.
- Nasal congestion, anterior and/or posterior rhinorrhoea, facial discomfort, hyposmia/anosmia.
- Examination may show inflamed nasal mucosa, oedematous middle meatus sometimes with discharge streaming into the postnasal space, and nasal polyps.

Investigations
- Skin-prick tests or RAST to exclude an allergic element to chronic symptoms.
- ESR, ANCA, and ACE levels to confirm or exclude granulomatous disease.
- Immunoglobulin levels to exclude hypogammaglobinaemia.
- CT scan of paranasal sinuses to delineate extent of disease and plan surgical treatment. Coronal images are the most useful for anterior sinus disease but axial cuts are essential for posterior ethmoidal and sphenoidal disease.
- Mucociliary clearance test: (see 📖 p. 538).
- Electron microscopy to exclude primary ciliary dyskinesia.

Treatment
Like acute sinusitis, most cases settle with full medical treatment. Even if surgery treatment is offered, most patients need prolonged post-operative medical treatment.

Medical treatment for at least 3 months
- Intranasal steroids: for mild cases, an intranasal steroid spray, e.g. fluticasone 2 puffs each nostrils od. In more severe cases, especially if there is associated nasal polyps, more potent intranasal steroid drops are used, e.g. betamethasone 2 drops each nostril bid for 6 weeks followed by nasal steroid sprays.
- Oral antihistamines, e.g. desloratidine 5mg od especially if positive allergy tests or symptoms of rhinorrhoea.
- Oral antibiotics, e.g. macrolides such as erythromycin or clarithromycin, especially if mucopus is present.

Surgical treatment if prolonged medical treatment fails
- FESS surgery ± septoplasty to relieve obstruction of the osteomeatal unit and to restore natural mucociliary drainage and ventilation of the sinuses.
- External sinus procedure are rarely performed now but can be considered if there is a complication of sinusitis or if repeated FESS surgery fails suggesting the mucosa is irreversibly diseased. External procedures remove all the diseased mucosa with the hope that new healthy mucosa will regrow.

Nasal polyps

Definition

Nasal polyps are the oedematous sino-nasal mucosa prolapsing into the nasal cavity. Simple nasal polyps are part of the spectrum of chronic rhinosinusitis and are formed by the sino-nasal lining becoming progressively more inflamed and thicker and then pedunculating into the nasal cavity.

Aetiology

Essentially unknown, but the following factors may contribute to polyp formation:

- Allergy, e.g. house-dust mite allergy where polyps are usually multiple and bilateral.
- Vasomotor: as above but no allergen identified.
- Inflammatory: occasionally, polyps can occur following acute viral or bacterial infections. Polyps tend to be single, soft, and slightly haemorrhagic.
- Genetic: especially if the patient has aspirin intolerance, late onset asthma, and nasal polyps (Samter's triad). These patients have extensive nasal polyposis that tend to recur quickly following treatment. A low salicylate diet may be helpful in improving symptoms.
- Paediatric polyps: polyps are rare in healthy children. If present, the child should be investigated for cystic fibrosis, Kartagener's syndrome, immunodeficiency, or coeliac disease.

Clinical features

Symptoms usually occur gradually over years but occasionally may occur more rapidly after an acute infection. The predominant symptom is nasal obstruction but patient may also have anosmia, postnasal drip, clear or mucopurulent rhinorrhoea depending on aetiology, and facial pains.

Simple nasal polyps are usually benign and have a characteristic translucent appearance. They are insensate on probing and mobile; this can help differentiate them from the inferior turbinate for the inexperienced. They tend to occur predominantly in the ethmoidal sinuses with the frontal and maxillary sinuses less affected. Gross nasal polyposis causes expansion of the nasal bones with broadening of the nasal bridge resulting in a characteristic 'frog face'.

- Unilateral antrochoanal polyps tend to occur in young adults following a viral infection (see 📖 p. 582).
- Unilateral nasal polyps should be considered neoplastic until proved otherwise. Neoplastic polyps tend to be solid, haemorrhagic, and show evidence of bone erosion on CT scanning.

Investigations

- Similar to chronic rhinosinusits.
- CT scan of paranasal sinuse, especially if endoscopic sinus surgery is going to be considered.
- Biopsy of unilateral polyps to exclude neoplasia. If there is a possibility that the unilateral polyp is a meningocele, then CT/MRI is performed first and biopsy avoided.

Treatment

Medical polypectomy

- For gross nasal polyps, oral prednisolone 40mg od for 1 week is prescribed. Warn patient of the side-effects of short-term course of steroids, especially gastric irritation, euphoria, and risk of avascular necrosis of the hip.
- For smaller polyps, a 1-month course of betnesol drops or flixonase nasules is prescribed followed by long-term intranasal steroid spray. Intermittent courses of oral steroids or steroid drops can be prescribed whilst on maintenance spray. Those with positive allergy tests should also be given antihistamines.
- Patients with Samter's triad are often treated with long-term topical steroid, montelukast, a mast-cell stabilizer, and a low salicylate diet (see Table 21.1).

Surgical polypectomy

- For large nasal polyps or patients that fail medical treatment, endo-scopic polypectomy with the microdebrider, combined with FESS, if operative conditions are favourable, is performed.
- In patients with recurrent polyps, CT scan of sinuses prior to surgery is mandatory to outline the bony anatomy of the sinuses, especially of the medial orbital wall and cribriform plate area. If the anatomy is grossly distorted, it may be safer to perform just an endoscopic polypectomy to improve the nasal obstruction.
- Rarely, external sinus procedures may be indicated, especially in multiple revision cases where the anatomy may be distorted.

Table 21.1 Foods high in salicylates

Drinks	Carbonated drinks, e.g. beer, distilled drinks (whiskey, vodka, gin), tea, wine.
Fruits	Apples, apricots, berries, cherries, currants, dates, grapes, melon, plums, pomegranates, avocadoes.
Vegetables	Potatoes, cucumbers, green peppers, radishes, tomatoes, olives, canned mushrooms.
Fats	Olive oil, salad dressing.
Desserts	Pies and cakes made with fruit.

▶ This list is by no means exhaustive. Nearly everything in the modern diet contains at least a trace of salicylate!

Antrochoanal polyps

Definition

A large unilateral inflammatory sinonasal polyp, arising from either the anterior or lateral wall of the maxillary sinus, and prolapsing through an accessory ostium, enlarging it over time, into the nasal cavity and postnasal space. ∴ it tends to have three components: large antral and posterior choanal parts; and a smaller anterior nasal part.

Clinical features

Antrochoanal polyps tend to occur in young adults, usually following a viral infection. They cause predominant symptoms of unilateral nasal obstruction, occasionally causing a 'ball valve' effect with nasal blockage on expiration only. They can also cause snoring, clear or mucopurulent rhinorrhoea, glue ear, globus symptoms, anosmia, and rarely facial pains. Nasal endoscopy will show the nasal component, which may obstruct further advancement of the endoscope. Oropharyngeal examination or posterior rhinoscopy will show the larger choanal part.

Investigations

- CT scan of paranasal sinuses will demonstrate all three components of the antrochoanal polyps. It will also show expansion of the maxillary sinus ostia. If there is significant bone erosion, then neoplasia should be suspected. (See Box 21.1).
- MRI scan of paranasal sinuses will show high signal on T2 due to the water content of the polyps and may help differentiate an antrochoanal polyp from other causes of unilateral paranasal sinus opacification.
- Representative biopsy to exclude neoplasia.

Treatment

As antrochoanal polyps are very symptomatic, and because the diagnosis may be in doubt, most antrochoanal polyps should be removed surgically unless the patient is medically unfit.

Surgery

FESS polypectomy

Most antrochoanal polyps can be removed endoscopically. Aspirating the contents of the antral component with a Tilley Lichwitz trocar may assist its delivery into the nasal cavity. The polyp should be grasped as it prolapses through the maxillary sinus ostium with Tilley Henckel forceps and the antral component is gently delivered into the nasal cavity by pushing the Tilley Henckel forceps into the postnasal space. The whole polyp is then removed either transnasally or from the oropharynx with a Boyle Davis gag. As the maxillary sinus ostium is widened, it is usually very easy to inspect the antrum with a 30-degree scope to check if any there are any remnants of the antral component. These must be removed to reduce risk of recurrence.

Caldwell Luc procedure combined with endoscopic clearance

This may be performed for recurrent antrochoanal polyps and it provides better access to anterior and lateral maxillary sinus walls to remove the points of attachment of the polyps. The canine fossa is infiltrated with 2ml xylocaine 2% with 1 : 80 000 adrenaline. A horizontal mucosal incision is made and the anterior maxilla bone is exposed (Fig. 21.3a and b). It is perforated by a large trocar or drill. Care must be taken to avoid the roots of the teeth, ∴ it is better to stay a little high (but avoid traumatizing the infra-orbital nerve). At the end of the procedure, ensure there is a large intranasal antrostomy and the sublabial mucosal incision is accurately sutured with vicryl.

Medical

Oral or topical steroids may provide temporary relief of symptoms. However, high doses are often required and symptoms return rapidly as the dose is reduced. Steroids are not ∴ considered to be an effective long-term treatment option.

Box 21.1 Differential diagnosis of unilateral polyp

- Inverting papilloma.
- Fungal sinusitis: CT scan may show areas of microcalcification.
- Paranasal sinus malignancy: CT may show bone erosion.
- Antrochoanal polyp.
- Nasal polyp secondary to odontogenic infection: CT may show a premolar or molar tooth root on the floor of the maxillary sinus.

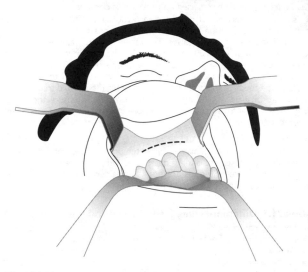

Fig. 21.3 a Caldwell Luc procedure: incision over canine fossa.

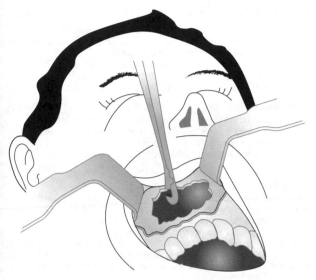

Fig. 21.3 b Caldwell Luc procudure: enlargement of antral opening.

Fungal sinusitis 1

Fungal infections have recently been implicated in the majority of cases of chronic rhinosinusitis. Fungi have been discovered in the mucus and may cause a florid inflammatory reaction in the mucosa.

Classically, fungal infections have been classified into:
- Non-invasive: allergic fungal sinusitis and sinus ball/mycetoma.
- Invasive: acute fulminant type and chronic invasive sinusitis.

Aetiology
- Non-invasive fungal sinusitis usually occurs in immunocompetent individuals, whilst invasive fungal sinusitis occurs in the immunocompromised, e.g. diabetics, AIDS, transplant patients.
- The most common pathogens are from the *Aspergillus* and *Mucor* species.

Pathophysiology
Allergic fungal sinusitis is linked to allergic rhinitis and type 1 (IgE) and type 3 (immune complex) hypersensitivity reactions. Histologically, the allergic mucin has intact and degenerate eosinophils (Charcot–Leyden crystal) with sparse hyphae. Patients often have asthma, eosinophilia, and have a pansinusitis. Sinus mycetoma is usually unilateral and involves the larger maxillary sinus. Allergic conditions are less common. Although the mucous membrane is chronically inflamed in non-invasive sinusitis, there is no evidence of fungal invasion.

Acute fulminant fungal sinusitis and chronic invasive sinusitis are caused by spread of fungus into the vascular channels with invasion into the orbit and CNS with associated bone destruction. Histologically, there is evidence of necrosis of the mucosa and submucosa with vascular thrombosis.

Clinical features
- Non-invasive fungal sinusitis presents with symptoms of chronic rhinosinusitis with/without polyposis. The thick mucin of allergic fungal sinusitis has been likened to 'peanut butter' or 'axle grease'. A mycetoma is more often 'clay-like'.
- Patients with potentially fatal acute fulminant fungal sinusitis are unwell with fever and headache. Examination and radiology show evidence of tissue and bone destruction and, in advanced cases, cavernous sinus thrombosis.
- Chronic invasive fungal sinusitis patients are not usually unwell and have symptoms of chronic rhinosinusitis. However, examination may reveal an orbital apex syndrome characterized by decrease in vision and ocular immobility due to a mass in the superior orbit.

Investigations
- Blood tests may show elevated fungus-specific IgE levels in patients with allergic fungal sinusitis. Inflammatory markers are usually elevated in the acute fulminant form.
- Skin-prick test may be positive to fungus in the non-invasive form.

- CT scans of the sinuses may show microcalcification of the opaque fungal mass in the non-invasive form, due to accumulated heavy metals, e.g. calcium, manganese (see box 21.2). There may be evidence of bone expansion. The invasive type, however, will show evidence of bone destruction with spread of disease outside the confines of the sinuses. MRI scanning may further help delineate fungal mucin from reactive inflammation and shoud be performed in addition to CT scanning if invasive sinusitis is suspected.
- Microbiology of any secretions and tissue to identify fungus and direct antimicrobial therapy.
- Biopsy to exclude neoplasia.

Box 21.2 Differential diagnosis of calcification in a paranasal sinus

- Infective: rhinolith, fungal sinusitis.
- Neoplastic: benign—osteoma, chordoma, chondroma, inverted papilloma.
- Malignant—chondrosarcoma.
- Other: fibrous dysplasia, meningioma.

Fungal sinusitis 2: treatment

The mainstay of treatment for all forms of fungal sinusitis is surgery to restore ventilation of the sinuses, but medical treatment may be started pre-operatively to make surgery easier and continued post-operatively. Invasive fungal sinusitis should be jointly managed with a microbiologist and, if necessary, neurosurgeons and ophthalmologists.

Medical

- Allergic fungal sinusitis: pre-operative topical steroids should be used to improve operative conditions and oral steroids commenced post-operatively along with nasal saline douching. Post-operative immunotherapy has also been advocated, although it is not widely available.
- Sinus mycetoma: once the fungal ball has been surgically removed, no further medical treatment is needed.
- Chronic invasive fungal sinusitis: once surgical debridement has been performed, amphotericin B or itraconazole is commenced. FBC, U + E and LFTs should be monitored.
- Acute fulminant fungal sinusitis: the patient's underlying immunodeficiency should be stabilized and urgent treatment with high-dose amphotericin B should be started. When the patient is stable, this is changed to itraconazole. Black mucosa, due to infarction, suggests need for urgent intervention.

Surgery

This is performed endoscopically if possible, but if there is extensive bone destruction and distortion of surgical landmarks, it may be safer to perform this externally. All secretions and diseased mucosa are removed and sent for analysis. In the invasive form, radical debridement is performed until healthy tissue is reached.

Prognosis

- Allergic fungal sinusitis carries a good prognosis following surgery and post-operative steroid treatment. Long-term topical steroids control relapses and prolonged follow-up is required.
- Sinus mycetoma has an excellent prognosis following surgery, with no need for long-term therapy or follow-up.
- Acute fulminant fungal sinusitis carries a poor prognosis with mortality rates of 50%, even with aggressive intervention.
- Chronic invasive fungal sinusitis has a good prognosis but patients often require long-term systemic antifungals to prevent relapse.

Complications of sinusitis (1)

This occurs when infection spreads outside the confines of the paranasal sinus. Broadly divided into:
- Acute:
  - Local:
    — Orbital.
    — Intracranial.
    — Bony.
    — Dental.
  - Distant:
    — Toxic shock syndrome.
- Chronic:
  - Mucocoele/pyocoele.
- Associated diseases:
    — ?Otitis media.
    — Adenotonsillitis.
    — Bronchiectasis.

Spread of infection
- Local:
  - Bone weakness:
    — Lamina papyracea.
    — Infra-orbital canal.
    — Dental roots.
  - Diploic veins into anterior cranial fossa.
  - Olfactory fila to subarachnoid space.
- Distant:
  - Haematogenous causing septicaemia.

Microbiology
- Organisms likely to cause sinusitis complications are: *Streptococcus pneumonia*, *Haemophilus influenza*, and *Staphlococcus aureus*. Invasive fungal sinusitis can occur in the immunocompromised.
- Broad-spectrum antibiotics with anaerobic cover are usually used until microbiology culture and sensitivity results are available, e.g. IV Augmentin® 1.2g tds or IV Cefuroxime 1.5g tds with Metronidazole 500mg tds.

Investigations
- Microbiology swab of any mucopus in the middle meatus.
- CT scan of paranasal sinuses, preferably with IV contrast to differentiate abscess (ring enhancement) from an inflammatory tissue.
- MRI scan of paranasal sinuses, especially if intracranial complications are suspected and initial CT scan was inconclusive.

Complications of sinusitis (2)
Periorbital cellulitis

Chandler's classification
I. Preseptal cellulitis (i.e. superficial to tarsal plate).
II. Orbital cellulitis without abscess (postseptal cellulitis).
III. Orbital cellulitis with subperiosteal abscess.
IV. Orbital abscess.
V. Cavernous sinus thrombosis.

Clinical features
- Usually an ill child with spiking pyrexia.
- Chemosis.
- Diplopia.
- Proptosis and painful restricted eye movement suggest possible abscess.
- Engorgement of retinal veins on fundoscopy.
- Colour blindness, especially red/green, detected by Ishihara charts, indicates impeding risk to sight.

▶ If optic nerve decompression is not achieved in 2h, irreversible neuropathy may occur.

Treatment
- If there is no suggestion of a subperiosteal abscess or orbital abscess, then the patient is given IV antibiotics, nasal decongestants, and topical Betnesol nasal drops for 24h. Expert nursing is essential during this time with regular observations including visual tests. If he/she fails to improve, CT scanning must be performed.
- However, if an abscess is clinically evident or seen on CT scanning, it must be drained urgently. This is usually done externally through a Lynch–Howarth incision and a drain is left *in situ* in the ethmoid cavity (see 🕮 p. 608). Bilateral antral washouts must be performed at the same time as drainage of any abscess. Some rhinologists may favour an endoscopic approach, although this can be challenging because of the gross inflammation present in the nasal cavity. However, following thorough decongestion, some pus can usually be seen draining from the ethmoid and antrum and this can be traced back to the relevant sinuses.
- If the patient fails to settle following initial surgical treatment, repeat scanning must be performed to exclude further collections.

Complications of sinusitis (3)

Osteomyelitis

Infection enters the marrow spaces of diploic bone (frontal bone in adolescents and adults or maxilla in infants only) and then into venules crossing suture lines. Isolated areas of infection and sequestrae can ∴ occur all over the calvarium. Osteomyelitis can be precipitated by sinusitis, trauma or operations on anterior wall of sinus.

Clinical features
- Dull local pain and headache.
- Oedematous area on forehead due to subperiosteal abscess (Pott's puffy tumour).

Treatment
- Prophylaxis: antibiotic cover for procedures on frontal sinus.
- Full medical treatment: IV antibiotics, nasal decongestants, and topical Betnesol nasal drops.
- If there is failure to improve with medical treatment, BAWO ± frontal sinus trephine through non-diploic bone of frontal sinus floor.
- If there is still no improvement, or sequestrae seen or if intracranial complications, radical surgery may be indicated. An osteoplastic procedure (MacBeth operation) involves a bicoronal incision, elevation of forehead tissue, and allows inspection of infected frontal bone and sequestrae. Dead tissue is debrided and the resulting defect may need plastic surgical reconstruction, once infection settles.

Intracranial complications

Usually associated with frontal, ethmoidal, and sphenoidal sinusitis. They are very rarely associated with maxillary sinusitis via ascending infection of the pterygoid plexus.
- Meningitis.
- Extradural abscess.
- Subdural abscess.
- Frontal lobe abscess.
- Otitic hydrocephalus via sagittal sinus thrombosis.
- Cavernous sinus thrombosis associated with sphenoid sinus sinusitis.

Mucocoeles and pyocoeles

If the dependant ostium of the frontal sinus is blocked, sterile mucus accumulates within it and its contents become increasingly viscous. The cyst expands gradually and thins the anterior and inferior wall. If there is superadded infection, the cyst is termed a pyocoele. Mucocoeles can also rarely affect the ethmoid, maxillary and sphenoid sinuses.

Clinical features
- Pain and swelling over the frontal sinus, occasionally with egg-shell cracking felt on palpation.
- Diplopia, proptosis and displacement of the globe laterally and inferiorly.

Treatment
Drain sinus and evacuate its content. This can be done endoscopically or externally via a Lynch–Howarth incision or bicoronal incision.

Secondary effects of suppurative sinusitis

- Effects of mucopus in the nasopharynx: otitis media, pharyngitis, adenotonsillitis, laryngitis, bronchitis, and bronchiectasis.
- Exacerbation of asthma due to inflammation spreading down the aerodigestive tract.

Functional endoscopic sinus surgery (FESS)

Theory

The most important area for normal mucociliary drainage of the paranasal sinuses is the osteomeatal complex (Fig. 21.4a). This is a 3D functionally crucial area of the middle meatus bounded by the inferior-lateral part of the middle turbinate, uncinate process, and the ethmoid bulla. A small amount of disease in the osteomeatal complex can obstruct the narrow drainage pathways of the frontal, ethmoid, and maxillary sinuses, producing a much more florid disease within the cavity of the sinuses.

The aim of FESS is to eradicate disease in the ostiomeatal complex by removing as little mucosa as possible, thereby restoring natural ventilation and mucocilary drainage of the frontal, ethmoid, and maxillary sinuses, and reversing any mucosal change within the sinuses.

Indications

- Chronic sinusitis with or without polyposis unresponsive to medical treatment.
- Significant recurrent acute sinusitis.
- Complications of sinus disease, e.g. subperiosteal abscess, mucoceles.
- For certain benign malignancies, e.g. inverting papillomas.

Surgical technique

Preparation

The procedure is usually performed with a hypotensive general anaesthesia, with an endotracheal tube and throat pack. Alternatively, a laryngeal mask can be used. The patient is placed supine on a head ring in the reverse Trendelenburg position. The nasal-cavity mucosa is vasoconstricted with Moffatt's solution (1ml of 1 : 1000 adrenaline, 2ml of 10% cocaine and 2ml of 8.4% sodium bicarbonate) either sprayed in the nasal cavity or applied on pledgets. Additional xylocaine 1% with adrenaline 1 : 80 000 can be infiltrated endoscopically at the root of the middle turbinate and at the anterior edge of the uncinate process.

Procedure

- If there is significant septal deviation impeding access to the middle meatus, then a septoplasty or SMR septum should be performed.
- The middle turbinate is gently medialized and the uncinate process is palpated with Freer elevator. The ball-tip seeker is useful for locating the free posterior edge of the uncinate process.
- An uncinectomy is performed with a sickle knife or sharp Freer elevator or paediatric back biter, taking care not to enter the orbit superiorly (Fig. 21.3b). The sickle-shaped uncinate bone is removed with Blakesley–Wilde forceps (Fig. 21.4c).
- The ethmoid bulla is exenterated by entering the air cells at its inferior and medial point, and then carefully working laterally and superiorly. Laterally, the lamina papyracea and posteriorly, the basal lamella is identified.

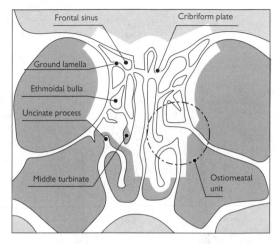

Fig. 21.4 a Coronal section through paranasal sinuses at level of ostiomeatal unit.

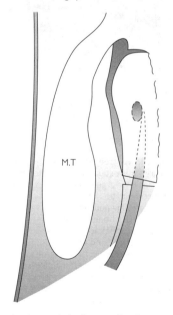

Fig. 21.4 b Left uncinectomy: anterior fracture of uncinate process.

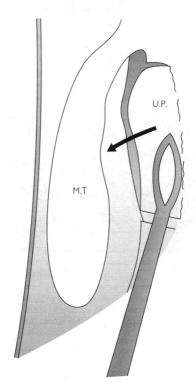

Fig. 21.4 c Left uncinectomy: removal of uncinate process.

- Just posterior to the lower free edge of the uncinate process is
  the natural maxillary sinus ostium, which is often best seen with a
  30-degree scope. This is enlarged to create a middle meatal
  antrostomy with a combination of forward biting Blakesley–Wilde
  forceps, back and side biting punches. Care is taken not to remove
  the anterior thick maxillary bone overlying the nasolacrimal duct.
- If required, the posterior ethmoid cells are entered by piercing
  the basal lamella at its lowest and most medial point. Alternatively, the
  posterior cells can be entered via the superior meatus. The skull base
  is seen in the roof of the posterior ethmoid cells and a curette can be
  used to remove tissue from posterior to anterior along the skull base
  taking care not to damage the anterior and posterior ethmoidal arteries, which can sometimes be seen in the roof of the ethmoid sinuses.

- If required, the sphenoid sinus is entered through the inferiomedial portion of the posterior ethmoid cells. Alternatively, it is safer to find the sphenoid sinus ostium approximately 10–15mm above the posterior choana in the sphenoethmoidal recess and enlarge it inferiorly with a sphenoid mushroom punch. The superior and lateral areas of the sphenoid, and sometimes the posterior ethmoid cells, are in close relation to the optic nerve and internal carotid artery respectively.
- If required, the frontal recess can be cleared and explored. This again is often best seen with a 30-degree scope. It is located at the anterior superior attachment of uncinate proces. Care should be taken not to strip mucosa circumferentially in this area, as it may create stenosis and subsequent mucocele formation. Disease in the frontal sinus is best cleared with giraffe forceps.
- If required, the nasal cavity is packed with non-adherent dressing, e.g. Telfa or Merocel®. If there is heavy bleeding, BIPP packing is occasionally necessary.

Post-operative management

Nasal packing is removed after 24–48h and the patient discharged. There may be sero-sanginous nasal discharge for up to 2 weeks post-operative. Nasal saline douche or oxymetazoline drops are often prescribed after surgery to help clear the nasal cavity. Occasionally topical or oral steroids or systemic antibiotics are given post-operatively depending on intraoperative findings. The patient is advised to remain off work for 2 weeks.

Complications

See 📖 p. 602.

Endoscopic approach to the frontal sinus

Aims

To provide a wide and patent frontonasal communication, prevent recurrent obstruction, and create conditions favourable for re-epithelialization.

Indications

- Acute or chronic frontal sinus disease unresponsive to medical treatment.
- The main advantage of the endoscopic approach is the lack of any visible incision. Also the lateral bony support of the frontal recess is preserved, preventing soft tissue prolapsing medially and later obstructing the frontal sinus outflow.

Surgical technique

Preparation

See 📖 p. 594. In addition, the head may need to be extended further to gain access to the frontal recess, if it cannot be visualized in the standard position. Image-guidance systems can be very helpful with frontal-sinus work, especially in revision cases.

Procedure

- Punches rather than forceps should be used in frontal-sinus work to avoid stripping mucosa, minimizing the risk of synechiae, as well as reducing bleeding.
- An uncinectomy, anterior ethmoidectomy, agger nasi removal, and resection of the anterosuperior attachment of the middle turbinate may all need to be removed to visualize the frontal recess. Before the middle turbinate attachment is removed, an 'axillary' flap may be created preserving mucosa at the root of the turbinate (Fig. 21.5a and b).
- An ostium probe or ball-tip seeker is used to locate the outflow tract. A 30-, 45-, or even 70-degree scope will need to be used.
- Once the frontal recess is located, the anterior nasofrontal beak, a shelf-like bony process anterior to the frontal recess, is removed with a Kerrison rongeur, drill or bony curette (Fig. 21.5c and d).
- Further drainage is achieved by removing the superior aspect of the nasal septum. The mucosa of the posterior table of the sinus must be preserved to allow re-epithelialization. If there is no healthy mucosa present, e.g. revision cases, stents may be left *in situ*.
- Endoscopic approach of the frontal sinus can be combined with trephination in difficult cases to locate the frontal recess via a retrograde approach.
- Extended drainage of the sinus can be achieved by resecting the frontal-sinus floor, lower inter-sinus septum, and anterosuperior nasal septum, leaving just a thin rim of bone around the frontal sinus outflow in the region of the glabella (modified Lothrop procedure).

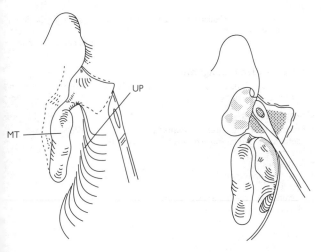

Fig. 21.5 a–b Left endoscopic frontal sinus approach: creation of axillary flap.

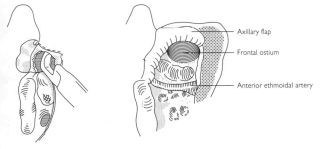

Fig. 21.5 c–d Left endoscopic frontal sinus approach: opening the frontal recess.

Closure

If a middle turbinate 'axillary' flap has been raised, it is swung back down to the raw area over the root of the turbinate. If stents are to be left, they are sutured onto the membranous septum. Nasal packing is rarely necessary.

Post-operative management

See 📖 p. 597. Crusting is minimized by regular douching. Stents are left *in situ* for 2–3 months.

Complications

- Bleeding from the anterior ethmoidal vessels with possible orbital haematoma due to the artery retracting into the orbit.
- Infection.
- Adhesions.
- Surgical emphysema.
- CSF leak.
- Restenosis of the frontal sinus outflow tract with recurrent symptoms.
- Mucocoele and pyocoele.

Complications of functional endoscopic sinus surgery

These can be:
- Rhinological.
- Orbital.
- Neurological.
- General: relate to general anaesthesia.

Rhinological
- Epistaxis: may be due to injury to sphenopalatine artery, anterior ethmoidal artery or internal carotid artery. Severe bleeding may necessitate abandoning procedure and packing the nasal cavity. Mild bleeding maybe controlled by suction bipolar cautery.
- Infection: risk minimized by not leaving any bony fragments in the FESS cavity and irrigating thoroughly at end of procedure. Some surgeons see post-operative patients weekly for endoscopic decrusting until the FESS cavity has healed but most surgeons will instruct the patient to saline douche for 2 weeks post-operatively.
- Synechia: risk minimized by accurate dissection and not leaving any loose tags of mucosa. It tends to occur where there are two denuded surfaces in close proximity, e.g. anterior end of inferior or middle turbinate, and the adjacent nasal septum. Post-operative splints may reduce synechia formation. Alternatively, they may be divided in clinic under LA in the early post-operative period.
- Recurrence of disease.
- Mucocele, especially if there is circumferential damage in region of frontal recess.

Orbital
- Orbital haematoma: due to damage to anterior ethmoidal vessels with retraction of vessels into orbit or damage to orbital periorbita. A tense haematoma causing proptosis requires immediate drainage via a lateral or medial canthotomy with pre-operative steroids and urgent ophthalmological opinion (see Box 21.3 and Fig. 21.6).
- Diplopia due to damage to extra-ocular muscles, especially medial rectus and superior oblique. This can occur if lamina papyracea is breached during ethmoidectomy. Ophthalmology consultation should be obtained.
- Surgical emphysema around eye, if lamina papyracea breached. This usually settles spontaneously within a week but most patients are given oral broad-spectrum antibiotics. Patient is advised not to blow nose post-operatively.
- Epiphora, if nasolacrimal duct damaged. This is avoided by not enlarging the middle meatal antrostomy too far anteriorly. The thick bone of the maxilla should not be nibbled with the back biting forceps.
- Blindness, if optic nerve is damaged. Take care in the sphenoid sinus or Onodi cells.

Neurological

- CSF rhinorrhoea if skull base is breached and dura is torn. Occasionally, it can occur if the middle turbinate is fractured medially. An intra-operative CSF leak should be repaired immediately. A free mucosal graft is used from the septum or inferior turbinate or a local flap graft from middle turbinate mucosa is used. The graft is held in place with tissue glue and gelfoam is packed on top of that to create a 'sandwich repair'. The nasal cavity is packed with BIPP for 5–7 days. A lumbar drain is considered and the patient confined to bed rest for 5–7 days. Straining is avoided.
- Meningitis, encephalitis, subdural abscess, and frontal lobe abscess.

General

- Cardiorespiratory problems, e.g. MI, pneumonia, pneumothorax.
- Thrombo-embolic problems, e.g. PE, DVT.

Box 21.3 Lateral canthotomy and inferior cantholysis
(See Fig. 21.6)

- Inject 1–2ml of 2% lignocaine with 1 : 80 000 adrenaline into the lateral canthus.
- Apply an artery clip from the lateral canthus towards the bony orbit to devascularize the area for 30–90s.
- Remove the clip and cut the demarcated area laterally down to the bone of the orbital rim, taking care not to damage the conjunctiva.
- Using forceps to pull the lower lid down, the inferior lateral canthal tendon is visualized and divided. The globe and orbital fat should prolapse forwards.
- The wound and lateral canthal tendon can be sutured after 24–48h.
- If further decompression is required, medial decompression can be achieved with an external ethmoidectomy or endoscopically removing the lamina papyracea.

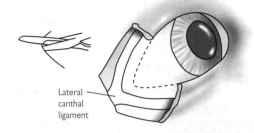

Fig. 21.6 Lateral canthotomy and inferior cantholysis (Lateral canthal ligament with superior and inferior limbs).

Lateral canthal ligament

Endoscopic dacrocystorhinostomy (DCR)

Indications
- Epiphora due to lacrimal sac or nasolacrimal duct obstruction, especially if conservative treatment of massaging, compression, and probing the duct fails.
- Main advantage of the endoscopic procedure is that it provides good exposure of the medial wall of sac without a visible external incision.

Pre-operative management
Thorough evaluation by an ophthalmologist is essential prior to considering the procedure. Proximal obstruction at the level of the common canaliculus, failure of lacrimal pump, and neuromuscular disorders should be all be excluded. Rhinology examination should exclude active infection and identify the presence of rhinitis, polyps, and septal deviation, which may necessitate additional treatment prior to the DCR.

Surgical technique
Preparation
Standard FESS preparation (see 📖 p. 594). The procedure can be performed under LA or GA.

Procedure
- The anterior edge of the uncinate process is identified. A lateral, nasal wall-flap, based on the anterior edge of the uncinate, is fashioned with a sickle knife and raised gently with a Freer elevator to expose the ascending process of the maxilla and the lacrimal bone. The flap is tucked under the middle turbinate out of the way.
- The exposed lacrimal bone is gently curetted or thinned with a diamond drill. If the dissection is too anterior, the thick maxillary bone will be encountered. The lacrimal sac should be exposed as widely as possible. The inferior canaliculus should now be cannulated with a silver lacrimal probe or light 'pipe' to confirm the position of the sac.
- As the medial wall of the sac is tented with the inferior canaliculus cannula, the lacrimal sac is opened and the medial sac wall is excised as widely as possible.
- If necessary, a O'Donoghue silastic stent is inserted via the superior and inferior canaliculi and tied in the nasal cavity.

Post-operative management
Nasal packing is rarely necessary and the patient can usually go home the same day. Nasal douching should be performed regularly. The stents are removed at 6–8 weeks by cutting the loop at the medial canthus and grasping the knotted ends in the nose.

Complications
- Haemorrhage.
- Orbital injury.
- Infection.
- Restenosis of lacrimal sac.

Frontal sinus trephine

Indications

- Treatment of acute frontal sinusitis refractory to medical treatment by allowing pus to be obtained for microbiology to help direct antibiotic therapy.
- As an adjunct to endoscopic sinus surgery when there is difficulty locating the frontal recess and sinus.

Pre-operative management

Frontal sinus trephine is contraindicated in an aplastic/very hypoplastic frontal sinus. ∴ CT scan of sinuses, or at least plain X-rays (occipitofrontal view) of the frontal sinus, should be performed to show degree of aeration of the frontal sinuses.

Surgical technique

Preparation

The procedure is usually performed with a hypotensive general anaesthesia, with an endotracheal tube and throat pack. The patient is placed supine on a head ring in the reverse Trendelenburg position. The incision line is marked and then infiltrated with xylocaine 2% with 1 : 80 000 adrenaline. The skin is cleaned with aqueous chlorhexidine, head draped and a temporary tarsorrhaphy performed.

Incision

A 1cm incision is placed parallel and medial to the normal position of the eyebrow (Fig. 21.7a). The incision is deepened to the periosteum.

Procedure

- The periosteum is stripped of the floor of the frontal sinus.
- The floor is perforated by a burr or small gouge and hammer.
- If no pus is encountered, a frontal ethmoidal (Kuhn) cell has been opened and the roof of this cell should be opened to enter the frontal sinus (Fig. 21.7b).
- If intracranial complications are suspected, the posterior wall of the frontal sinus should be exposed and inspected by further removal of bone from the frontal sinus floor and anterior wall.

Closure

A small drainage tube is inserted into the sinus and secured onto the skin. An additional skin stitch may be necessary.

Post-operative management

The frontal sinus is irrigated via the indwelling drainage tube for 48h. Antibiotic therapy is modified when the results of the pus microbiology are available.

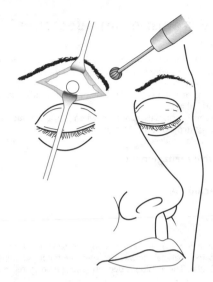

Fig. 21.7 a Frontal sinus trephine: exposing the floor.

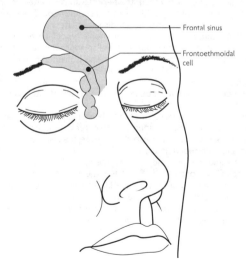

Fig. 21.7 b Frontal sinus trephine: relationship of frontoethmoidal (Kuhn) cell to frontal sinus.

External fronto-ethmoidectomy

Indications

Endoscopic sinus surgery has largely reduced the number of external sinus procedures. However, external fronto-ethmoidectomy may still have a role in the following situations:

- Complications of acute ethmoiditis and frontal sinusitis, e.g. subperiosteal and orbital abscess.
- Recurrent chronic sinusitis, especially when previous endoscopic sinus surgery has destroyed surgical landmarks.
- Frontoethmoidal mucoceles.

Pre-operative management

See 📖 p. 606.

Surgical technique

Preparation

See 📖 p. 606.

Incision

A curvilinear incision, often with a 'v' or 'w' to prevent post-operative webbing, is placed parallel midway between the medial canthus and nasal bridge (Fig. 21.8a). The incision is deepened to the periosteum.

Procedure

- Periosteal elevation (Fig. 21.8b): the periosteum is elevated off the ascending process of the maxilla with a Freer elevator. The lacrimal sac is elevated out of its groove and displaced laterally.
- Division of ethmoidal arteries: the anterior ethmoidal artery will be seen as a tethering of the subperiosteal flap approximately 24mm posterior to the anterior lacrimal crest. This is diathermied or ligated with surgical clips and divided. The posterior ethmoidal artery is approximately 12mm behind the anterior ethmoidal artery and is similarly divided. Care must be taken not to inadvertently injure the optic nerve.
- Opening of the ethmoidal sinuses: The lamina papyracea will now be fully exposed and is easily penetrated to enter the ethmoidal sinus. The cells are progressively cleared to expose the insertion of the middle and then superior turbinates. The cribriform plate is defined superiorly and the sphenoid sinus may be opened at this stage.
- Opening of the frontal sinus (Fig. 21.8c): the medial floor of the frontal sinus is removed and this is continued laterally if required. The skin incision may need to be extended under the eyebrow taking care not to damage the supratrochlear neurovascular bundle. The trochlea may need to be carefully dissected from its niche.

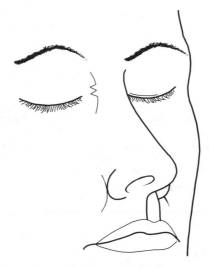

Fig. 21.8 a External fronto-ethmoidectomy: skin incision.

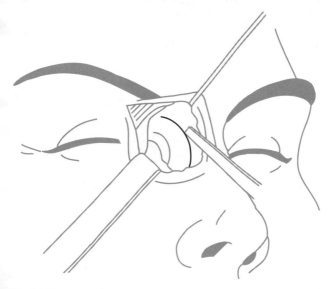

Fig. 21.8 b External fronto-ethmoidectomy: periosteal elevation.

- Removal of frontal sinus mucosa: All diseased mucosa is removed but, if possible, some mucosa should be preserved at the frontal sinus osteum to prevent stenosis. Also, if bone lateral to this area can also be preserved, this will prevent prolapse of orbital contents and subsequent obstruction.
- Frontal sinus drainage (Fig. 21.8d): the main drawback of frontal sinus procedures is stenosis of the outflow tract with subsequent recurrent disease and/or mucoceles formation. ∴ a 1cm silastic tube is placed in the frontal sinus and trimmed so its lower end sits in the middle meatus. If the frontal recess can be clearly seen endoscopically, intra- and post-operatively, it may be best to avoid stenting the outflow tract.

Closure

The periosteum, fat, and skin are all accurately closed. The trochlea is re-attached with a non-resorbable suture, e.g. prolene. Pressure dressing over the eye overnight will reduce post-operative oedema.

Post-operative management

The skin sutures are removed at 5 days. Nasal douches should be used regularly until the sinus re-epithelializes. The sinus cavity is cleaned regularly in outpatients by rigid endoscopy and the patency of the frontal recess assessed. The frontal sinus stents are removed after 3–6 months.

Complications

- Wound problems, including infection and webbing.
- Diplopia, especially if the trochlea is not re-attached.
- Epiphora, which is usually temporary.
- CSF leak due to defect in cribriform plate or posterior table of frontal sinus caused by disease or surgery.
- Obstruction of frontal sinus resulting in recurrent disease and/or mucocele formation.

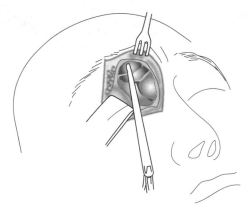

Fig. 21.8 c External fronto-ethmoidectomy: entering the frontal sinus via the ethmoid air cells.

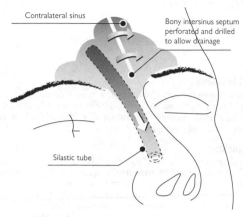

Fig. 21.8 d External fronto-ethmoidectomy: drainage of the frontal sinus.

CSF rhinorrhoea

Aetiology
- Iatrogenic following FESS surgery or tumour surgery.
- Head injury involving anterior cranial fossa.
- Spontaneous.

Clinical features
Any unilateral watery rhinorrhea should arouse suspicion of a CSF leak, especially if nasal discharge is increased by leaning forward, or it occurs following FESS or head injury. Persistent CSF leaks should be repaired because of the risk of meningitis.

Investigations
- β2 transferrin analysis in nasal secretions: this protein is highly specific to CSF. (It is also found in much smaller quantities in perilymph.)
- CT scan anterior cranial fossa: may show small defects in anterior skull base or sphenoid sinuses with opacification in the adjacent air cell. Intrathecal contrast will confirm the site of an active leak.
- MRI scan of anterior cranial fossa (T2W) may further help by showing CSF in ethmoidal cells or sphenoid but MRI lacks the bony detail provided by CT scans.
- Intrathecal fluoroscein with endoscopic evaluation with a blue or standard cold light. This is usually done in theatre, with 0.2ml of 5% fluoroscein mixed with 5–10ml of CSF, re-injected slowly into the subarachnoid space 30min prior to examination. If a leak is seen, endoscopic repair is performed.

Treatment
Conservative
- Most cases resolve with conservative management. This includes bed rest in a head-up position, stool softeners, avoidance of straining and decreasing CSF pressure by using a lumbar drain.
- Use of prophylactic antibiotics is controversial with opponents arguing that it may mask the signs of meningitis and promote infection with more resistant organisms.

Transnasal endoscopic surgical repair (Fig. 21.9a–d)
- If conservative measures fail, then endoscopic repair is the preferred option. Success rates vary on the size of the bony and dural defect.
- FESS techniques provide excellent visualization of the defect.
- The mucosa is elevated from the surrounding bone and free abdominal fat or temporalis fascia graft is tucked into the defect so that it lies intracranially adjacent the frontal lobe.
- Free or pedicled nasal mucosal grafts are then placed over the defect and held in place with fibrin glue.
- Finally the graft materials are further supported by gelfoam and BIPP packing.

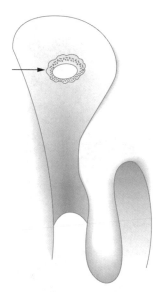

Fig. 21.9 a Endoscopic approach to the skull base defect in ethmoidal roof.

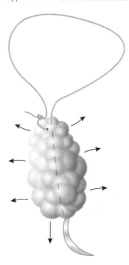

Fig. 21.9 b Suture placed through fat graft and secured so that as the suture is tightened, once the graft is inplace, it expands to fill the dural defect.

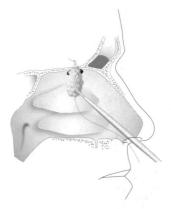

Fig. 21.9 c Fat graft gently pushed through the defect.

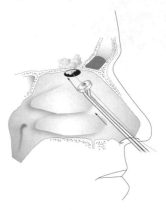

Fig. 21.9 d Mucosal graft slides up the suture to its final position.

External extracranial repair (Fig. 21.9e)

Standard external incisions are used to open the ethmoid and frontal sinuses (Lynch Howarth, bicoronal or eyebrow) and the defect repaired using vascularized pedicled pericranium or septal mucosa, which is glued into position. The frontal sinus may need to be obliterated with abdominal fat.

Neurosurgical repair (intracranial)

The intracranial technique visualizes the defect from above via a craniotomy and frontal lobe retraction but it does carry all the expected risks of a neurosurgical procedure. The entire anterior skull base can be inspected so it is a useful technique if investigations cannot locate the defect.

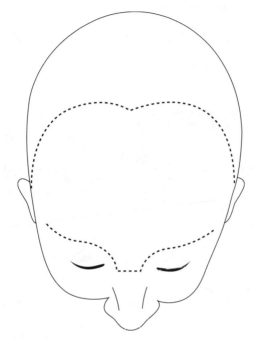

Fig. 21.9 e External extracranial repair: frontal sinus exposure via bicoronal (above) or eyebrow (below) incisions.

Sinonasal malignancy

This includes tumours of the columella, nasal vestibule, as well as the nasal cavity and paranasal sinuses. Commonest malignancies are:
- basal cell carcinomas,
- squamous cell carcinomas,
- tumours of minor salivary glands,
- sarcomas, and
- malignant melanomas.

Less common tumours are:
- esthesioneuroblastoma, and
- adenocarcinomas.

Aetiology
- Hardwood dust predisposes to adenocarcinomas of the ethmoids, whilst softwood dust predisposes to squamous cell carcinomas. High Wycombe was the centre of the wood-working industry in the UK for many years and there was a high incidence of sinonasal malignancy in the area until the end of the last century.
- Other occupations at risk include nickel (for undifferentiated and squamous carcinomas) and chromium workers, shoe and textile workers, and those working with volatile hydrocarbons.
- Human papilloma virus 16 and 18 may be a cofactor in the development of squamous cell carcinomas.

Clinical features
- Tumours of the columella and nasal vestibule tend to cause destruction of the anterior nose and face.
- Nasal-cavity melanomas are characteristically dark, polypoid masses.
- Antral tumours can cause: nasal obstruction, epistaxis, infra-orbital anaesthesia, dental pain, facial pain and swelling, and trismus.
- Ethmoidal tumours can cause: nasal obstruction, epistaxis, CSF rhinorrhoea, diplopia, and proptosis.

Investigations
- CT scan paranasal sinuses, neck and chest will give some information on size of the primary tumour, extent of bone erosion, presence of lymphadenopathy and distant metastasis. However, presence of oedema and inflammation secondary to sinus obstruction may overestimate extent of disease.
- MRI scan of sinuses, anterior cranial fossa, orbit and neck will help differentiate tumour from oedema. Critical areas are cribriform plate, fovea, pterygopalatine fossa, medial orbit, and sphenoid. It may also help characterize retropharyngeal and cervical nodes.
- Specific tests, if indicated, for multiple myeloma (plasma protein electrophoresis, Bence Jones proteins), esthesioneuroblastoma (urinary catacholamines), CSF analysis ($\beta 2$ transferrin).

- Biopsy of the sinonasal mass, if necessary, via an antrostomy. Immuno-histochemistry will be required for 'anaplastic or small cell tumours' to differentiate between a poorly differentiated carcinoma, esthesioneuroblastoma, melanomas and lymphomas. FNA of any cervical nodes.

Classification

- Ohngren line extends between medial canthus to the angle of the mandible.
- Tumours below this line a better prognosis presenting earlier than tumours above the line, which have a tendency to invade the orbit and anterior cranial fossa.
- TNM classification for tumours arising from the maxillary and ethmoid sinus is shown in Box 21.4.

Treatment

Any treatment decisions should be made in the context of a multidiscipli-nary team clinic, involving surgeons, oncologist, prosthodontist, ophthal-mologist, and professionals allied to medicine. About half of all patients will be incurable. Surgery may still have a palliative role in these patients. Nodal disease is a very poor prognostic sign.

- Treatment of basal and squamous cell carcinomas of the nasal vestibule and columella is the same as other skin cancers although rich lymphatic drainage bilaterally may lead to neck metastases early. There appears to be little difference in survival in patients treated by primary surgery, primary radiotherapy, or combined modality treatment. Surgical exci-sion often leaves a complex defect, needing local flap reconstruction. Occasionally if there is a large cutaneous malignancy, the only solution is total rhinectomy, osseointegrated implants, and prosthesis post-operatively.
- Nasal lymphomas are usually treated with radiotherapy with/without chemotherapy.
- Malignant melanomas are characteristically unpredictable and are best treated with wide local excision, possibly with a neck dissection, if node-positive. The role of sentinel node dissection is currently being evaluated.

Surgical treatment of paranasal sinus malignancies may also require an orbital exenteration, if there is invasion of the orbit and orbital perio-steum has been breached. If the tumour has invaded the pterygoids, it is difficult to completely clear the disease, as there is no surgical plane of dissection here. Tumour removal in this case is often piecemeal.

Surgery of paranasal sinus malignancies
Medial maxillectomy
This is performed for low-grade malignancies confined to the lateral nasal cavity and medial antral wall. The ethmoid sinuses can also be cleared, preserving the fovea and skull base. Medial maxillectomy can be carried out via a lateral rhinotomy incision or a mid-facial degloving procedure.

Box 21.4 TNM staging of sinonasal malignancy

Maxillary sinus
T1—Tumour limited to antral mucosa.
T2—Tumour causing erosion or destruction into hard plate/lateral nasal wall.
T3—Tumour eroding posterior wall/subcutaneous/cheek/medial orbit.
T4—Intracranial extension/orbital apex/skin of nose.

Ethmoid sinus
T1—confined to ethmoid.
T2—Extends to nasal cavity.
T3—Extends to anterior orbit/maxillary sinus.
T4—Intracranial extension.

Total maxillectomy

If the tumour affects more than the medial wall of the antrum, then a more extensive maxillectomy is indicated. If the floor of the antrum and hard palate is involved, then an inferior maxillectomy is performed, preserving the orbital floor. However, a tumour involving most of the antrum requires a total maxillectomy, with/without an orbital exenteration. Occasionally, if cheek skin is involved, this has to be resected and the cutaneous defect is reconstructed with a free flap.

Craniofacial resection with a neurosurgeon

If the tumour has involved the fronto-ethmoidal complex extensively, with destruction of the cribriform plate and dura, then a craniofacial resection, possibly combined with a maxillectomy and orbital exenteration, may be indicated.

Radiotherapy for paranasal sinus malignancies

Given pre- or more commonly post-operatively for advanced disease, especially if microscopic clearance has not been achieved. The whole of the maxilla area, ethmoid sinus, nasal cavity, pterygopalatine fossa, and often the orbit are included in the field. If there is nodal disease, the ipsilateral neck is also irradiated. Radiotherapy is usually given after wound healing has taken place at about 6–8 weeks post-operatively, and approximately 60 Gray is fractionated over 6 weeks.

Chemotherapy for paranasal sinus malignancies

Usually reserved for patients with disseminated lymphoma or for sarcomas, where it is given with radiotherapy.

In some centres, topical 5-FU has been used post-operatively following radiotherapy in the management of squamous cell and adenocarcinomas. The cavity is decrusted and packed with 5-FU cream on ribbon gauze weekly for up to several months. Good results are claimed especially for adenocarcinomas.

Palliation

Considered if frontal lobes involved extensively or if both optic nerves, nasopharynx, posterior wall of the sphenoid, ICA or cavernous sinus involved. Other reasons to consider palliation include: distant metastasis, poor surgical risk, and a patient with undifferentiated carcinoma.

Lateral rhinotomy with medial maxillectomy

Definitions

- Lateral rhinotomy is the external skin incision, also called Moure's incision, starting superiorly midway between the medial canthus and dorsum, lateral border of the nose in the nasomaxillary groove and curving medially in the alar groove to the midline.
- Medial maxillectomy is the removal *en bloc* of the lateral nasal wall, including the middle and inferior turbinate, ethmoid labyrinth, and the medial wall of the maxilla (Fig. 21.10a).

Indications

- Resection of a tumour confined to the lateral nasal wall and ethmoid sinuses, e.g. inverting papillomas, small ethmoidal tumours, mucosal malignant melanomas.
- Access to the anterior septum, e.g. to repair septal perforation, or to the posterior nasal cavity, e.g. juvenile angiofibromas.
- As a palliative procedure to allow debulking of large tumours prior to chemo/radiotherapy.

Pre-operative management

- CT/MRI scan of the paranasal sinuses, orbits and anterior cranial fossa will identify those patients whose disease has spread from the nasal cavity and ethmoid sinuses and who are unsuitable for this procedure. MRI is preferred for adenoid cystic tumours to detect perineural, skull base and intracranial spread.
- Biopsy of the lesion. Aggressive malignancies are unsuitable for this procedure.
- Exclude distant metastases with CXR, CT scan.

Surgical technique

Preparation

- The procedure is usually performed with a hypotensive general anaesthesia with an endotracheal tube and throat pack.
- The patient is placed supine on a head ring in the reverse Trendelenburg position.
- The nasal cavity mucosa is vasoconstricted with Moffatt's solution (1ml of 1 : 1000 adrenaline, 2ml of 10% cocaine and 2ml of 8.4% sodium bicarbonate) either sprayed in the nasal cavity or applied on pledgets.
- The incision line is marked and then infiltrated with xylocaine 2% with 1 : 80000 adrenaline.
- The skin is cleaned with aqueous chlorhexidine, head draped, and a temporary tarsorrhaphy performed.
- Prophylactic broad-spectrum antibiotics, e.g. IV Augmentin® 1.2g are given.

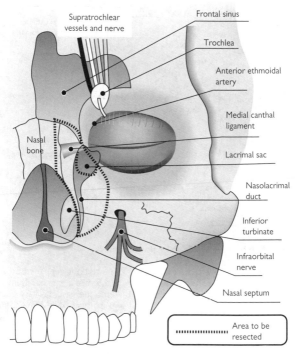

Fig. 21.10 a Medial maxillectomy: relevant anatomy.

Tip: Study a dry skull immediately pre-operatively to familiarize yourself with the bony anatomy and position of the osteotomies.

Incision (Fig. 21.10b)

The incision is marked and cross-hatches placed to aid accurate stitch placement during closure. The incision line starts from midway between the medial canthus and the bony nasal dorsum and runs inferiorly along the nasomaxillary groove, and curves medially in the nasal alar groove to enter the nostril. The upper part of the incision can be extended laterally just beneath the medial eyebrow (for ethmoid clearance) or superiorly onto the forehead (for frontal sinus clearance). The lower part of the incision can be extended vertically to split the lip along one side of the

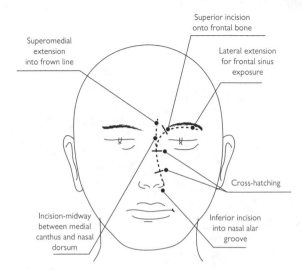

Superior incision
onto frontal bone

Superomedial
extension
into frown line

Lateral extension
for frontal sinus
exposure

Cross-hatching

Incision-midway
between medial
canthus and nasal
dorsum

Inferior incision
into nasal alar
groove

Fig. 21.10 b Medial maxillectomy: skin incisions.

philtrum (to remove the hard palate). The incision is deepened down to bone through the periosteum. Superiorly the medial canthal ligament is avoided as the incision is medial to it. Along the nasomaxillary groove, the angular vein may be encountered and is usually diathermied. Inferiorly, the incision enters the nasal cavity and is deepened to the pyriform aperture.

Elevation of periosteum (Fig. 21.10c)
- The periosteum over the nasal bones and ascending process of the maxilla is elevated laterally with a Freer's elevator. Adrenaline-soaked pledgets, copper malleable retractor, and Belluci sucker are helpful in the dissection.
- Superiorly, the trochlea is encountered and is carefully prised out of its bony fossa.
- In the medial orbital area, the lacrimal sac is elevated out of its bony fossa. The duct leaves inferiorly from the sac to enter its bony canal. The bone overlying the duct is nibbled with a Hajek's punch and the duct is transacted as low as possible.
- The periorbita is elevated further to expose first the anterior and then the posterior ethmoidal arteries. These arteries mark the level of the skull base and the osteotomies must be below this level. The arteries are clipped or cauterized and then divided.
- Inferiorly, in the nasomaxillary area, the border of the pyriform apertures is encountered. The periosteum is elevated laterally as far as the infra-orbital nerve to expose the anterior face of the maxilla.
- The nasal mucosa is elevated medially off the pyriform aperture.

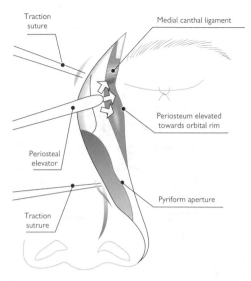

Fig. 21.10 c Medial maxillectomy: elevation of periosteum.

Osteotomies (Fig. 21.10d)

- Osteotomies are performed with a fissure burr or oscillating saw with irrigation.
- A medial vertical osteotomy is made along the nasal bone to the level of the ethmoidal arteries.
- A superior-lateral horizontal osteotomy is made along the level of the skull base or below.
- An inferior-lateral horizontal osteotomy is made just below the inferior turbinate to the anterior face of the maxilla.
- An oblique osteotomy is made from the level of the skull base and along the orbital floor.
- A lateral vertical osteotomy connects to the other osteotomies and is placed medial to the infra-orbital nerve.
- Heavy curved Mayo scissors are used to free the specimen from its remaining attachments, especially superiorly along the skull base and middle turbinate attachment, and inferiorly along the floor of the nose. The block of tissue is fractured medially, inferiorly, and anteriorly, and then removed. Bleeding is usually encountered from branches of the maxillary artery which are cauterised.
- Any further ethmoidal, frontal, or maxillary sinus tissue is removed under vision. Bone around the frontal recess is removed widely to prevent stenosis and subsequent mucocele formation.

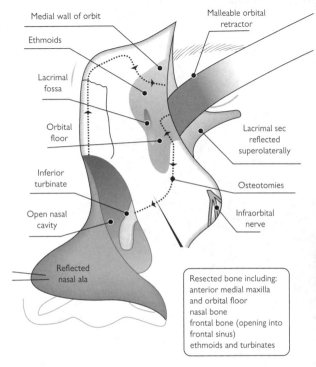

Medial wall of orbit

Ethmoids

Lacrimal fossa

Orbital floor

Inferior turbinate

Open nasal cavity

Reflected nasal ala

Malleable orbital retractor

Lacrimal sec reflected superolaterally

Osteotomies

Infraorbital nerve

Resected bone including:
anterior medial maxilla
and orbital floor
nasal bone
frontal bone (opening into
frontal sinus)
ethmoids and turbinates

Fig. 21.10 d Medial maxollectomy: osteotomies.

Closure (Fig. 21.10e)
- The lacrimal duct is spatulated and stitched to the surrounding tissues to prevent stenosis. Alternatively, the duct can be stented for 6 weeks with O'Donoghue silastic stents by cannulating the superior and inferior cannaliculus and tying a knot in the nasal cavity.
- The trochlea is re-attached to its bony fossa to reduce post-operative diplopia.
- If the medial canthal ligament has been divided, it is resutured to the periosteum.
- If the orbital periosteum has been damaged, it should be sutured.
- The maxillectomy cavity is packed with a Whitehead varnish pack.
- The incision is closed accurately in two layers with the aid of the previously made cross hatches. Great care must be taken, especially around the medial canthus, to prevent webbing and around the alar rim to prevent stenosis. The tarsorrhaphy suture is removed.

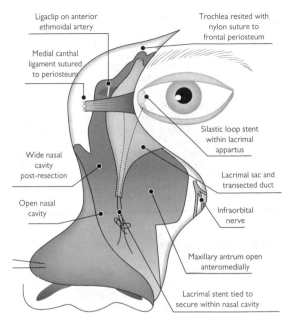

Fig. 21.10 e Medial maxillectomy: closure.

Post-operative management

The patient is nursed in a head-up position to reduce post-operative oedema. The nasal pack is removed under GA after 7–10 days and the cavity cleaned. The lacrimal stents can be removed in the clinic after 6–8 weeks by dividing the silastic loop at the inner canthus and withdrawing the knot endoscopically via the nasal cavity.

Complications

- Epistaxis from the ethmoidal arteries or sphenopalatine artery.
- CSF rhinorrhoea due to superior horizontal osteotomy being placed too high.
- Optic nerve damage due to osteotomies being carried too far posteriorly.
- Diplopia due to malalignment of the medial canthal ligament and trochlea.
- Epiphora due to nasolacrimal duct stenosis.
- Facial paraesthesia due to excessive retraction of the infra-orbital nerve.
- Frontal sinus mucocele.
- Cavity infection due to excessive crusting.
- Cosmetic problems related to incision.

Total maxillectomy

Indications

To remove malignancies involving the maxillary sinus. It is often combined with orbital exenteration, ethmoidectomy, and/or resection of skin, depending on the extent of disease. If there is destruction of the cribriform plate, then it is combined with a craniofacial resection (see 📖 p. 632).

Pre-operative management

- The tumour should be adequately staged clinically, and up to date CT ± MRI scans should be available delineating the exact extent of the lesion and the appropriateness of radical surgery.
- Generally, neck metastases are an extremely bad prognostic sign.
- The patient should be consented for orbital exenteration as often the orbital periosteum is involved either macroscopically or on frozen section.
- If the hard palate is mainly involved, then the patient should be seen pre-operatively by a prosthetic orthodontist, so that a dental plate can be made and fitted at time of surgery.
- Depending on the method of reconstruction, the thigh or abdomen should be prepared for donor graft material (split skin graft, lateral thigh flap or rectus flap).

Surgical technique

Preparation (see also 📖 p. 620)

- The procedure is usually performed with a hypotensive general anaesthesia with an nasotracheal tube inserted into the opposite nostril.
- If hard-palate resection is required, a temporary tracheostomy is preferred.
- The patient is placed supine on a head ring in the reverse Trendelenburg position.
- The nasal cavity mucosa is vasoconstricted with Moffatt's solution (1ml of 1 : 1000 adrenaline, 2ml of 10% cocaine and 2 ml of 8.4% sodium bicarbonate) either sprayed in the nasal cavity or applied on pledgets.
- The incision line is marked and then infiltrated with xylocaine 2% with 1 : 80 000 adrenaline. The skin is cleaned with aqueous chlorhexidine, head draped, and a temporary tarsorrhaphy performed. The neck may also need to be prepared if a free flap is planned.
- Prophylactic broad-spectrum antibiotics, e.g. IV Augmentin® 1.2g are given.

Incisions

- For maxillectomy without orbital exenteration, the Weber–Fergusson incision is used (Fig. 21.11a).
- Skin incision: this starts 1cm lateral to the outer canthus and skirts 3mm below the lower eyelid to the medial canthus. Here, the incision turns inferiorly along the nasomaxillary groove and then curves medially in the nasal alar groove. The skin incision ends by vertically splitting the upper lip from the columella to the central incisors. Cross-hatching the incision line will aid later closure.

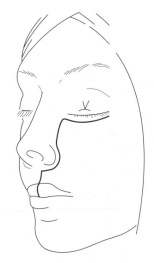

Fig. 21.11 a Total maxillectomy: skin incision.

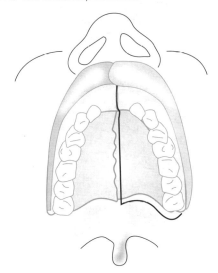

Fig. 21.11 b Total maxillectomy: intra-oral incision.

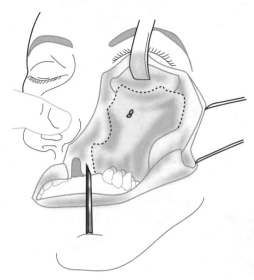

Fig. 21.11 c Total maxillectomy: anterior osteotomies.

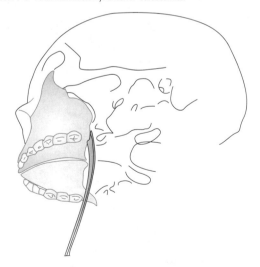

Fig. 21.11 d Total maxillectomy: final posterior osteotomy between maxillary tuberosity and pterygoid plates.

- Intra-oral incision (Fig. 21.11b): the midline lip-splitting incision is extended along the alveolar buccal sulcus and around the maxillary tuberosity, then across the palate at the junction of the soft and hard palate. The palatine arteries are coagulated. Finally, a midline incision, 3mm on the side of the resection, connects the cuts from the incisors and the palate-splitting incision.
- If orbital exenteration is planned, a superior supraconjunctival incision is also made 3mm above the free edge of the upper eyelid, so that the skin of both eyelids is preserved to facilitate fitting of an ocular prosthesis.

Procedure

Elevation of facial skin

- With the aid of skin hooks, the soft tissue over the maxilla is elevated, leaving the orbicularis oculi on the globe if the eye is to be preserved, but otherwise exposing the anterior maxillary bone and the zygomatic arch.
- The masseteric attachment is cleared of the zygoma. The infra-orbital nerve and vessels are ligated. The periosteum is incised over the inferior orbital rim and the tissue in raised of the orbital floor as far as the inferior orbital fissure.
- Medially in the orbit, the lacrimal sac is elevated from its fossa and its duct is transected low as possible. The anterior and posterior ethmoidal arteries are identified and coagulated.
- If the tumour is adherent to orbital periosteum, frozen sections are sent and, if necessary, orbital clearance performed.
- As the globe is removed, the branches of the ophthalmic artery in the optic canal and superior orbital fissure are clamped using a curved clip and then transfixed *en masse*.

Osteotomies (Fig. 21.11c and d)

- The zygoma is divided with an oscillating saw or fissure burr and the cut is extended medially to the inferior orbital fissure and then across the orbital floor.
- Next, the pyriform aperture is cleared at the level of the middle turbinate and a vertical, then horizontal, osteotomy is made, staying below the ethmoidal arteries and ∴ skull base, and this cut is joined with that of the orbital floor.
- The hard palate is divided initially from the anterior nasal spine to the incisors, then intra-orally just lateral to the midline (to avoid the lower nasal septum) from anterior to posterior.
- The final bony cut involves inserting a curved osteotome in a groove between the maxillary tuberosity and the pterygoid plates.

Removal of the maxilla

- The maxilla is now only held in place by nasal mucosa at the posterior end of the middle turbinate, and muscle fibres in the pterygopalatine area, which is divided by turbinectomy or heavy Mayo scissors.
- The branches of the maxillary artery are coagulated or tied. Any bleeding from the pterygoid plexus of veins is coagulated and controlled by surgicel.
- The ethmoids can also now be completely exenterated.

Closure (Fig. 21.11e)
- Prior to skin closure, the inner raw surface of the cheek flap may be lined with a split-skin graft to reduce contracture, although this is not always necessary.
- The facial incision is closed in two layers with vicryl to the subcutaneous tissues and 6/0 prolene to skin.
- The cavity is packed lightly with Whitehead's Varnish pack.
- The palatal prosthesis is fitted to close off the maxillectomy cavity from the oral cavity, to allow post-operative feeding to commence early and to maintain the facial contour.
- If the eye has been excised, the eyelashes are removed, as are the tarsal plates, and the eyelids sutured together. The orbital socket is packed.
- If there has been significant skin loss, a free flap reconstruction may be required. If the eye has been preserved, the orbital floor can be reconstructed with iliac crest bone.

Post-operative management
- The patient is nursed in a head-up position to reduce post-operative oedema.
- Nasogastric feed are commenced the following day and oral fluids slowly start on day 2.
- Sutures are removed on day 5–7.
- The nasal and orbital pack is removed under GA after 10–14 days.

Complications
- Bleeding from the branches of the maxillary artery or pterygoid plexus.
- Ectropion, if subconjunctival incision is placed too close to the eyelashes.
- Lid lymphoedema, if subconjunctival incision is placed too inferiorly.
- Necrosis of facial skin, particularly by the medial canthus, if the skin incision turns too sharply into the nasomaxillary groove.
- Facial depression due to an ill fitting prosthesis.
- Diplopia due to lack of support for the globe.

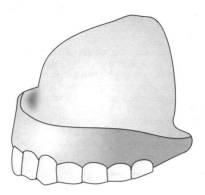

Fig. 21.11 e Total maxillectomy: closure with palatal prosthesis.

Craniofacial resection

Indications

- To resect tumours involving the ethmoid cribriform plate and/or posterior table of the frontal sinus (Fig. 21.12a), e.g. esthesioneuroblastoma, carcinomas, inverting papillomas, olfactory groove meningiomas.
- It is a combined neurosurgical procedure with the neurosurgeon dissecting disease in the anterior cranial fossa and closing the resultant dural defect.
- Craniofacial procedures may be performed as a transfacial approach with vertical forehead incision, as described below, or alternatively with a combined bicoronal, transfacial approach avoiding the forehead incision.

Pre-operative management

- All the points outlined previously for medial and total maxillectomy should be considered, in particular the importance of adequately staging the disease clinically, and with both CT and MRI scan of paranasal sinuses and anterior cranial fossa.
- Involvement of the ICA, optic chiasma, and posterior sphenoidal wall negates surgery.
- Consent should be obtained for orbital exenteration, if necessary, and the patient should be seen by a prosthedontist, especially if a maxillectomy is also going to be performed.

Surgical technique

Preparation

- The procedure is usually performed with a hypotensive general anaesthesia, with an endotracheal tube and throat pack.
- The patient is placed supine on a head ring in the reverse Trendelenburg position.
- When the frontal craniotomy is performed, the table should be levelled out to prevent air embolism.
- The nose, skin, and incision line are prepared as for total maxillectomy. Bilateral tarsorrhaphy is performed.
- Anti-epileptics, antibiotics, and steroids are routinely administered because a craniotomy is performed to allow retraction of the frontal lobe.
- The thigh is shaved and prepared for harvesting of fascia lata graft to repair the dural defect.

Incision (Fig. 21.12b)

A lateral rhinotomy incision is made (see p. 621) and continued onto the forehead with a vertical extension either in the midline or in a paramedian forehead crease.

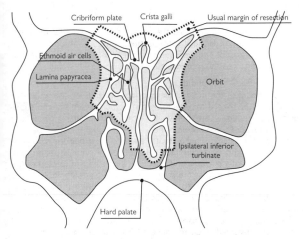

Fig. 21.12 a Craniofacial resection: relevant anatomy.

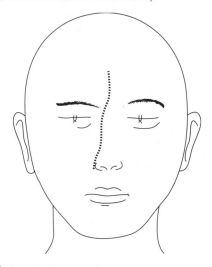

Fig. 21.12 b Craniofacial resection: skin incision.

Procedure

Soft-tissue dissection (Fig. 21.12c)

The soft tissues of the facial bones are dissected, as with medial maxillectomy. The nasal bones, lacrimal fossa, lamina papyracea, anterior face of the maxilla are exposed. The periosteum of the frontal bones is preserved and cleaned laterally to the supraorbital vessels.

Bony dissection (Fig. 21.12c and d)

Specific positioning of the inferior osteotomies depends on the extent of tumour. A total or medial maxillectomy can be performed but the superiomedial cuts generally are below the ethmoidal foramina to ensure complete removal of the ethmoid bone.

A 3cm by 2.5cm shield-shaped frontal craniotomy is performed. Inferiorly, the anterior and posterior table of the frontal sinus is penetrated. The bone flap is gently elevated and the underlying dura is dissected of the flap. Care is taken not to tear the sagittal sinus. The posterior table of the frontal sinus is nibbled down to the level of the cribriform plate. Dural elevation is then continued by sharp dissection along the cribriform plate posteriorly to the sphenoid and laterally over the orbital plates. If the dura is involved with tumour, a margin of normal dura is resected. If frontal lobe is directly involved, then the affected brain tissue can be resected. The ethmoidal vessels are clipped or coagulated.

The cranial osteotomies are outlined with a rosehead burr to encompass both ethmoids and the anterior wall of the sphenoid sinus. A fissure burr completes the anterior osteotomy through floor of the frontal sinus.

Removal of tumour bloc

The bony specimen is now mobile and is gently delivered into the face and removed. Any soft tissue attachments are freed with Mayo scissors. Care is taken not to damage the internal carotid arteries and optic nerves in the sphenoid sinus. Complete ethmoidal excision is ensured and frozen sections may be sent to confirm microscopic clearance.

Closure

- Any dural and orbital defects are repaired with fascia lata graft held in place with fibrin glue and sutures.
- All exposed soft tissue in the maxillectomy and orbital cavity are lined by split-skin graft to prevent contracture.
- The maxillectomy cavity is packed with Whitehead varnish pack.
- The bone from the frontal craniotomy is replaced and held in place with steel wire or plates.
- The frontal periosteum is closed and the skin is then closed in two layers. A firm forehead bandage is applied.

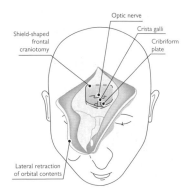

Fig. 21.12 c Craniofacial resection: soft tissue and bony dissection.

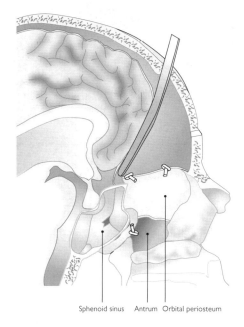

Fig. 21.12 d Craniofacial resection: retraction of frontal lobe to exposure cribriform plate (clips on ethmoidal and sphenopalatine arteries).

Post-operative management
- The patient is nursed flat for 5days and then gradually allowed to sit up.
- Full HDU and neurological monitoring is required.
- Oral feeding can be commenced on the day of surgery.
- Sutures are removed after 5–7 days and nasal packing is removed on day 10–14 under a short GA.

Complications
- CSF leak.
- Meningitis.
- Haemorrhage.
- Cerebrovascular accident.

Facial plastics

Principles of facial plastic surgery

The role of facioplastic surgery in ENT can be divided into:
- Aesthetic surgery to the face, eyelids, nose, and ears (rhytidectomy, blepharoplasty, rhinoplasty, and pinnaplasty).
- The repair of cutaneous defects following excision of facial lesions, e.g. BCC, SCC, melanomas.

Ladder of reconstruction (Fig. 22.1a)

A basic principle of wound closure is to use the simplest, most reliable method to cover a cutaneous defect. This is at the bottom of the reconstructive ladder. However, healing by secondary intention can take a long time and is somewhat unpredictable and ∴ where the defect is small and there is enough lax tissue, direct closure is preferred. The higher one climbs up the ladder, the more complex the surgery.

Relaxed skin tension lines (Fig. 22.1b)

These are essentially skin wrinkles and are lines of election for the placement of surgical incisions. They run perpendicular to the underlying facial muscles and the contractions of these muscles are responsible for the creasing of the skin. Relaxed skin tension-lines are not quite the same as Langer's lines, which are produced by rigor mortis and have a slightly different pattern on the face. Elsewhere Langer's lines correspond fairly well to relaxed skin-tension lines.

Facial cosmetic units (Fig. 22.1c and d)

The skin colour, thickness, and texture vary in each facial unit. It is generally accepted that if more than 50% of a facial unit is excised during removal of a skin lesion, a better camouflage is achieved if the whole unit is removed and replaced, if possible, with a neighbouring unit.

Grafts vs flaps

- Grafts are essentially dead tissue that relies on the recipient site for its survival. Angiogenesis occurs into the free graft over 10–14 days.
- Flaps bring their own blood supply to the recipient site from the donor site, and tend to be more robust. Pre-operative planning and drawing are essential. Flaps are preferred over grafts, if exposed cartilage or bone need to be covered.

(a)

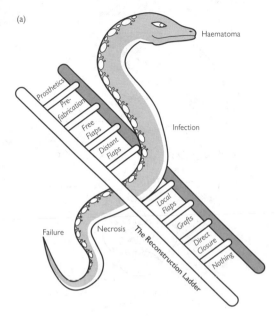

Haematoma

Infection

Prosthetics

Pre-fabrication

Free Flaps

Distant Flaps

Local Flaps

Grafts

Direct Closure

Nothing

The Reconstruction Ladder

Failure Necrosis

Fig. 22.1 a Ladder of reconstruction.

(b)

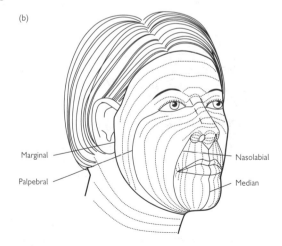

Marginal

Palpebral

Nasolabial

Median

Fig. 22.1 b Relaxed skin tension lines.

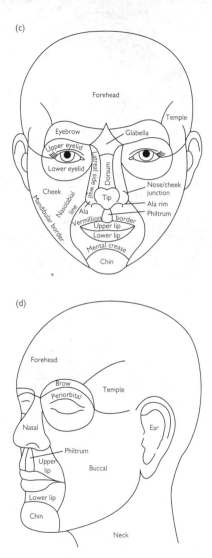

Fig. 22.1 c and **d** Facial cosmetic units.

Blood supply to the skin

A detailed knowledge of the musculocutaneous blood circulation is important for the planning and survival of skin flaps.

- Segmental blood vessels run below the muscle mass and keep myocutaneous flaps viable (e.g. acromiothoracic artery and pectoralis major flap) (Fig. 22.1e).
- Musculocutaneous perforators supply a skin angiosome.
- Direct cutaneous arteries run on top of a muscle and keep axial flaps viable (e.g. facial artery and nasolabial flap) (Fig. 22.1f).
- Anastomosis in the dermal-subdermal plexus keeps random pattern flaps alive (Fig. 22.1e). The length : width ratio for a random flap is usually 1.5 : 1 but on occasions in the head and neck can be extended up to 3 : 1, especially if the flap is 'delayed'.
- The tip of an axial flap usually has a random pattern of blood supply.

(e)

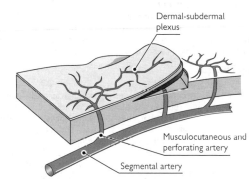

(f)

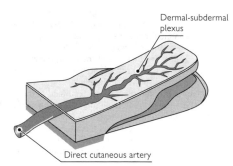

Fig. 22.1 e Axial pattern flap and random pattern flap.

Pinnaplasty/otoplasty

Indications

Protrusion of the external ear causing parents or child significant concern. The ideal time for surgical correction is the year before starting school (usually age 4 or 5) in order to prevent teasing by peers. After the age of 6, the child develops body-image awareness.

There are two techniques for pinnaplasty:

- Cartilage-splitting, which involves breaking the tension in the cartilage by scoring the lateral surface (Senstrom and Converse). This is discussed below.
- Cartilage-sparing, utilizing permanent sutures to fold create the antihelical fold (Mustarde). This works well in the young child with soft, pliable cartilage but there is a higher risk of infection.

Pre-operative management

The patient is assessed with the parents. Realistic expectations of surgery should be discussed. When the pinna is examined, the under development of an antihelical fold or presence of large, deep conchal bowl is noted, as these are the most common causes of prominent ears deformity.

Surgical technique

Preparation

The operation is usually performed under a general anaesthesia delivered through an endotracheal tube. In the older child or adult, the procedure can be performed under local anaesthesia. The patient is placed supine, head-up, and slightly rotated to the opposite side. The pinna is prepared and draped. The pinna is folded back and the line of the new antihelical fold is tattooed with a needle laden with methylene blue. The amount of conchal-bowl reduction and posterior-skin excision is assessed. The incision line is infiltrated with xylocaine 2% with 1 : 80 000 adrenaline.

Procedure

- Skin excision (Fig. 22.2a): a dumb-bell ellipse of skin is excised from the medial aspect of the pinna. All soft tissue is excised leaving the peri-chondrium and methylene blue marks clearly visible. The skin and soft tissues are elevated towards the free edge of the helix.
- Cartilage incision (Fig. 22.2b): the cartilage of the pinna is incised approximately 5mm proximal to the rim of the pinna. Care is taken not to incise the skin on the lateral surface of the pinna.
- Lateral cartilage exposure: the skin on the lateral surface of the pinna is elevated in a subperichondral plane until all the tattooed marks of the new antihelix have been passed by approximately 5mm.
- Lateral cartilage scoring: using a no.15 blade, the lateral cartilage is repeatedly scored parallel to the new antihelical fold. A full-thickness incision may be required just above the earlobe to produce a sharper edge to the concha near the antitragus.
- Conchal-bowl reduction: once the pinna is folded back following scoring, the conchal depth will be reduced. If further reduction is required, a strip of cartilage can be excised from edge of the incised cartilage.

(a)

(b)

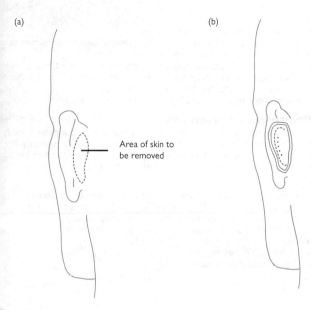

Area of skin to be removed

Fig. 22.2 a and **b** Pinnaplasty: skin and cartilage incisions.

Closure
- The skin is redraped over the cartilage.
- Immaculate haemostasis is important to prevent haematoma formation.
- The skin incision is closed with a subcuticular suture.
- Proflavine wool is used to pack the conchal bowl, scaphoid, and triangular fossae, and more proflavine wool and gauze is placed in the post-auricular sulcus and laterally over the pinna.
- A firm crepe bandage is applied and secured with elastoplast.

Post-operative management

The procedure can be done as a day-case but the patient/parents must be advised to return to the ward if there is uncontrollable pain or if the bandage slips. The head bandage is removed on day 10–14 and an elastic headband can be worn at night for a further month.

Complications
- Subperichondrial haematoma. This should be suspected if there is excessive uncontrollable pain in the first week. The head bandage should be removed and the haematoma drained urgently.
- Skin necrosis due to excessive pressure or ineffective packing.
- Infection and chondritis.
- Asymmetry of pinnae.
- Hypertrophic/keloid scar.

Rhinoplasty

Indications

- Cosmetic: patients who are unhappy about the appearance of their nose, e.g. to correct a dorsal hump, dorsal saddle, too wide or too narrow dorsum, under- or over-projected nasal tip.
- Functional: to improve nasal obstruction or snoring. If the nasal pyramid is deviated as well as the nasal septum, better realignment of the septum will be achieved if a septoplasty is combined with a rhinoplasty.

A rhinoplasty can be performed via a closed or open approach.

Closed

Hump reduction, medial osteotomies, and limited-tip work is performed internally without any external skin incisions. Lateral osteotomies can be performed internally or via tiny percutaneous incisions. Because of limited dissection, there tends to be less scarring and a more predictable result using the closed method. However, it is difficult to master.

Open

With a stepped transcolumellar incision and bilateral rim incisions. The dorsal skin is elevated to expose the alar cartilages and nasal bones. It provides great exposure for tip work and difficult cases, and is ideal if complex grafts need to be accurately secured.

Pre-operative management

A thorough pre-operative consultation is important before any facial plastic surgery. The patient must have realistic expectations of surgery. Five steps of beauty have been described, with the most ugly nose at the bottom and the perfect nose on top. With a good result, one can hope to rise one, possibly two steps, but it will be impossible to create a beautiful nose from an extremely deformed nose.

If a patient displays any obsessive neurosis or seems very preoccupied with the most minor defect in their nose, a clinical psychology consult should be sought. The face should be assessed as a whole. Occasionally, the nose looks more prominent because of a receding chin. What the patient would then benefit from is a mentoplasty rather than a rhinoplasty. Similarly, the premaxilla can be under-developed and can be augmented.

If the patient has nasal obstruction or the cartilaginous dorsum is deviated, a septoplasty is combined with a rhinoplasty. Significant sinusitis may need to be addressed at the same time. Pre-operative photographs must be taken for medicolegal documentation.

A basic closed reduction rhinoplasty is described below.

Surgical technique

Preparation

- The patient is prepared as per septoplasty (see 📖 p. 548).
- The head drapes and endotracheal tubes are secured in the midline.
- The eyes are protected by steristrips.

- Further local anaesthetic infiltration is applied externally at the site of the percutaneous osteotomies, and internally at the lateral edge of the returning of the upper lateral cartilages, internal nasal valve area, and over the dorsum.
- Vestibular hairs are plucked with artery clips or trimmed with iris scissors whose tips have been smeared with Vaseline.

Incisions

Intercartilaginous incision (Fig. 22.3a)

A two-prong alar retractor is inserted under the alar rim and the ring finger of the same hand pushes the upper lateral down to clearly define the junction between the upper and lower lateral cartilages. A no.15 blade is used for the incision, which is deepened to reach a plane immediately lateral to the upper-lateral cartilages and the incision can be joined medially with a hemitransfixion or transfixion incision used for the initial septoplasty. Care must be taken not to transect the feet of the medial crura.

External percutaneous incisions (Fig. 22.3b)

Two stab incisions are made with a no.15 blade on each side of the external lateral osteotomies. The first horizontal stab is placed midway between the medial canthus and the dorsum. The second vertical stab is in the nasomaxillary groove midway between the medial canthus and pyriform aperture. Troublesome bleeding may be encountered from the angular vein, so the incisions should pierce skin only and not the deeper tissues.

Procedure

- Elevation of skin and SMAS of dorsum: a no.15 blade is inserted into the inter-cartilaginous incision, and the skin and SMAS layer is elevated gradually by pinching the overlying skin and rotating the knife onto the surface of the upper lateral cartilages, and then the surface of the nasal bones. Alternatively, curved, blunt-ended scissors can be used. Care must be taken not to dissect under the nasal bones in the keystone area. Also do not dissect too laterally to preserve soft tissue support for the nasal bones, which will be infractured later. The skin and SMAS sleeve is elevated through both inter-cartilaginous incisions and an Aufrecht retractor, and McIndoe scissors are used to complete the dissection. A Howarth elevator is used to scrap the procerus muscle and the periosteum of the nasal bones.
- Cartilaginous dorsum reduction: an Aufrecht retractor elevates the skin of the dorsum and then a no.11 blade is placed parallel to and hugging the nasal septum. The upper laterals are freed from the septum by cutting onto an Aufrecht retractor, which protects the skin of the dorsum. The upper lateral cartilages and nasal septum are then trimmed individually, with a no.11 blade or Foman scissors, to gradually lower the cartilaginous dorsum. Removal of small slivers of cartilage will have a dramatic effect on the nasal profile. Reduction of the cartilaginous dorsum will result in an obvious step deformity, which can be seen if the nose is viewed from the lateral profile.

- Bony dorsum reduction: a sharp, Robin T-shaped chisel is engaged at the lower end of the nasal bones. It is advanced steadily in a cephalic direction to the root of the nose with aid of a mallet. The direction of the chisel is constantly checked with each tap of the mallet. The bony fragment is grasped with heavy artery forceps and the fragment is further advanced into the nose before it is removed. Any remaining irregularities are excised or removed with a rasp.
- External lateral osteotomies (Fig. 22.3b): the superior osteotomy runs horizontally and anteriorly, and also slopes inferiorly to the nasomaxillary groove. Approximately three osteotomies can be made through the superior incision. The inferior osteotomy joins the superior osteotomy above and then runs in the nasomaxillary groove, curving slightly anteriorly before connecting with the pyriform aperture. Approximately four osteotomies can be made through the inferior incision. If possible, the osteotomies should not go all the way through the bone, to allow a 'green-stick' fracture of the bones. Also, the inferior fracture should be low on the face to avoid a step deformity.
- Internal medial osteotomies (Fig. 22.3c): a wide 10–13mm osteotome is used to create two vertical and slightly laterally curved medial osteotomies, which connect with the superior external lateral osteotomies. It is usually extremely easy to advance the osteotome cranially following removal of a large dorsal hump, but care should be taken not to go further than the intercanthal line, to avoid penetrating the skull base.
- The bones are then fractured into the required position. If the bones resist fracture, it is worth checking the osteotomies are complete and then using Walsham forceps.

Closure
- The inter-cartilaginous and any septal incision is accurately closed with vicryl.
- The nose is packed, if necessary.
- Half-inch steristrips are applied to the dorsum and tip of the nose until it is fully covered. This will reduce post-operative oedema.
- The dorsum is then covered with a plaster of Paris cast, which has been pre-cut to a shield shape. The cast is secured to the forehead and cheek area with Micropore tape. Friar's Balsam will help secure the tape on the skin.

Post-operative management
- The patient is nursed head-up 30 degrees to minimize facial oedema.
- The nasal packs are removed after 4–24h.
- The procedure can be performed as a day-case and the patient is seen 10–14 days later for removal of plaster cast.
- Peri-orbital swelling and blood-stained nasal discharge is normal for 2 weeks.
- Post-operative photos should be taken at 6–12 months.

(a)

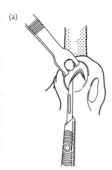

Fig. 22.3 a Intercartilaginous incision.

(b)

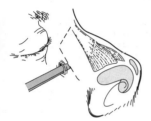

Fig. 22.3 b Lateral osteotomies.

(c)

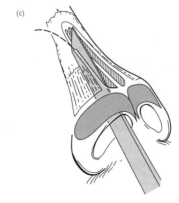

Fig. 22.3 c Medial osteotomies.

Complications

As per septoplasty (see 📖 p. 552). Additional complications are:

- Patient dissatisfaction with final result. The revision rate for rhinoplasty is 10–20% but it does vary for each surgeon, and depends on the nature of the initial problem, patient selection, and the patient's expectations. Further refinement should be delayed for 12 months to allow any scarring to mature and for the patient to get used to their 'new' nose.
- Polly-beak deformity because of inadequate reduction of the cartilaginous dorsum.
- Open-roof deformity because of failure to infracture nasal bones following dorsal hump removal.
- Pinching of nose because the nasal bones have fallen medially following infracturing.

Additional rhinoplasty techniques

- External approach (Fig. 22.3d): a step incision or w or inverted v is marked at the midpoint of the columella. This is continued laterally along the alar rim at the lower edge of the lower lateral cartilage. The area is infiltrated with xylocaine 2% with 1 : 80 000 adrenaline. A no.15 blade is used to make the incision, and the skin elevated off the medial and lateral crus of lower lateral cartilage, using blunt-ended tenotomy scissors. Two skin hooks and an alar retractor help open up the planes. The columellar branch of the superior labial artery may need to be cauterized. This approach provides superb exposure of upper and lower lateral cartilages. The nasal bones are further visualized by placing an Aufrecht retractor under the soft-tissue sleeve. Multiple fractures in the anterior septum can also be corrected with the external approach in an 'open' septoplasty. Following completion of the rhinoplasty, the rim incision is precisely closed with vicryl and the columella incision is closed with 6/0 prolene.
- Cephalic trimming of lower lateral cartilage to rotate tip upwards (Fig. 22.3e, f, g). In the closed approach, after the inter-cartilaginous incision has been made, the caudal end of the lower laterals is identified by palpation and a cartilage splitting incision is made preserving at least 5mm of caudal lower lateral cartilage. Sharp, pointed scissors elevates the skin and SMAS overlying the cephalic strip. A Freer elevator assists in 'bucket handling' the cephalic strip and the vestibular skin is freed from the cartilage. The cephalic strip is then resected and care is taken to remove symmetrical pieces from both sides. The cartilage splitting incision is closed with Vicryl.
- Intermediate osteotomies. If the nasal bones are very bulbous and convex, additional intermediate osteotomies may be required to vertically fracture the middle of the nasal bones, narrowing the nose. This can be performed through the external lateral osteotomy incisions or through a separate incision.

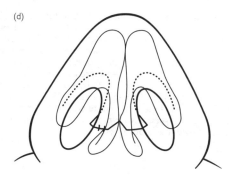

(d)

Fig. 22.3 d External rhinoplasty: skin incision.

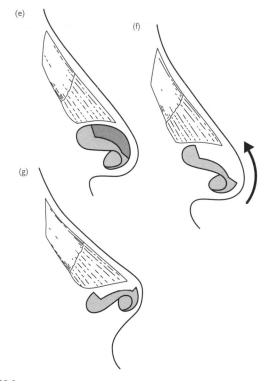

(e)

(f)

(g)

Fig. 22.3 e–g Cephalic trimming of lower lateral cartilages.

- Augmentation rhinoplasty. Undoubtedly the best tissue to augment the dorsal profile is autologous cartilage, e.g. septal, auricular, or even costal cartilage. Occasionally, this may not be practical, and synthetic implants, e.g. silicone, is used but they carry the risk of infection and extrusion. In the closed approach, the graft is placed in a precise pocket in the dorsal skin. In the open approach, it is accurately stitched in place with non absorbable Prolene under direct vision.
- Correction of the 'boxy' bifid tip: this is best performed via the open approach. The domes of the intermediate crus of the lower lateral cartilages are approximated to each other using several non absorbable prolene sutures (with the knots buried).

Local facial flaps: an overview

Local facial flaps are used to repair cutaneous defects following excision of skin lesions, e.g. BCC, or following trauma. During tumour surgery, it is imperative that the lesion is completely excised without any compromise. The resultant defect can then be closed with a variety of techniques using skin from a neighbouring area to reconstruct the defect. Most reconstructive flaps rely on a degree of elasticity in the skin and they are ∴ easier to perform in younger patients. Older patients, however, do have more lax skin, even though it may not stretch, and have easily visible RSTLs.

Types of flaps
- Local:
  - Random: receiving blood supply from dermal-subdermal plexus.
  - Axial: receiving blood supply from a named vessel lying on underling facial muscle.
- Regional.
- Free microvascular.

Local flaps
- Advancement, e.g. V-Y (Fig. 22.4a), cervico-facial.
- Pivot: around a pivot point to leave a defect that is closed primarily or grafted:
  - Rotation (using an arc of a circle) (Fig. 22.4b).
  - Transposition, e.g. Z plasty.
- Interpolated: pedicle of flap rests across a bridge of intervening tissue, e.g. forehead flap.
- Interposition: pedicle does not rests across intervening tissue, e.g. bilobed (Fig. 22.4d and e), rhomboid (actually a special type of transposition flap) (Fig. 22.4c).

Poor flap patients
- Advancing age.
- Peripheral vascular disease.
- Blood dyscrasias, e.g. aspirin, warfarin.
- Smokers.
- Diabetics.
- Previous surgery/radiotherapy.
- Untreated infection.

Fixed points
These are points that should not be displaced in the reconstruction, as it will leave severe functional or cosmetic problems:
- Eyebrows.
- Medial and lateral canthi.
- Alar rim.
- Hairline.

(a)

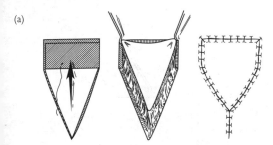

Fig. 22.4 a V–Y advancement flap.

(b)

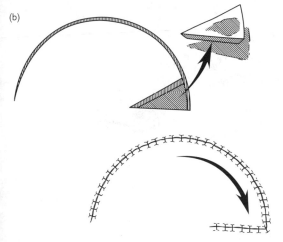

Fig. 22.4 b Rotation flap.

(c)

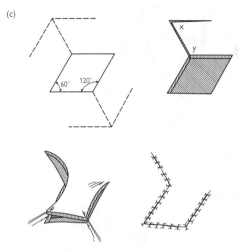

Fig. 22.4 c Rhomboid flap.

(d)

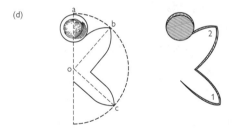

Fig. 22.4 d Bilobed flap (1)

(e)

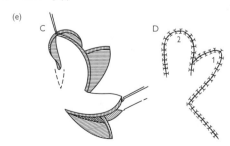

Fig. 22.4 e Bilobed flap (2)

Surgical technique

Preparation

- Patient is placed in reverse trendelenburg position with 30-degree head-up.
- The lines of excision are marked, ensuring complete tumour clearance. It is often helpful to also mark the reconstructive local flap, although this is usually easier to do once the lesion has been excised. If possible, plan the flap so the pedicle is inferiorly placed to reduce post-operative oedema.
- Most local-flap surgery is performed under local anaesthesia ± sedation. A dental syringe is used to slowly inject xylocaine 2% with 1 : 80 000 adrenaline. The surgeon should then wait 10min before commencing surgery.

Procedure

The skin should be incised perpendicular to underlying tissues. Try and camouflage all incisions by placing them parallel to RSTNs, at junctions of aesthetic units or in hair bearing areas. Skin hooks or fine toothed forceps should be used to handle the flap and tissue crushing should be avoided. The subcutaneous flap and dermis layer should be grasped and the epidermis should not be pinched. The plane of dissection for flap raising is at the level of the subcutaneous fat (onto of the facial muscles to avoid damage to the facial nerve branches). The thickness of the flap is tailored to the recipient site by trimming subcutaneous fat but the dermal–subdermal plexus must be left intact. Adequate undermining must be performed to release tension of the flap, but there is little benefit in undermining >2cm (except on the forehead and scalp). Meticulous haemostasis should be performed.

Closure

- Deep dermal sutures will reduce dead space and tension on the flap.
- Monofilament sutures, e.g. 5/0 or 6/0 Prolene should be used for skin closure.
- Drains are not usually required, except for large flaps, e.g. cervical advancement.
- Most of the time, dressings are not needed.

Post-operative care

- Sutures are removed early at 3–5 days and, if needed, the wound re-inforced with steristrips.
- Wound should be kept dry until it has healed.
- After suture removal, the wound is massaged with aqueous cream to reduce oedema.

Complications

- Nerve damage, e.g. branches of facial nerve, supratrochlear and supraorbital nerves.
- Haematoma and flap failure.
- Infection.
- Hypertrophic/Keloid scar.

Specific local facial flaps

Glabellar flap (Fig. 22.5a–c)

Axial flap used to reconstruct defects on upper nasal bridge and medial canthus. It can sometimes pull the medial end of the eyebrows inferiorly. Longer paramedian forehead flaps can be raised, based on supratrochlear artery, to reconstruct larger nasal defects and can reach all the way down to the nasal tip.

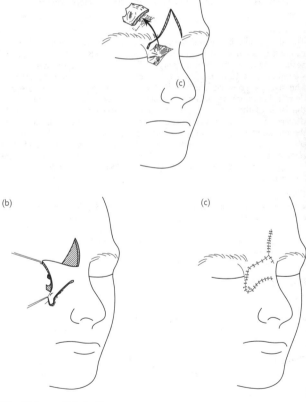

(a)

(b)

(c)

Fig. 22.5 a–c Glabellar flap.

Nasolabial flap (Fig. 22.5d–f)

Axial flap used to reconstruct defects on lower half of nose, lips, and cheek. It can be superiorly or inferiorly based, and is based on branches of the facial artery.

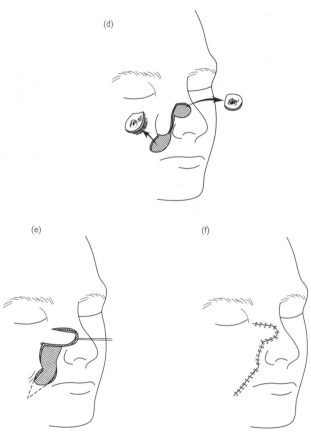

Fig. 22.5 d–f Nasolabial flap.

Romberg (limberg) flap (Fig. 22.5g–i)

An interposition flap used to reconstruct a rhomboid defects on flat areas of the cheek and temple. This is a flap with a pure geometric design closing the recipient defect with exactly the same area of tissue from a donor defect. Four flaps are available to close the recipient defect and choice depends on position of donor defect and RSTLs.

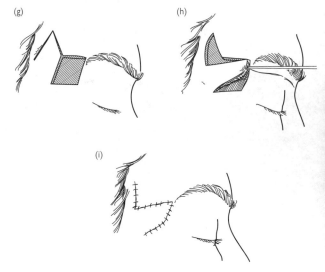

Fig. 22.5 g–i Romberg flap.

Bilobed Flap (Fig. 22.5j–l)

This interposition flap is useful for repairing defects in contoured areas, e.g. around the lower nose and cheek. A primary flap is used to repair the surgical defect and a smaller secondary flap fills the gap left by the primary flap. The secondary defect is closed primarily.

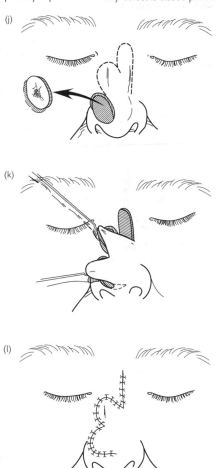

Fig. 22.5 j–l Bilobed flap.

Note flap

This flap allows closure of small circular defects up to 1.5cm in diameter. A neighbouring triangular flap closes the circular defect. The tip of the flap is trimmed.

Single or double-pedicled advancement flap (Fig. 22.5m)

Horizontal advancement flaps can be used to reconstruct defects on the forehead (if double-advancement flap, it is called an H-plasty). Single-pedicled vertical advancement flaps can be used to reconstruct defects on the dorsum of the nose (Rintala flap). Burrow's triangles may be needed to removed 'dog ears' at the base of the flap.

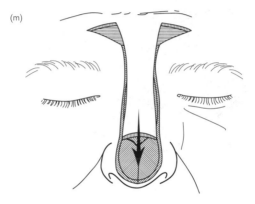

(m)

Fig. 22.5 m Single advancement flap.

Cheek rotation flap

Used to reconstruct a triangular defect on the medial area of the cheek near the alar-cheek function. Care is taken to plan the flap carefully to prevent lower-lid ectropion.

V-Y island advancement flap

Used to reconstruct defects on the cheek especially near the alar-facial area.

Z-plasty (Fig. 22.5n–p)

Used to change the direction of a scar, to make it more in line with an RSTL by rotating the contracting diagonal of the new scar by a right angle. It can also be used to interrupt scar linearity, making it less noticeable and to lengthen scar contractures, e.g. around the eye where a scar is causing ectropion.

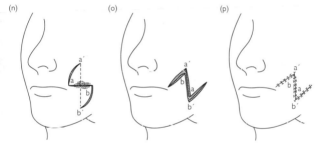

Fig. 22.5 n–p Z-plasty.

Paediatric otolaryngology

General considerations

Paediatric consultation

Setting
- Bright cheerful room with simple quiet toys.
- Large enough to accommodate child, both parents, siblings, buggies, and so on.
- Play area for waiting.
- Try to stick to clinic times and inform parents of delays so that they can plan feeding, toilet trips, and so on.
- Avoid across-the-desk consultation.
- Have a nurse to occupy patient or siblings.
- Keep only small proportion of instruments on view.

Optimize the consultation
- Always introduce yourself to the patient and the child.
- Listen carefully to the parents as they are the best witnesses.
- Allow older children to speak for themselves.
- A good deal of the examination can be performed by inspection and listening to breathing and voice.
- Allow younger patients to sit on parents lap.
- Let children touch the instruments and avoid sudden movements.
- If possible use cameras to allow parents and children to see the findings.
- If child is uncooperative, try reassuring them or rebook appointment.
- Only consider restraining when absolutely necessary and with parents full consent.
- It is important to know the procedures to be followed in the event of concerns about child protection issues, i.e. who to call. If concerned, it is our duty to act—at least call a paediatrician for advice.

Discussing the management
- Summarize the history and findings.
- Explain current knowledge-base for every proposed intervention.
- Give all the alternatives.
- Listen to the views of the parents and child.
- Beware of consent issues.

Children and consent

(See also 📖 p. 11).

Doctors who care for children need to be familiar with the law relating to parental responsibility and consent within the jurisdiction in which they practice.

Competency

Competence implies that a child has the capacity to comprehend and retain information material to a decision, and the ability to weigh this information in decision making.

At 16 years of age, children are deemed competent to give consent. Below 16 years, the consent is given by parents or guardian. There are certain circumstances where this may change:

- If a child <16 is thought to have sufficient understanding of what an intervention involves, they are deemed competent and can consent themselves. This is colloquially known as 'Gillick competence'.
- If a child 16–18 is not felt to be competent, a person with 'parental responsibility' may consent instead.

Key points in UK Law

Unless adopted a mother will always have parental responsibility for her child.

A father has parental responsibility if:
- He is married to the mother at the time of the child's birth.
- He has a parental-responsibility agreement, court order, or residence order.
- He is appointed as the child's guardian.

After 1 December 2003, a father named on the birth certificate has parental responsibility, regardless if he is married to the mother.

Others may acquire responsibility by
- Appointment as the child's guardian.
- Residence order.
- Adoption order.
- Some responsibilities can be transferred by the mother to another person (Section2(9) Children's act 1989).

The local authority can acquire it by
- Emergency court order.
- Care orders.

Further reading

www.doh.gov.uk (National Service Framework for children including issues such as consent).
Gallic vs Norfolk and Wisbech AHA (1985) 3 WLR 830, 3 All ER 402.
www.bristol-inquiry.org.uk (Set of recommendations for provision of health care services for children).
Department of Education and Skills. *Every Child Matters* (2003). www.dfes.gov.uk/everychildmatters.

Imaging in children

Imaging should only be performed if absolutely necessary for the present management of the patient. Unnecessary irradiation should be avoided.

It is difficult to get children to sit still in order to comply with imaging. Depending on their age, sedation or a general anaesthetic may be required. Babies up to 6 months should be imaged straight after feeding, as they usually sleep.

Pitfalls to be aware of in paediatric imaging
- Positioning is vital, a lateral C-spine X-ray in expiration can look like retropharyngeal swelling.
- CXR for FB has to be taken on inspiration and expiration.
- Do not image if airway-obstruction is suspected without securing airway first.
- Retropharyngeal nodes in a child are not usually pathological, unlike in an adult.
- Benign reactive lymphadenopathy in children can be impressive reaching >2cm. This size in adults is almost always neoplastic.

Feeding disorders

Dysphagia may be divided into three categories:
- Structural abnormalities.
- Neurological abnormalities.
- Behavioral abnormalities.

Or a combination of all three.

History
- Is type of feeding appropriate for age?
- Duration of feed.
- During a feed is there evidence of:
  - Gagging.
  - Coughing.
  - Apnoea.
  - Cyanosis.
- Delayed feeding or periods of cessation due to illness?
- Respiratory disorders.
- Poor speech.
- General delayed development.

Examination
- Look for integrity of the lip and palate.
- Craniofacial abnormalities, such as macroglossia and retrognathia.
- Absence of gag reflex may suggest neurological problems.
- Flexible laryngoscopy—look for any structural abnormalities, pooling retained secretions.
- Observation of a feeding session.

Investigation
- Barium swallow looking for fistulae, vascular rings, and general coordination of the movement of the bolus.
- Video swallow.
- Fibreoptic endoscopic evaluation of swallowing.
- Endoscopy.
- Manometer.

Management
- Correction of structural abnormality.
- Speech therapy targeting methods to prevent aspiration.
- Behavioural therapy.
- Prosthetics to aid pharyngeal feeding, e.g. in cleft palate.
- Consider alternative to oral feeding where:
  - Temporary measure during assessment or treatment.
  - Non-correctable structural and neurological abnormalities make it impossible.
  - Aspiration is too great to allow child to clear airway with cough and cilliary flow.
  - To supplement when oral feeding so slow that unpractical for child and carer's life.

Alternatives

- NG.
- Peg.
- Parenteral feeding.

Box 23.1 Structural causes of feeding disorders

- Cleft lip/palate.
- Macroglossia.
- Tracheo-oesophageal fistula.
- Oesophageal atresia/stricture.
- Vascular ring.
- Pierre Robin syndrome.

Willing et al. (1999).[1]

Box 23.2 Disorders affecting suck–swallow–breathe coordination

- Brainstem dysfunction.
- Choanal atresia.
- Laryngomalacia.
- Bronchopulmonary dysplasia.
- Cardiac disease.
- Tachypnoea.

Willing et al. (1999).[1]

Box 23.3 Neuromuscular causes of feeding disorders

- Cerebral palsy.
- Bulbar atresia.
- Familial dysautonomia.
- Bulbar atresia.
- Tardive dyskinesia.
- Muscular dystrophy.
- Oculopharyngeal dystrophy.
- Arnold-Chiari Malformation.

Willing et al. (1999).[1]

---

1 Willinging J P, Miller C K, Rudolph C D (1999). Feeding disorders in children. In: *Practical Pediatric Otolaryngology*, Chapter 37 □ pp. 606–7. Lippingcott-Raven, USA. 227, East Washington Square, , Philadelphia PA 19106–3780.

Paediatric gastro-oesophageal reflux disease (GORD)

Incompetence of the lower oesophageal sphincter in newborn infants is a common occurrence and reflux of a small amount of gastric fluid may be regarded as physiological. It is only when it becomes prolonged, associated with complications, that it becomes pathological or GORD.

Presentation

Older children may have the classic general and ENT symptoms seen in adults (see 📖 p. 208). Younger children can present with recurrent vomiting, night vomiting of mucus, and failure to thrive. GORD can also be associated with significant upper and lower respiratory problems. These can occur without the obvious gastroenterological symptoms, giving rise to the term 'silent reflux'.

Respiratory disorders thought to be associated with GORD include:
- Upper respiratory tract disorders:
  - Otitis media.
  - Sinusitis.
  - Laryngitis.
  - Laryngmalacia.
  - Stridor.
  - Recurrent croup.
  - Chronic cough.
  - Laryngotracheomalacia.
- Lower respiratory tract disorders:
  - Chronic bronchitis.
  - Recurrent pneumonia.
  - Asthma.
  - Bronchopulmonary dysplasia.

Upper or lower respiratory tract symptoms that are atypical in their course or in their response to standard therapy should arouse suspicion for silent GORD.

Investigations

Often if the history suggests GORD, a therapeutic trial of anti-reflux medication is commenced and the diagnosis is made retrospectively on improvement of symptoms.

The gold standard for the diagnosis is oesophageal pH monitoring for 18–24h, looking at the episodes when the pH level <4. Although this is considered the most accurate measurement of reflux available, it still has some limitations such as, it does not take into account alkaline reflux.

Other investigations include:
- Barium swallow looking for reflux and anatomical abnormalities, such as cleft larynx, tracheooesophageal fistulas, and gastric outlet obstruction.
- Oesophageal manometry looking at lower oesophageal sphincter pressures.

- Endoscopy looking for oesphagitis, arytenoid erythema, cobblestoning of trachea.
- Scintiscanning can look at GORD and identify delayed gastric emptying and aspiration of gastric contents.
- Bronchoalveolar lavage can identify lipid laden macrophages suggestive of aspiration.

Treatment

Conservative treatment

- Prone positioning.
- Multiple small feeds.
- Thicken feeds.
- In older children avoid citric juices.
- Antacids.
- Prokinetic agents, e.g. domperidone.
- H$_2$ antagonists.
- Proton-pump inhibitors.

Surgical treatment

- If possible, repair any congenital structural abnormality, e.g. laryngeal cleft.
- Fundoplication.

Drooling

All babies drool, especially when teething, this usually ceases by 18 months to 2 years of age.

Persistent chronic drooling is usually due to a failure of coordination of the muscles of the tongue, palate, and face that act in the first stage of swallowing. This is most commonly seen in neurologically impaired children, such as those with cerebral palsy. Drooling usually presents because of social problems—children may be shunned by their peers or teased. There is constant soiling of clothes that increases the laundry burden. Excoriation of the skin over the chin and upper chest can occur. Very rarely, excessive drooling can lead to dehydration or electrolyte disturbance.

Conservative treatment

The aim of the treatment is to improve swallowing or reduce the flow of saliva.

Speech therapy

Speech therapy is aimed at improving voluntary control of the oral phase of swallowing with exercises to improve jaw and lip closure, and enhance tongue and palatal movement. Improved head and neck posture can also help.

Anticholinergic drugs

Anticholinergic drugs, such as atropine and hyoscine, can be used to reduce saliva flow but have the unwanted side-effects of constipation, urinary retention, restlessness, or even xerostomia.

Radiotherapy

Radiotherapy has been used in the past but it is difficult to get the dosage right to avoid xerostomia and there is a potential longer term risk of dysplastic or neoplastic change within the salivary or thyroid glands.

Surgery

Conservative treatment to improve oromotor skills should be tried for at least 6 months before considering surgery. Avoid surgery in children under the age of 5–6 years as there is a natural tendency for drooling to improve.

Consider adenotonsillectomy if there is marked adenotonsillar hypertrophy increasing the drooling by causing a 'mouth-open' facies.

Salivary gland surgery aimed at redistribution of saliva.

Bilateral submandibular duct transposition

This is probably the most common operation used for drooling. Each submandibular duct is dissected out and rerouted through a submucosal tunnel to open posteriorly in the tonsillar fossa.

Some surgeons also remove the sublingual glands to reduce the risk of ranula formation but the deeper dissection can increase the risk of underling lingual nerve damage.

Salivary gland surgery aimed at reducing flow of saliva.
These include:
- Direct injection of botox into salivary glands.
- Submandibular gland excision.
- Parotid duct ligation.
- Dennervation procedures including tympanic neurectomy and chorda tympani nerve section.

Management of haemorrhage in children

The main haemorrhage that an ENT surgeon will encounter is secondary to tonsillar or adenoidal surgery.

A knowledge of the normal circulatory blood volume in children, recognition of the clinical signs of major haemorrhage, and ability to adequately fluid resuscitate a child is essential.

History

The child and their parents will present with a history of bleeding from the nose or mouth. The parents may be able to estimate the amount of blood loss but it is important to bear in mind that a significant amount of blood may have been swallowed.

Examination

Children with significant haemorrhage will display the following signs:
• Tachycardia.
• Pallor.
• Decreased skin perfusion.
• Reduced capillary refill time >2s.
• Hypotension.

Hypotension is an important sign but it is important to know that children often maintain their blood pressure despite severe hypovolaemia until they are on the point of collapse.

Management

Intravascular fluids should be administered to restore circulatory volume and ensure adequate perfusion of vital organ tissues.

Access

If the child is severely compromised and IV access is difficult then the intraosseous route is the emergency circulatory access route of choice.

The usual site of insertion for an IO cannula is 2–3cm below the tuberosity on the anteromedial surface of the tibia. Other sites that can be used include the lower end of the tibia (approximately 3cm above the medial malleolus) or on the lateral aspect of the distal femur (approximately 3cm above the lateral condyle). These sites specifically avoid growth plates of the bones.

Generally it is recommended that size 18 gauge is used for a newborn–6 months of age, 16 gauge for a child 6–18 months of age, and 14 gauge for children >18 months.

IV access should also be obtained as soon as possible and FBC, clotting, G and S ± crossmatch should be urgently performed.

Fluid replacement

Initial resuscitation fluid should be administered as a bolus of 20ml/kg. The child circulatory status should be reassessed and if signs of failure persist, this should be repeated. The infusion of large amounts (60–80ml/kg) of fluid in the first hour of resuscitation may be required.

Types of fluid

In the initial phase of resuscitation, balanced salt solutions should be used. There is no clear advantage of using colloids. Glucose-containing solutions (such as dextrose saline) should never be used for volume-replacement, as they can cause hyponatraemia and hyperglycaemia. The administration of blood products should be considered for extreme loss but the risk of giving a child potentially contaminated blood must always be borne in mind.

Box 23.4 Useful information

- A child's blood volume is approximately 80ml/kg.
- Maintenance fluid requirements in a child are:
  - 100ml/kg/24h—1st 10kg.
  - 50ml/kg/24h—2nd 10kg.
  - 20ml/kg/24h—for any weight after 20kg.

Paediatric airway assessment

When assessing the paediatric airway it is important to remember how it differs from an adult's airway:

- Narrow nares.
- Relatively large tongue can obstruct pharynx.
- Relatively large occiput makes head positioning more difficult.
- Smaller, less rigid airway—more easily obstructed in response to infection, inflammation, or foreign body.
- Poor collateral pulmonary circulation.
- ↓ chest-wall compliance allowing collapse.
- Horizontal rib position yields ↑ intercostals movement.
- Easily fatigable respiratory muscles.
- Greater susceptibility to upper respiratory infections.
- Deceptively good at maintaining respiration and circulation in the face of impending collapse.

Management of the paediatric airway

History

It is important to ask specific questions even if not volunteered re.:

- Neonatal intubation.
- Previous stridor/stertor.
- Abnormal voice/cry.
- Feeling difficulties.
- Cough/cyanotic attacks.
- Failure to thrive.
- Other related abnormalities.
- Birth trauma.
- Upper respiratory tract infection.

Examination

Look for signs of respiratory distress and failure to maintain own airway:

- Stridor, stertor (see Table 23.1 for the difference between these noises).
- Pallor, cyanosis.
- Tracheal tug.
- Sternal, intercostal, and subcostal recession.
- Pectus excavatum, Harrison's sulci.
- Abnormal voice/cry.
- Cough.
- Drooling.
- Pyrexia suggesting acute infection.
- Cutaneous haemangioma suggesting possible subglottic haemangioma.
- Craniofacial abnormalities.

Table 23.1 Different sites of airway obstruction lead to different clinical presentations

	Stridor	Voice	Cough
Nasal/oropharyngeal region	Stertor	Muffled	–
Supraglottis, glottis	Inspiratory	hoarse	Barking
Subglottis, extrathoracic tracheal	Biphasic	Normal	Brassy
Intrathoracic tracheal, bronchi	Expiratory	Normal	+

Stertor vs stridor vs wheeze

Stertor is a low pitched noise caused by the partial obstruction of the airways at the level above the level of the larynx (nasal, oro and nasopharyngeal regions). Pharyngeal (stertor) tends to be worse when asleep. Stridor is a high pitched noise caused by the partial obstruction of the airways at or below the level of the larynx. Laryngeal, tracheal or bronchial (stridor) tends to be worse when awake especially if stressed. Wheeze is the expiratory sound produced by turbulant airflow through the bronchioles.

Investigations

> ▶ In an emergency situation the priority is to maintain the child's airway and minimize distress, ∴ investigations may not be appropriate.

In the elective patient (not emergency) consider:
- Soft-tissue lateral neck X-ray looking for lesions or foreign bodies obstructing the nasopharynx and pharynx, e.g. adenoidal hypertrophy, retropharyngeal mass.
- PA chest X-ray looking for cardiopulmonary anomalies.
- Cincinnati (high-kV filter) view looking for subglottic stenosis.
- Barium swallow/echo looking for vascular anomalies, such as double aortic arch.
- Air bronchogram looking for tracheobronchial anomalies.
- Spiral CT and virtual endoscopy looking for abnormailities in the tracheobronhial tree and cardiovascular abnormalities.

Management
- Keep the child calm.
- If maintaining own airway:
  - Humidified oxygen.
  - Nebulized adrenalin (1 in 1000) with 2ml n/saline.
  - Heliox.
  - Dexamethasone (1–1.5mg/kg) but avoid cannulation if distressing the child could increase risk of airway obstruction.

If failing to maintain airway, an appropriate level of ventilatory support is required. Consider:
- Bag and mask.
- Nasopharyngeal airway.
- Laryngeal mask.
- Endotracheal intubation.
- Tracheostomy.

For acute infections such as croup and acute epiglottis see pp. 708–12 and remember to think of bilateral choanal atresia (see p. 768).

Endoscopy

This may be performed using a flexible, fibre-optic endoscope or a rigid endoscope as part of a microlaryngobronchcoscopy.

Flexible, fibre-optic endoscopy

Advantages

- Outpatient procedure.
- Suitable for infants using simple restraint.
- Dynamic investigation ∴ helpful for laryngo-malacia and assessing vocal cord function.

Disadvantages

- Difficult to perform in toddlers and small children.
- Only gives a view of supraglottis.
- Does not exclude coexisting lower airway pathology.
- A diagnostic procedure only.

Microlaryngobronchoscopy (MLB)

This is the gold standard.

Advantages

- It allows a complete view of the larynx, subglottis, trachea, and proximal bronchial tree.
- It can be therapeutic as well as diagnostic.

Disadvantages

- This procedure requires a general anaesthetic.
- An experienced paediatric otolaryngologist and anaesthetist are essential.
- It is less reliable for dynamic airway problems such as vocal cord paralysis.

Box 23.5 List of diagnoses found on MLB in a five year period at Great Ormond Street, London, UK

(752 in 5 years).
- Subglottic stenosis 158.
- Laryngomalacia 125.
- Vocal cord palsy 44.
- Tracheomalacia 36.
- Foreign body 29.
- Subglottic haemangioma 28.
- Respiratory Papillomatosis 28.

(Bailey et al. 2006. Unpublished data taken from a presentation at the British Paediatric Otolaryngology Course 2006, London, UK).

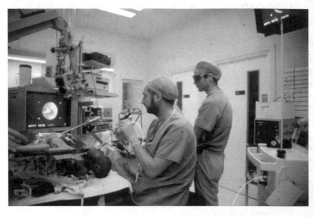

Fig. 23.1 Photograph of typical microlaryngobronchoscopy set up.

MLB operative notes

Close liason between the surgeon and anaesthetist is required at all times during the procedure. It is important for the surgeon to understand the anaesthetic technique.

Place the child in slightly extended position. A Spontaneous respiration anaesthetic technique is used.

- IM Atropine premedication.
- Inhalational induction of anaesthesia—sevoflurane and oxygen.
- Metered dose of lignocaine spray.
- Nasotracheal intubation.
- IV access, full monitoring.

Use a laryngoscope to assess the supraglottis and glottis. Using a probe, assess mobility of crico-arytenoid joints and palpate for the presence of a laryngeal cleft.

Then either pass a 0-degree rigid endoscope through the laryngossope or use a bronchoscope to assess subglottis, tracheal, and bronchi. A 30 or 70-degree rigid scope can be used to give a more angled view, if required. The laryngoscope can be suspended to allow further instrumentation of the airway.

Equipment

- Head ring and shoulder bag.
- A selection of paediatric laryngoscopes.
- Age-appropriate ventilating bronchoscopes (Table 23.2).
- A selection of rigid endoscopes, size 2.7 and 4mm (0, 30, and 70 degrees).
- Metal and flexible suction tubes.
- Saline-soaked gauze to protect mouth and teeth.
- 1 in 10 000 adrenaline on neuro patties.
- Photo and video documentation system.

Tools for endoscopic treatment

- Cold steel.
- Microlaryngoscopy instruments.
- Optical forceps, peanut and alligator.
- Endoscopic needles for injection/aspiration.
- CO_2 and KTP lasers.

Table 23.2 Paediatric tube sizes

Age		Preterm	<1 month	1–6 months	6–18 months	18 months –3y	3–6y	6–9y	9–12y	>12y
Trachea*			5	5–6	6–7	7–8	8–9	9–10	10–13	13
cricoid*			3.6–4.8	4.8–5.8	5.8–6.5	6.5–7.4	7.4–8.2	8.2–9.0	9.0–10	10.7
ETT tube (portex)	ID (mm)	2.5	3	3.5	4	4.5	5	6	7	8
	OD (mm)	3.4	4.2	4.8	5.4	6.2	6.8	8.2	9.6	10.8
Bronchoscope	Size		2.5	3	3.5	4	4.5	5	6	6
	ID (mm)		3.5	4.3	5	6	6.6	7.1	7.5	7.5
	OD (mm)		4.2	5	5.7	6.7	7.3	7.8	8.2	8.2
Shiley tracheostomy tube	Size		3	3.5	4	4.5	5	5.5	6	6.5
	ID (mm)		3	3.5	4	4.5	5	5.5	6	6.5
	OD (mm)		4.5	5.2	5.9	6.5	7.1	7.7	8.3	9
	Neonatal length		30	32	34	36				
	Paediatric length		39	40	41	42	44 or 50	46 or 52	54	56

* Transverse diameter (mm).

Paediatric tracheostomy

A paediatric tracheostomy places considerable burden on patients and parents, and makes social and verbal development more difficult. It should be considered in the following circumstances where no other alternative is available.

Indications
- Upper airway obstruction.
- Maintenance of long term ventilation.
- Pulmonary toilet.

Operative notes
See adult tracheostomy (Chapter 8) and note the differences for children.

Preparation
Select and check an age-appropriate and one-size smaller tube prior to embarking on surgery. See table 23.2.

Positioning
Avoid hyperextension to avoid mediastinal structures presenting in the neck; ensure head taped in the midline. Use shoulder roll to extend the neck, bringing the trachea more anterior and superior but avoid hyperextension as this can cause mediastinal structures to enter the neck (see Fig. 23.2). Tape the chin in midline position.

Landmarks
Soft cartilages, landmarks of laryngeal framework more diificult to feel. Mark midline, cricoid cartilage, suprasternal notch, and sternocleidomastoid muscles.

Surgery
- Vertical incision, 1cm below cricoid to 1cm about suprasternal notch (author's preference but horizontal can be used).
- Remove excess subcutaneous fat with diathermy.
- Retract straps in midline.
- Divide isthmus with diathermy.
- Identify tracheal rings and place two 4.0 nylon stay sutures either side of midline. These are left uncut, labelled left and right, and taped to the child's chest.
- Vertical tracheal incision 3–5 rings avoid removing cartilage to prevent later stenosis.
- Place four 4.0 vicryl sutures from edge of trachea to skin edge (see Fig. 23.2). This is an extra set of sutures that secures trachea to skin surface to reduce risk of decanulation followed by incorrect re-insertion. There is an argument that it renders the stoma more permanent but most paediatric tracheostomies are inserted for mid- to long-term problems. The risk of tracheocutaneous fistula on subsequent extubation occurs, regardless of technique, because a well-established tract will form around the tube over a few weeks.
- Tracheostomy tube is inserted and position of distal tip above carina is checked with flexible or rigid scope.
- Tracheostomy tube is secured by suturing it to skin with 3.0 nylon and with tapes.

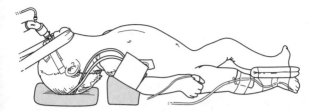

Fig. 23.2 Position of a neonate for tracheostomy. Note the chin straps to ensure extension and correct head positioning.

Early complications

Bleeding
Usually due to capillary ooze but beware of the potential for vascular anomalies and upward movement of the inominate artery on neck extension.

Surgical emphysema
Leave skin incision loosely open to avoid surgical emphysema. Stay in the midline when dissecting of the pre-tracheal fascia to prevent damaging apex of the lung.

Damage to lateral structures
Make sure that always dissecting in the midline, it is relatively easy to push the larynx laterally and damage the underlying oesphagus, recurrent nerves, or even carotid arteries.

Tracheotomy tube problems
Ensure that the correct tube is used. If too small it can be dislodged, if too large it can lead to pressure necrosis. If it is too long it can damage the carina or intubate only one bronchus. Mucous plugs can obstruct the tube leading to respiratory arrest.

Respiratory arrest
This can be caused by loss of ventilatory drive due to rapid change in CO_2 levels or tube displacement.

Pulmonary oedema
This is thought to be cause by rapid influx of fluid across the alveolar wall because of the sudden change in airway pressure following tracheostomy.

Late complications
- Bleeding secondary to tracheal wall erosion, Massive haemorrhage secondary to inominate artery erosion.
- Tracheostomy tube problems.
- Mucous plugs, excessive crusting.
- Tracheitis.
- Pseudomonas and Staph are the most common culprits.
- Swallowing difficulties.
- Splinting of larynx and compression of the oesophagus.
- Cosmesis.

- Fistula or scar.
- Aphonia.
- Can be a problem if tube inserted pre-lingually and child unable to speak around it. Need planned speech development.

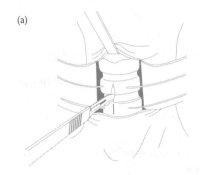

Fig. 23.3 a Vertical incision.

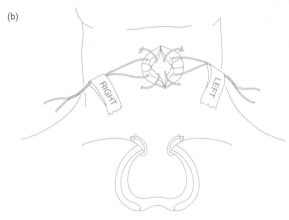

Fig. 23.3 b Positioning of sutures.

Congenital abnormalities of the larynx

These patients may present to any ENT surgeon/unit but the management of these abnormalities is complex and referral to a regional paediatric supraspeciality unit is the norm.

Laryngomalacia

- This is the commonest congenital laryngeal abnormality.
- Its hallmark is inspiratory stridor. Boys are affected twice as much as girls. It is generally a self-limiting condition starting around 2 weeks of age, getting progressively worse over the first few months, then resolving by the age of 2 years.
- Some infants develop severe obstruction requiring surgical intervention.

Aetiology

Most theories suggest immaturity of either the cartilaginous framework or the neuromusculature coordinating the laryngeal movement. However, this is not borne out by histological studies, nor is laryngomalacia increased in premature infants. Laryngomalacia has been classified into five types based on the following key anatomical features:[1]

- Type 1—inward collapse of aryepiglottic folds secondary to floppy enlarged cuneiform and corniculate cartilages.
- Type 2—long, tubular epiglottis (exaggerated normal omega shaped).
- Type 3—anterior medial collapse of the cuneiform and corniculate cartilages.
- Type 4—posterior inspiratory displacement of the epiglottis against the posterior pharyngeal wall or inferior collapse to the vocal cords.
- Type 5—short aryepiglottic folds.

Presentation

- Inspiratory stridor worse on exertion or supine positioning.
- Normal cry.

More severe cases may be complicated by:

- Delayed feeding.
- Gastro-oesophageal reflux.
- Failure to thrive.
- Airway obstruction.
- Pes excavatum.
- Cor pulmonale.

1 Hollinger L D (1997). Congenital laryngeal anomalies. *Pediatric Laryngology and Bronchoesophagology*, Chapter 10, 📖 p. 140. 227, East Washington Square, Lippingcott-Raven, Philadelphia PA 19106–3780.

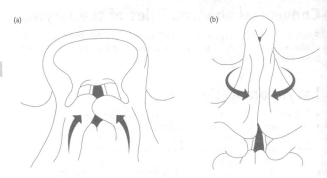

Fig. 23.4 The mechanism of airway collapse in laryngomalacia.

Investigations

- A dynamic study is required to assess the extent of laryngeal collapse.
- Flexible laryngoscopy in unanaesthetized patient in upright position gives most accurate assessment but may be difficult to achieve.
- Microlaryngobronchcoscopy has the advantage of allowing full assessment of airway for additional pathology. The child is slowly woken with a laryngoscope and telescope in place allowing observation and camera recording.
- Plain X-rays of the chest and airway may show medial and inferior displacement of the arytenoids and epiglottis if taken during inspiration with full neck extension but are most helpful to investigate associated cardiopulmonary anomalies.

Treatment

In mild cases, reassurance and correction of gastro-oesphageal reflux may be all that is necessary. Severe cases require surgical intervention.

Operative notes

Aryepiglottoplasty

This is term used to describe an operation to modify the floppy tissues of the supraglottis.

The child undergoes a microlaryngobronchoscopy to confirm the diagnosis. The most common problems are:

- tight aryepiglottic folds, which can lead to inspiratory collapse of the associated structures
- excessive mucosa and cartilage in the region of the cuneiform, corniculate, and arytenoid cartilages
- A combination of the above.

The tight aryepiglottic folds can be released by removing a wedge of tissue from aryepiglottic folds. The excessive mucosa of the arytenoids cartilages can be trimmed. Both procedures can be performed endoscopically using cold steel or CO_2 laser.

Complications

If surgery is over-aggressive, aspiration can result, ∴ it is better to be cautious when removing excessive mucosa from the arytenoids and consider trimming only one side first. Laser has fallen out of favour more recently, as there is an increased risk of collateral scarring leading to the difficult problem of supraglottic stenosis.

Other procedures performed for more severe laryngomalacia have been described including tracheostomy, hyomandibulopexy, and epiglottoplasty.

Vocal cord palsy

Vocal cord palsy is the third most common congenital laryngeal abnormaility after laryngomalacia and subglottic stenosis. 50% are bilateral. Of the bilateral palsies:
- 50% are acquired.
- 50% recover spontaneously.
- 50% need a tracheostomy.

Unilateral

This is most commonly caused by birth trauma. Occasionally it is a complication of surgery for other congenital abnormalities.

Presentation
- Breathy voice/cry.
- Weak cough.
- Aspiration problems.
- Can be asymptomatic.

Investigations
- Flexible laryngoscopy.
- MLB is an important procedure to differentiate palsy from crico-arytenoid joint fixation by palpation of the joint.
- MRI/CT scan to exclude a lesion of the larynx or the recurrent laryngeal or vagus nerves along their tracts from skull base to arch of aorta.
- Ultrasonagraphy can be used to detect asymmetrical vocal movement.
- Laryngeal electromyography, this is a difficult procedure in children.

Management
- Speech therapy to encourage vocal exercises to increase compensation.
- Thickened feeds.
- NG feed if aspiration.
- If there is no resolution, a medialization procedure should be considered when the child is older, such as injection of cord gelfoam paste or fat or thyroplasty (see 📖 p. 176).

Bilateral

This is often associated with underlying neurological abnormality such as Arnold–Chiari malformation.

Presentation
- Severe inspiratory stridor.
- Strong cry.
- Dysphagia and aspiration, particularly when associated with other neurological problems.

Investigations
- Flexible laryngoscopy.
- MRI brain.
- Neurological assessment.
- MLB is important to differeniate palsy from crico-arytenoid joint fixation.

Management
- Tracheostomy.

If there is no long-term recovery of vocal cord function then lateralization procedures can be considered. The observation period for recovery varies from 2 to 12 years, depending on the surgeon views. Lateralization procedures include:
- Cordopexy.
- Cordotomy.
- Partial arytenoidectomy.
- Complete arytenoidectomy.

Laryngeal cleft

Failure of the interarytenoid cartilage or cricoid cartilage to fuse in the posterior midline during embryogenesis will result in a laryngeal cleft. Incomplete formation of the tracheoesphageal septum produces a tracheoesophageal fistula (TOF) or cleft.

This is a rare abnormality and most cases are sporadic. Over 6% of children with tracheooesphageal fistulas will have a coexisting laryngeal cleft. Other syndromes with laryngeal clefts include G syndrome, Opitz Frias syndrome, and Pallister Hall syndrome.

- Type 1—intra-arytenoid.
- Type 2—partial cricoid.
- Type 3—complete cricoid.
- Type 4—laryngotrachealoesophageal.

Presentation

The severity is related to extent of cleft.

- Aspiration and cyanosis during feeding.
- Respiratory diffculties.
- Recurrent pulmonary infections.
- Gastro-oesphageal reflux.
- Increased tracheal secretions.
- Occasional stridor.
- Weak voice.

Investigations

- MLB—type 1 may be difficult to detect, palpation is essential using a probe.
- CXR—may detect associated aspiration pneumonia.
- Water soluble contrast swallow to look for TOF and may detect cleft.

Management

The management is determined by the extent of cleft.

- In severe cases, tracheostomy to protect from aspiration and respiratory obstruction.
- Aggressive anti-gastro-oesphageal reflux treatment and postural care.
- Optimize nutritional and pulmonary status.
- Consider repair of cleft.
- Investigate and manage associated congenital anomalies.

Surgery

For milder cases consider endoscopic repair by trimming the cleft edges encouraging them to close by secondary intention or using a single layer of sutures.

More extensive clefts require open procedure usually involving anterior laryngofissure, freshening margin of cleft, and layered closure.

For type 4 clefts, extending to carina, a posterolateral approach allowing two-layer closure, avoiding intra-operative bypass, should be considered. Type 4 clefts are associated with a poor prognosis.

Complications
- Laryngeal nerve injury.
- Breakdown of repair.
- Excessive granulation tissue.
- Posterior glottic stenosis.

Saccular cysts and laryngoceles

These are rare lesions arising from saccule of the ventricule of the larynx.

Saccular cysts can be classified according to their position into anterior and lateral cysts. Laryngoceles are classified into internal (within the thyrohyoid membrane), external or mixed.

Presentation

• Smooth obstructing laryngeal swelling.
• Respiratory distress often at birth with saccular cysts, later with laryngoceles.
• Muffled cry.
• Dysphagia.
• External laryngoceles may present as a neck mass especially during crying.

Investigations

• Flexible layngoscopy.
• Lateral soft tissue neck X-ray.
• MRI/CT neck.
• MLB.

Treatment

• Endoscopic de-roofing and marsupilization for small internal cysts.
• Endoscopic excision for small internal cysts.
• External lateral cervical approach to remove recurrent cysts or large external laryngocele.

Laryngeal webs

These are uncommon and represent failure of canalization of the larynx during embryogenesis. Most are posterior glottic extending into the subglottis. Complete laryngeal atresia is incompatible with life. They are classified type I–IV according to the extent of glottic involvement.

Presentation

- Variable voice, weak breathy to aphonia.
- Stridor.
- Airway obstruction.

Investigations

- Flexible laryngoscopy.
- MLB.
- Lateral neck X-ray/CT to assess the degree of cricoid abnormality and subglottic extent.

Treatment

- Mild cases may respond to endocscopic incision or dilatation.
- A tracheostomy may be necessary due to airway obstruction.
- A more severe web may require endoscopic or open incision with keel insertion or even laryngotracheal reconstruction.
- In severe cases definitive surgery may be delayed until 3–4 years old with covering tracheostomy whilst the child grows.

Subglottic cysts

These are usually a result of intubation. They are caused by mucous gland obstruction within the larynx, secondary to damage to the mucosa in this area. They can occur upto 5 months after the intubation.

Presentation
- Biphasic stridor.
- Airway obstruction.

Investigations
- MLB—may be associated with an underlying subglottic stenosis.

Management
- Endoscopic de-roofing/marsupialization.
- Recurrent cysts may require open excision via a laryngofissure.

Vocal cord granuloma

These can occur following intubation. They result from trauma causing granuloma formation on the endolaryngeal surface of the true vocal cords. They can vary in size from a tiny red polyp to a large ulcerative obstructing lesion. They can be a cause of failed intubation.

Granulomas may resolve by reducing the trauma from intubation, downsizing or removing endotracheal tube, and steroid therapy. In severe cases, a tracheostomy may be necessary to allow laryngeal rest.

Subglottic haemangioma

The histology of haemangiomas is dicussed on □ p. 748.

Presentation

- Increasing biphasic stridor around 6 weeks old.
- There may be altered cry and feeding difficulties.
- Barking cough and croupy symptoms are common.
- Symptoms worsen for first year then start to regress and usually resolve by the age of 6.
- 50% are associated with cutaneous hamangioma (only 10% with cutaneous haemangioma have subglottic haemangioma).

Investigation

- CXR high KV may show a large mass narrowing subglottis.
- MLB, diagnosis is made on endoscopy. A smooth, compressible mass is usually seen arising from the posterior-lateral subglottis, often on the left-hand side. It is usually submucosal and may have a slightly blue colour. More superficially, lesions will appear more red. Biopsy is usually not necessary but if performed some bleeding may occur, which can usually be controlled by compression with an endotracheal tube.
- MRI/CT can be used to delineate the lesion looking for further extension into the neck or mediastinum.

Management

Historically the lesion was bypassed by a tracheostomy, which was subsequently removed when the lesion underwent involution. Several therapies are now in use either in isolation or combined to try and avoid a tracheostomy.

Steroids

Oral steroids are thought to decrease the size of haemangiomas by blocking estradiol-induced-growth or modifying capillary vasoconstriction. The risks of growth retardation and immunosuppression associated with long-term steroid use have to be taken into consideration.

Intralesional injection with steroids with short-term intubation has been described to be successful.

Endoscopic debulking

Haemangiomas can be debulked endoscopically with a CO_2 laser. There is a risk of subglottic stenosis associated with this technique ∴ it should be reserved for lesions no greater than 30% of the diameter of the subglottis. Endoscopic debulking using a microdebrider is now being trialled in the hope that it will produce less scarring and stenosis than the CO_2 laser.

Open excision

Open surgical excision should be considered for isolated posterior subglottic lesions causing airway obstruction not controlled by steroids lesions. A cricoid split is performed and the lesion is excised trying to maintain mucosa. The remaining cricoid/trachea can then be supported by a small cartilage graft.

Tracheomalacia

Tracheomalacia is an abnormal collapse of the trachea that can result in airway obstruction. It accounts for almost half of the congenital tracheal anomalies that present with stridor. It can be primary or secondary.

- Primary tracheomalacia can occur in both normal and premature babies. The defect is intrinsic to the trachea. The cartilage to membranous trachea ratio decreases from a normal 4.5 to 1 to 3 to 1 or even 2 to 1. The flattened posterior membranous trachea collapses inward during expiration particularly with coughing.
- Secondary tracheomalacia is caused by other associated malformations, such as a tracheo-oesophageal fistula or external compression due to a vascular/cardiac anomaly. A localized area of tracheomalacia can also be associated with a tracheostomy.

Presentation

The symptoms depend on the site, length and severity of the pathology. They include:

- Stridor, which develops in the weeks following birth; it is often episodic with impressive acute exacerbations.
- The stridor can be associated with attacks of acute airways obstruction or 'dying spells', often precipitated by severe crying, coughing, and feeding.
- Tracheobronchomalacia can produce an expiratory stridor or wheeze that can mimic asthma.
- Harsh barking cough.
- Grunting, this action may provide some positive airways pressure to limit the collapse seen in tracheomalacia.
- Hyperextension of the neck.
- Recurrent chest infections.
- Attacks of reflex apnea when associated with an anomalous innominate artery.

Investigations

These include:

- Lateral X-ray of the chest, which may show narrowing of the trachea during expiration.
- Microlaryngobronchoscopy/spontaneous respiration technique can demonstrate the collapse of the trachea on expiration. When using a bronchoscope be careful to avoid splinting open the trachea, thus missing the diagnosis. The shape and site of narrowing of the trachea can suggest the cause of extrinsic compression. An aberrant innominate artery compresses the right anterior trachea just above the carina. A double aortic arch surrounds the trachea and main bronchi, producing a crescentric or triangular compression. A pulmonary artery sling compresses the right main bronchus to the extent that the lumen may be a thin slit.
- Barium swallow can be used to identify vascular anomalies, such as double aortic or tracheo-oesphageal fistula.

- Echocardiography can detect vascular anomlies.
- CT/MRI neck and chest can detect anomalies of the tracheobronchial tree, causes of extrinsic tracheal compression and further delineate vascular anomalies.
- CT angiogram may be required.

Treatment

Secondary tracheomalacia due to vascular anomalies needs referral to a cardiologist/cardiothoracic surgeon.

Mild tracheomalacia

This is self-limiting and usually requires no treatment. Parents should be given lots of support and should be taught resuscitation, delivering positive airway pressure using mouth-to-mouth or with a bag and mask, if the child suffers from apnoeas or dying spells. Treat any gastro-oesphageal reflux, which may be an exacerbating factor.

Severe tracheomalacia

The patient may require long-term CPAP. Surgical intervention may include tracheostomy, stenting an area of collapse, segmental resection, or cartilage grafting.

Subglottic stenosis

The subglottis is the narrowest part of the airway. Any additional narrowing can cause stridor and airway obstruction.

Diagnosis

Endoscopic appearance of subglottic stenosis and no air leak with age-appropriate tube at normal ventilation pressures.

Classification

Congenital

- Membranous subglottic stenosis is usually circumferential and consists of soft-tissue thickening caused by increased fibrous connective tissue or hyperplasia of the submucous glands.
- Cartilaginous type usually results from a thickened or deformed cricoid cartilage.

Membranous subglottic stenosis is usually less severe than the cartilaginous type.

Acquired

Trauma to the subglottis most often following intubation causes mucosal ulceration and perichondritis. Healing is by secondary intention with granulation tissue proliferation and deposition of fibrous tissue. This results in a weak cartilage framework and a firm scar narrowing the subglottic airway.

Risk factors for acquired stenosis

Endotracheal intubation—exacerbated by:

- Prolonged intubation though no safe-period.
- Excessive tube movement, repeated.
- Intubations.
- Birth weight less than 1500g.
- Infection or inflammation.
- Compromised immune status.
- Presence of nasogastric tubes.
- Gastro-oesophageal or laryngotracheal reflux.
- Infection or inflammation.
- Thermal or caustic injuries.

Presentation

- Recurrrent croup.
- Biphasic stridor.
- Increased respiratory effort causing tracheal tug and intercostal recession.
- Failure to thrive.

Investigations.

- CXR/Cincinatti view.
- Microlarygobronchoscopy—gold standard (see p. 681).

Subglottic Stenosis grading system

Size of ET tube which will pass through the subglottis with normal ventilatory pressures/expected age-appropiate endotracheal tube × 100%. (Fig. 23.6)

I	<50% obstruction
II	51–70% obstruction
III	71–99% obstruction
IV	no detectable lumen

Meyer et al. 1994.

Classification of stenosis with actual endotracheal tube size									
Patient Age		ID 2.0	ID 2.5	ID 3.0	ID 3.5	ID 4.0	ID 4.5	ID 5.0	ID 5.5	ID 6.0
Premature		40								
		58	30		no obstruction					
0–3/12		68	48	26						
3/12–9/12	No Detectable Lumen	75	59	41	22					
9/12–2		80	67	53	38	20				
2yrs		84	74	62	50	35	19			
4yrs		86	78	68	57	45	32	17		
6yrs		89	81	73	64	54	43	30	16	
	Grade IV	Grade III				Grade II		Grade I		

Fig. 23.6

Myer CM III, O'Connor DM, Cotton RL. Proposed grading system for subglottic stenosis based on endotracheal tube sizes. *Ann Otol Rhinol Laryngol.* 1994; **108**: 319.

Management
- Dependent on the severity or grade of stenosis.
- Congenital stenosis tends to get better with age, acquired gets worse.

Medical
Adrenaline nebs, systemic steroids, Heliox inhalation, anti-reflux agents.

Surgical
Mild stenosis (grades I and II) can usually be treated with endoscopic techniques such as dilatation or radial cuts with a CO_2 laser.

Grade III or IV stenoses require laryngotracheal reconstruction. Tracheostomy maybe the first procedure in severe cases.

Anterior cricoid split
This can be performed for early or soft stenosis, most commonly in neonates after failed intubation. The criteria for anterior cricoid split includes:
- Extubation failure on two occasions due to laryngeal pathology.
- Weight >1500g.
- No assisted ventilation for 10 days prior to evaluation.
- Oxygen requirements <30%.
- No congestive heart failure for 1 month prior to evaluation.
- No acute respiratory tract infection.
- No antihypertensive medications 10 days prior to evaluation.

Technique
- Vertical midline incision through the cricoid cartilage, first two tracheal rings, and the lower-third of thyroid cartilage, avoiding the anterior commisure.
- Stented with age-appropriate endotracheal tube inserted in an endonasal or oral fashion.
- Drain.
- Intubation on ICU for 7–14 days then 'stent' removal.

Laryngotracheal reconstruction

Laryngotracheal expansion surgery involves scar division with distraction of the edges by interposition of graft material to widen the airway lumen. There are several techniques depending on the location and severity of the stenosis.

Anterior laryngofissure with anterior graft

This technique is used in cases of subglottic stenosis that do not involve the glottis or have significant loss of cartilage support. The patient's own costal cartilage is the material of choice. Many other materials have been used for grafting including auricular and thyroid cartilage and hyoid bone.

Technique (see Fig. 23.5a–e)

- Laryngofissure.
- Harvest free graft of costal cartilage.
- Shape graft to fit defect.
- Place into defect (perichondrium internally).
- Secure with 5/O ethilon suture.
- Drain.

Insertion of stent if tracheostomy is insitu or for single stage maintain intubation for 1 week post-operatively.

Posterior laryngofissure with posterior graft

If stenosis involves the posterior part of the glottis and interarytenoid fixation, the posterior cricoid lamina is divided and a posterior rib graft is inserted.

Combined anterior and posterior grafting can be performed for severe stenosis.

Crico-tracheal resection

Surgical resection of the cricoid cartilage with thyrotracheal anastomosis can be performed for severe stenosis limited to the subglottis or upper trachea. This technique can be technically difficult due to the close proximity of the vocal cords and recurrent laryngeal nerves.

Further reading

Myer C M III, O'Connor D M, Cotton RT (1994). Proposed grading system for subglottic stenosis based on endotracheal tube size. *Ann. Otol. Rhinol. Laryngol.* **108**: 31.

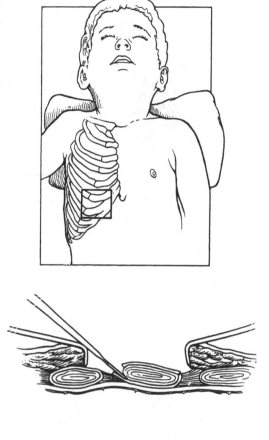

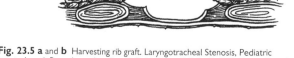

Fig. 23.5 a and **b** Harvesting rib graft. Laryngotracheal Stenosis, Pediatric laryngology & Bronchoesphagology. L.D. Holinger, R.P. Lusk, C.G. Green (1997) Lippincott-Raven Publishers, 277 East Washington Square, Philadelphia PA 19106.

(c)

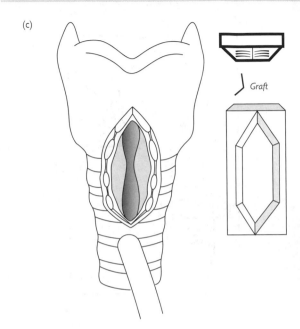

Fig. 23.5 c Laryngofissure.

(d)

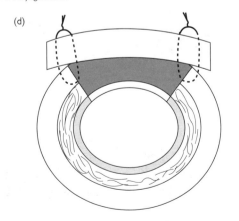

Fig. 23.5 d Insertion of Graft.

(e)

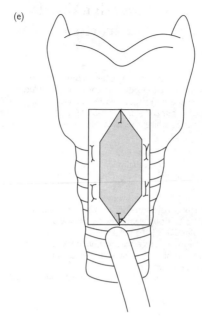

Fig. 23.5 e Securing of graft with sutures.

Inflammatory/infective diseases of the larynx and trachea

Epiglottitis

Definition

Inflammation of all the supraglottic tissues including the epiglottis. This disease used to be caused most commonly by *Haemophilus influenza* type B but since the HIB vaccine, other pathogens such as *Candida albicans*, *Haemophilus parainfluenza* and *Staphylococcus* have become more common culprits. The diagnosis is usually at the foot of the bed from the history and the following signs.

Presentation

- A child aged 1–5 years (usually 3).
- History of a mild URTI that rapidly progresses to severe throat pain and dysphagia.
- Respiratory stridor then follows within hours.
- Child looks toxic (pale and shocked) and is drooling.
- He/she prefers to sit up right and lean forward.
- Speech is muffled if able to talk at all.
- There is usually marked cervical lymphadenopathy.
- As the symptoms progress, the child will become quiet, floppy, and the respiratory rate will reduce.
- If no treatment is given, extreme fatigue will lead to respiratory and cardiac arrest.
- An X-ray is no longer indicated as it may increase the risk of airway obstruction by delaying treatment but classical appearance will show an epiglottic swelling, 'thumbprint sign'.

Management

- Do not distress the child by attempting intra-oral examination or IV cannulation.
- Allow the child to be comforted by parent who should hold him/her upright.
- Humidified oxygen should be given.
- Contact most senior anaesthetist and ENT surgeon.
- Proceed directly to the operating room in order to secure airway. Make sure that the necessary equipment is available (see Box 23.6).
- Breath the child down with halothane and oxygen in the upright position.
- Muscle relaxants are avoided.
- As soon as the child is asleep place him/her in supine or semi-prone position.
- Anaesthesia is deepened to allow CPAP.
- Avoid intubation too early as this will lead to laryngospasm. Insert laryngoscope to confirm the diagnosis.
- Swab epiglottis and suction pooled secretions.
- Aim at the anterior aspect of the laryngeal inlet using an age appropriate tube with a semi-rigid introducer to displace the epiglottis anteriorly.

- If intubation is unsuccessful, do not continue with repeated attempts as this will increase the oedema and can result in severe bradycardia and respiratory arrest.
- If first intubation fails, then intubate using an age-appropriate, ventilating bronchoscope. If not available, then use a Magill's nasal sucker.
- A bougie or suction catheter can then be inserted and used as a guide-wire to place an oral or nasal endotracheal tube. This is firmly secured.
- If unable to intubate, proceed to tracheostomy.
- IV access is obtained and cefotaxime, chloramphenicol is given.
- An NG tube is inserted to decompress the stomach.
- Transfer to PICU.
- Consider extubation with steroid cover when there is evidence of a leak around the tube with airway pressure of 20cm of water.

Box 23.6 Equipment required for epiglottitis and other emergency airways

- Resuscitation trolley.
- Naso and oro-tracheal tubes ranging from size 2.5 upwards.
- Introducers.
- Suction equipment.
- A selection of paediatric laryngoscopes.
- Age-appropriate ventilating bronchoscopes size 2.5 upwards.
- A selection of rigid endoscopes, size 2.7 and 4mm (0, 30, and 70 degrees).

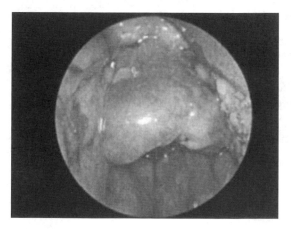

Fig. 23.7 Epiglottis in a 3-year-old.

Croup (acute laryngotracheobronchitis)

Croup is responsible for approximately 90% of acute infections causing respiratory distress. It is a viral condition caused by parainfluenza virus I and II, respiratory syncitial virus and influenza A and B. Affects children aged 6 months to 3 years (peak at 2).

Presentation
- Usually winter.
- ♂ : ♀, 2.1 : 1.
- URTI 1–3 days.
- Barking cough, low-grade fever, and hoarseness.
- Biphasic stridor.
- Airway obstruction.
- Airway films show hypopahryngeal distension, subglottic narrowing, thickened vocal folds with normal epiglottis.
- AP view shows narrowing known as the 'steeple sign' in subglottic region.

Management
- Primarily supportive.
- Observation and humidity.
- Nebulized adrenaline.
- IV Dexamethasone or nebulized budesonide.
- Heliox.
- Rarely ventilatory support.

If recurrent croup, consider microlaryngobronchoscopy looking for anatomical problem such as subglottic stenosis.

Bacterial tracheitis

Also known as membranous or pseudomembraneous croup. It is caused by bacteria such as *Staphylococcus aureus*, *Moraxella catarrhalis*, and *Streptococcus pneumoniae*.
- Age of onset slightly older than croup: 3.5y.
- More severe symptoms.
- Voice often normal.

Management
- Humidified oxygen.
- Nebulized adrenaline.
- Microlaryngobronchoscopy is required to remove thick obstructing mucus crusts within the trachea.
- Intubation may be necessary.

Juvenile respiratory papillomatosis (JVP)

Respiratory papillomatosis is a disease characterized by development of papillomatoma in the respiratory tract but most common where there is a change in epithelium in the larynx. It is caused by human papilloma virus 6 and 11. HPV6 is associated with a more severe form in younger children. Incidence is approximately 4 per 100 000. Maternal genital warts have been implicated in the development of JVP but the precise relationship remains unclear. The natural history is variable but there is a tendency for remission by adulthood. Malignant transformation is rare.

Presentation
- Age 2–3y.
- ♀ = ♂.
- Hoarseness.
- Stridor.
- Respiratory distress.
- Chronic cough.
- Respiratory Infections.
- Failure to thrive.

Investigations
- Flexible laryngoscopy if the child will tolerate it, if not MLB.
- CXR, CT chest, if suspect extensive lesions.

Management
Aim is to remove the papillomata that are blocking the lumen and restore normal airway, at the same time minimizing trauma to underlying tissues.

Surgical treatment
- Powered microdebrider.
- Cold-steel surgery.
- CO_2, KTP, Nd:YAG and pulse-dyed laser (themal damage can lead to extensive scaring).
- Photodynamic therapy.

Adjuvant therapy
Consider when >4 surgical procedures required per year, distal pulmonary disease, rapid regrowth, and/or airway compromise.
- Cidofovir (intralesional) is the most commnly used antiviral agent. There are some reports of use of ribaviran as an aerosol.
- Systemic α-interferon.
- Indole-3-carbinol derived from cruciferous vegetables ∴ increase dietary intake.
- Oral cimetidine.

In severe cases tracheostomy may be required however papilloma may then extrude through the trachestome.

Congenital ear deformities

External ear: auricle

Embryology

- Development of the auricle commences on the 38th day of foetal life.
- 6 nodules, the Hillocks of His, form on the margins of the 1st and 2nd branchial arch.
- These eventually fuse to form the auricle, which is originally positioned on the neck but migrates cranially during mandibular development (see Fig. 23.8).

Congenital malformations of the auricle

- Minor abnormalities include pre-auricular sinuses or skin tags.
- Arrested development of the hillocks leads to:
  - Anotia—total absence.
  - Microtia—malformed rudimentary and placed lower and more anterior than normal.

Skin tags

- These are small elevations of skin containing a bar of elastic cartilage.
- The can be single or mulitiple.
- They are commonly situated just anterior to tragus but can extend along a line towards the mouth.
- They can be associated with another 1st arch anomaly, most commonly macrostomia.

Excision is required for cosmesis only but remember the elastic cartilage can extend deep into underlying tissues.

Pre-auricular sinuses

- These are congenital sinuses lined by squamous epithelium commonly found in the pre-auricular region along ascending crus if the helix.
- They can become infected and discharge requiring antibiotics.
- Surgery is only required if repeated infections occurs. Complete excision of all possible sinus tracts must be performed to prevent recurrence.

Operative notes

- Probing and injecting methylene blue into the tract is unlikely to be helpful in identifying all branches and may be misleading or create false passages.
- Perform a wide elliptial incision around the sinus down to temporalis fascia and root of ascending helix. Rather than look for tract, excise all this tissue, including a slither of helical cartilage.
- Undermine skin edges.
- Close the deep fascia with interrupted 4.0 vicryl.
- Close the skin with interrupted 5.0 prolene.

Collaural sinuses/fistula

These are first arch system anomalies and are discussed in p. 746.

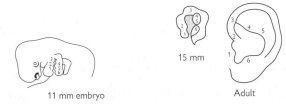

Fig. 23.8 Development of the auricle from the hillocks of his.

Microtia and anotia

Microtia and anotia are often associated with meatal atresia and other abnormalities of the middle ear. The extent of abnormality is usually proportional to the extent of external deformity. The incidence of microtia is 1 in 7500. Other features include:

- Unilateral > bilateral microtia.
- Right more than left.
- Higher incidence in Asians.
- Microtia is often graded according to severity.
- Fig. 23.9 describes one of the grading systems commonly used.

Investigation and management of microtia is discussed with external auditory canal abnormalities.

External auditory canal (EAC) malformations

Embryology

- The EAC develops on day 41 at the dorsal end of the first branchial cleft.
- The ectodermal diverticulum extends inwards towards the pharynx forming a meatal plug.
- The plug canalizes, a residual thin ectodermal layer forms the stratified squamous epithelia of canal and outer eardrum by week 18.

Congenital malformations

Failure in formation of the external auditory canal leads to stenosis or atresia. This can be unilateral or bilateral and is often associated with an auricular deformity. The resultant hearing loss is conductive.

Investigation

Hearing assessment is crucial, particularly if the problem is bilateral and should include:

- Age-appropriate behavioral audiology.
- Brain stem evoked reponses.

A CT scan of the temporal bones should be performed looking at the extent of stenosis and middle ear/inner ear abnormalities and to exclude cholesteatoma.

Management

Atresia/stenosis of EAC

No treatment may be a reasonable option for a unilateral malformation.

* Surgical reconstruction of the external ear canal is difficult and results are unreliable.
* Good results are achieved with a bone conducting hearing-aids in particular a bone anchored hearing-aid (see 📖 p. 420).

Microtia/anotia

* Unilateral/mild malformation may not require treatment.
* Bone conducting/bone anchored hearing-aid may be necessary for associated atresia/stenosis of the canal.

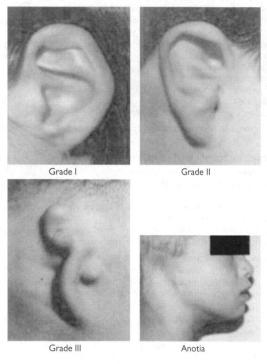

Grade I   Grade II

Grade III   Anotia

Fig. 23.9 Types of microtia: grade I all subunits present but misshapen; grade II, subunits either deficient or absent; grade III, rudimentary bar; IV, anotia.

- The decision regarding improving cosmesis should be delayed until the child is 12 years old. They can then decide whether they want any intervention. If so, the best options are a bone anchored auricular prothesis or surgical reconstruction of the auricle using sulptured cartilage harvested from a rib graft and incorporating some of the residual pinna elements.

Middle-ear malformations

Embryology
- Middle-tympanic cavity is derived from 1st pharyngeal pouch.
- 1st pharyngeal arch mesoderm forms the malleus and incus and tensor tympani muscle.
- 2nd pharyngeal arch mesoderm forms stapes and stapedius.

Ossicular-chain malformations
- These may be isolated or in association with other external- or inner-ear malformations.
- Malformations take on various forms:
  - Malformed malleus and/or incus.
  - Congenital fixation of stapes.
  - Stapes anchored to oval window.
  - Annular ligament fails to develop.
- Ossicular-chain malformations should be suspected in a child with a conductive loss, where glue ear has been excluded.
- A high-definition CT of the temporal bones may reveal the ossicular abnormalities.
- Exploratory tympanotomy will establish the diagnosis but proceeding with an ossiculoplasty on a congenital ossicular malformation has a higher risk of complications, such as perilymph gusher and dead ear, ∴ hearing-aid is usually the recommended first-line treatment in children.

Inner-ear malformations

Embryology
- At week 3 an otic placode forms on the surface ectoderm.
- This sinks into the mesoderm forming the otic vesicle or otocyst.
- The otocyst then divides into two sacs: the ventral sac develops into the cochlear duct and saccule, and the dorsal sac is transformed into the endolymphatic sac and duct, utricle, and semicircular canals.
- By the 10th week, the adult membranous labyrinth is recognized, and completely developed by week 26.
- The bony semicircular canals begin at the 6th week and are complete by week 22.
- The bony labyrinthine begins in the 4th week as a condensation of mesenchyme and forms a cartilage capsule around the developing membranous labyrinth. Its ossification begins at week 14 and is completed by week 23.

Congenital ear malformations result from a defect in the development of the membranous labyrinthine, the osseous labyrinthine, or both.

- **Michel's defect**, is complete labyrinthine aplasia, a rare defect caused by failure in development in 3rd week of gestation.
- **Cock defect/common cavity** is caused by failure of development in the 4th week; the cochlear and vestibule form one common cavity.
- **Cochlear aplasia** occurs because the cochlear fails to develop in the 5th week and forms a single cavity.
- **Mondini's dysplasia** is caused by incomplete partition of the cochlear in week 5–6; the cochlea is usually flat and has one and one-half turns instead of the normal two and one-half turns, Mondini also described an associated widened vestibular aqueduct and endolymphatic sac. Some hearing is usually present but deafness may be progressive. A true Mondini deformity is not associated with spontaneous CSF fistula.
- **Schiebe's dysplasia (Cochleosaccular dysplasia)** is characterized by a collapse of the cochlear duct and saccule. It is probably the most common form of inner-ear pathology in patients with congenital deafness.
- **Alexander's dysplasia** is characterized by cochlear base turn dysplasia. It is related to familial high frequency sensori-neural hearing loss.

The semicircular canals may be missing or dysplastic to varying degrees associated with the cochlear malformations. The commonest SSC abnormality is a solitary dilated dysplastic lateral semicircular canal often associated with normal cochlear function.

Spontaneous CSF fistula
Severe congenital dysplasia of the labyrinth can be associated with a fistulous communication with the subarachnoid space. A CT scan of temporal bones looking for this anomaly should be performed in a child with anacusis who develops meningitis.

Investigations
- An age-appropriate behavioural hearing assessment.
- Brain-stem evoked responses.
- CT temporal bones—looking for abnormalities of the bony labyrinth, IAM, and CSF fistulas.
- MRI temporal bone—looking for labyrinth patency, abnormalities of the endolymphatic duct and sac, cochlear, vestibular and facial nerves.

Management
- Multidisciplinary approach is required, aimed at encouraging communication by any means including input from teachers of the deaf and a paediatric developmental assessment.
- Minor dysplasia may require a hearing-aid or cochlear implant.
- Severe malformations are not suitable for cochlear implants ∴ communication should be encouraged using methods such as sign language.
- A malformation associated with a CSF fistula causing meningitis may need surgical exploration by an experienced neuro-otologist.

Paediatric audiology

Paediatric hearing assessment

Hearing is essential for normal speech and language development. Early detection of severe hearing loss and appropriate management with hearing-aids or cochlear implantation are essential, as the auditory pathway needs early stimulation for proper development. It is for this reason that most developed countries have implemented a screening mechanism for the early detection of hearing-impaired infants.

Pure-tone audiometry is not possible until a child is 4–5 years old ∴ an assessment of hearing is achieved by a number of objective and subjective tests. Parental and school concerns regarding hearing are also extremely valuable in raising awareness regarding a hearing problem.

Objective tests

These tests detect the reflex response to sound and do not require any cognitive or behavioural response from the patient.
- Tympanometry.
- Otoacoustic emissions.
- Evoked Response audiometry.

For more details see Chapter 14.

Subjective tests

These tests require cooperation from the child ∴ they are age-, cognitive-, and motor function-dependent. All subjective testing requires at least two testers. The best results are achieved at paediatric hearing assessment centres, where the appropriate time and expertise are available for each individual child's needs.

Newborn/neonatal screening

Since 2005, all UK babies are screened for congenital hearing loss. This occurs in the first few days after birth. It is performed by specially trained screeners, often paediatric nurses. It involves two objective tests:
- Oto-acoustic emissions (see Chapter 14).
- Auditory brain response test at 30dB (see Chapter 14).

If they fail either test in either ear then they are referred to a paediatric audiologist for a more detailed evaluation, including brain-stem evoked responses.

6–24months: distraction tests

Prior to neonatal screening this test was performed at 6–8 months by health visitors as a screening test. This set-up was often unsatisfactory and failed to pick up over half of the hearing problems.

Performed in an appropriate paediatric audiological setting with experienced paediatric testers, this test can be used to screen for hearing loss and gives an estimate of thresholds in the better-hearing ear. The child usually sits at a table on his or her parent's lap. Tester one also sits at the table playing with the child. Tester two introduces sounds of varying intensity to one side and behind the child. A positive response is denoted by the child turning to the sound. More frequency-specific information can be obtained using a sound-generating box producing warble tones.

6–24 months: visual response audiometry

This is performed in the same position as for distraction testing. Tester one distracts the child whilst tester two presents pure tones at calibrated loudness levels, free field via a loud speaker in front of the child, or with two speakers either side. A positive response with correct turning towards the noise is rewarded by a light flashing or a toy moving on top of the speaker.

>24 months: performance/play audiometry

This technique is essentially like a pure-tone audiogram but instead of a child pressing a button when they hear the sound, they are conditioned to perform a task such as put the marble in the cup. It can be performed free field or with head phones.

2–5 years: speech audiometry

This technique involves children pointing to or picking up the relevant toy when asked to 'show me the …'. The toys are tested so that they cover a range of speech patterns. The words can be presented at varying volume intensities free field or with head phones. One example is the McCormick toy test.

>5years: pure-tone audiometry

As for adults (see Chapter 14).

Congenital hearing loss

1 in 1000 children is born deaf and is usually detected by universal neonatal screening. A further 1 in 1000 become deaf during childhood, and parental or school concern may raise awareness of these children.

Management

The management of congenital hearing loss requires a multidisciplinary approach including:

- Paediatric audiologist
- Otolaryngologist
- Paediatrician
- Teacher of the deaf
- Speech therapist.
- parents.
- school involvement.
- self-help groups.
- deaf community.

The role of the ENT surgeon includes:
- Investigation of the cause of loss.
- Development of a support plan liaising with other MDT members.
- Consideration of surgical intervention for conductive loss.
- Evaluation for bone anchored hearing-aid, cochlear implantation.

Investigation

50% of congenital deafness is caused by environmental factors and 50% is caused by genetic factors. The investigations vary depending on whether the hearing loss is present at birth or late-onset.

Failed neonatal screening

- If a child fails neonatal screening, they are referred to a paediatric audiologist for further testing.
- If a severe hearing impairment is confirmed then the following management is recommended.

Environmental causes

Factors suggesting environmental causes of hearing loss include:
- Poor maternal health/difficult pregnancy.
- Perinatal infections, e.g. TORCH.
- Birth complications.
- History of SCBU, ventilation.
- Hyperbilirubinaemia.
- Ototoxic medications.

Genetic causes

Factors suggesting genetic causes of hearing loss include:
- Hearing loss in 1st- and 2nd-degree relatives.
- Hearing loss in a relative occurring before the age of 30.
- Consanguinity or parents from same ethnically isolated area.

Examination

Ear

The external, middle, and inner ear should be examined looking for abnormalities.

General

A complete physical examination should be performed by a paediatrician looking for features suggestive of syndromic hearing loss. A child with hearing loss should also have a developmental assessment.

- Hair colour: white forelock, premature graying.
- Facial shape.
- Skull shape.
- Eye: colour, position, intercanthal distance, cataracts, retinal findings.
- Ear: pre-auricular pit, skin tags, shape and size of pinna, abnormality of ear canal and tympanic membrane.
- Oral cavity: cleft.
- Neck: branchial anomalies, goitre.
- Skin: hyper/hypopigmentation, café-au-lait spots.
- Digits: number, size, shape.
- Neurological examination: gait, balance.

Infection screen

An infection screen may have already been performed, if general examination of the newborn raised concerns regarding perinatal infection.

Cytomegalovirus (cmV)

This is the most common intra-uterine infection causing hearing loss in the UK. Congenital cmV can cause a wide range of general and intracranial problems and is found in up to 0.5% of all births.

4% of those infected will be deaf. If untreated the deafness can be progressive and up to 8% of children will be significantly deaf by the age of 5. It is ∴ very important to screen for and treat any baby with perinatal cmV infection. For children <3 weeks of age, the virus can be cultured from the blood, urine, or throat. If congenital cmV is detected, antivirals should be considered to halt the progression of the disease.

▶ After 3 weeks of age, virus isolation could be due to postnatal infection which is not found to be associated with adverse outcome.

Other congenital infections causing hearing loss include rubella, toxoplamosis, syphilis, and herpes. Rubella infections have reduced markedly since most mothers are now immunized against it during their childhood. If infection is present, the diagnosis is confirmed by IgM rubella detected in first 3 months after birth.

Serological testing can also be performed to determine infection with toxoplasmosis, syphilis, and herpes, as dictated by clinical suspicion.

A variety of other blood tests can be performed to look for conditions associated with congenital hearing loss (see Table 23.3). Urine testing can also be used to detect certain conditions associated with congenital hearing loss (see Table 23.4).

Table 23.3 Tests used to detect congenital hearing loss

Test	Suspected Aetiology
Newborn heel prick, Tfts	Thyroid dysfunction, cretinism, Pendred's syndrome
FBC	Acute myeloid leuknaemia
Lipid profile	Hyperlipidaemia
Glucose	Diabetes
ESR	Vasculitis
Toxicology	Ototoxc drugs, chemicals
68-kd inner ear antigen	Autoimmune disorder

Table 23.4

Test	Suspected Aetiology
PCR—CMV virus	Congenital cmV infection
Dipstick—haematuria	Alport Syndrome (NB Haematuria may not manifest until later)
Metabolic screen	Where specific metabolic problem is suspected

ECG

This is performed to detect Jervell Lange–Nielsen syndrome.
- Autosomal recessive condition with hearing loss associated with a widened Q–T interval on ECG, syncope, and sudden death.
- Very rare 1 in 150–500K population.
- High incidence of consanguinity (prevalence in unrelated parents is extremely low).
- All children with severe to profound hearing loss, especially when associated with vestibular abnormalities, should have an ECG to look for this syndrome.
- Anyone found with a corrected Q–T interval > expected for their age should be referred to a paediatric cardiologist.
- Genetic defect is a mutation in either KVLQT1 or KCNE1 genes, both subunits of a potassium channel involved in endolymph haemostasis.

Imaging

A CT scan of the temporal bones will give information regarding malformations of the external, middle and inner ear (see 📖 pp. 717–18).

An MRI scan of the temporal bones can be used to look for suspected neurological lesions, such as congenital 8th nerve anomalies. It can also be used to determine the patency of the cochlear following meningitis.

It is worth remembering that a child may require sedation or general anaesthetic to perform any imaging ∴ it may be deferred to a later date if it is not going to change the immediate management.

Indications for early imaging include:
- Post or recurrent meningitis to look for evidence of labyrinthitis ossificans.
- Cochlear implant assessment to assess appropriate anatomy.
- Progressive or fluctuating hearing loss (e.g. widened vestibular aqueduct).
- When structural renal abnormalities are present there is a risk of synchronous otological abnormalities.
- If risk of abnormalities in future offspring/genetic diagnosis is important to parents and physicians.

▶ A renal ultrasound should also be considered if branchio-oto-renal syndrome is suspected or there are multiple abnormalities or family history of renal problems.

Ophthalmology

All children presenting with severe sensori-neural hearing loss should be seen by an ophthalmologist for two reasons:
- Often associated eye anomalies can help to confirm the type of syndromic hearing loss.
- Children with hearing problems often have visual problems, which need optimizing to ensure they reach their maximum potential.

Genetics

Parents have to give consent prior to any genetic testing ∴ they need appropriate counselling involving paediatricians and/or clinical geneticists.

Table 23.5 Ophthalmological manefestations of syndrmic hearing loss

Eye Abnormality	Syndrome or disease
Hypertelorism	Waardenburg's, Crouzon's or Apert's syndrome
Eyelid coloboma	Treacher Collins, Goldenhars, Charge syndromes
Iris/retina coloboma	Charge syndrome
Retinitis pigmentosa	Usher's, Alstrom's, Laurence-Moon syndrome
Cataract	Congenital Rubella
Interstitial keratits	Coogan's
Optic atrophy	Congenital syphilis
Keratoconus	Osteogenesis imperfecta

Table 23.6 Suggested tests to aid detection of genetic hearing loss

Clinical Findings	Genetic Test
Developmental delay/dimorphic child with multiple abnormalities	Chromosome Analysis
Non-syndromic sensori-neural hearing loss	Connexin 26, 30
Goitre, hypothyroidism, progressive sensori-neural hearing loss, widened vestibular aqueduct/Mondini malformation	Pendrin gene for Pendred's syndrome
Maternal family history, hearing loss with aminoglycoside exposure	A1555G mitochondrial test
Hearing loss, renal and 1st/2nd branchial arch anomalies	EYA1 test for branchio-oto-renal syndrome
Any severe hearing loss	Store DNA for further testing

Genetic hearing loss

Half of congenital hearing loss is genetic. Hereditary hearing loss can be split into syndromic (30%) and non-syndromic hearing loss (70%). The same gene can sometimes be responsible for both non-syndromic and syndromic loss. Detailed genetic information is beyond the scope of this chapter but further reading sites have been referenced.

Syndromic hearing loss

Hearing loss may be a minor or major part of the condition. Over 400 syndromic causes of deafness have already been identified.

The main ones are listed in Table 23.7.

Table 23.7 Examples of genetic hearing loss

Autosomal Recessive	Autosomal Dominant
Pendred's syndrome	Waardenburg's syndrome
Usher's syndrome	Treacher–Collins syndrome
Alport's syndrome	Pierre–Robin syndrome
Jervell–Lange–Neilsen syndrome	Crouzon's disease
Refsum's syndrome	Apert's syndrome

Pendred's syndrome
- Most common form of syndromal deafness (4–10%).
- Autosomal recessive disorder.

Clinical features
- Progressive sensori-neural hearing loss.
- Widened vestibular aqueduct/Mondini cochlear.
- Malformation.
- Hypothyroid or euthyroid.
- Goitre often not evident until late childhood.

Genetic defect
- Mutations in the Pendrin gene on chromosome 7q31.
- It encodes pendrin: an anion transporter expressed in the middle ear, thyroid and kidney.

Usher's syndrome
Autosomal recessive disorder.

Clinical features
- Sensori-neural hearing loss.
- Progressive loss of vision due to retinitis pigmentosa.
- Three different clinical types:
  - Profound congenital deafness, absent vestibular response, onset of retinitis pigmentosa in the first decade.

- Sloping congenital deafness, normal vestibular response, onset of retinitis pigmentosa in the 1st or 2nd decade of life.
- Progressive hearing loss, variable vestibular response, variable onset of retinitis pigmentosa.

Genetic defect

11 loci and 6 genes have been identified. MY07A, USH1C, and CDH23 encode proteins that form a transient functional complex in stereocilia.

Treacher-Collins syndrome

See 📖 p. 735.

Waardenburg syndrome

Usually autosomal dominant.

Clinical features

- Sensori-neural hearing loss.
- Four different clinical types.
  1. Dystropia canthorum, wide confluent eyebrow, high broad nasal root, heterochromia irides, sapphire eyes, white forelock, premature graying of hair, eyelashes. Eyebrows, vestibular dysfunction.
  2. Like type 1 but without dystopia canthorum.
  3. Klein–Waardenburg syndrome, like type 1 plus hypoplastic limbs and contactures of the upper limbs.
  4. Shah–Waardenburg syndrome, like type 2 plus Hirshsprung's disease.

Genetic defects

6 genes identified so far: PAX3, MITF, SNAI2, EDNRB, EAN3, SOXOA.

Jervell and Lange-Neilsen sydromes

See 📖 p. 724.

Alport syndrome

Inheritance can be autosomal dominant/recessive or X-linked.

Clinical features

- Sensori-neural hearing loss: mostly high tone.
- Microscopic haematuria.
- Glomerulonephritis, onset in childhood progressing to renal.
- Failure in adulthood.
- Increased risk of developing anti-GBM nephritis after renal.
- Transplantation.
- Occular abnormalities, lenticulus and retinal flecks.

Genetic defect

- Defective collagen type 4 causes abnormalities in the basement membranes of inner ear, kidney and retina.
- 3 genes have been isolated: COL4A3, COL4A4, COL4A5.

Brancho-oto-renal syndrome

Autosomal dominant disorder.

Clinical features
- Variable hearing loss (sensori-neural, conductive or mixed).
- Malformed pinna, pre-auricular pits.
- Branchial derived abnormalities: cyst, cleft, fistula.
- Renal malformations: renal dysplasia, agenesis.
- lacrimal duct abnormalities can also be a feature.

Genetic defect
2 genes found:
- EYA1—expressed in epithelium of branchial clefts 2–4 and pouches, role in inner, middle, external ear development.
- SIX1 regulatory gene for embryonic development of ear and kidney.

Neurofibromatosis NF2
Autosomal dominant disorder.

Clinical features
- Bilateral vestibular Schwannomas, or
- Family history of NF2. plus any two of:
  - Meningioma.
  - Glioma.
  - Neurofibroma.
  - Schwannoma.
  - Posterior subcapsular lens opacity.

Genetic defect
Defect in tumour suppressor gene on Chromosome 22, that produces a protein called Merlin.

Non-syndromic hearing loss

About 70% of hereditary hearing loss is non-syndromic. So far over 43 genes and 100 loci have been identified. The hearing loss can be classified according to the pattern of inheritance:
- Autosomal recessive (80%).
- Autosomal dominant (15%).
- X-linked (3%).
- Mitochondrial (2%).

The Identified genes can be classified according to the function of the protein they encode which includes:
- Unconventional myosin and cytoskeleton proteins, e.g. MYO3A.
- Extracellular matrix proteins, e.g. COCH.
- Channel and gap junction components, e.g. Connexin 26.
- Transcription factors, e.g. POU3F4.
- Proteins with unknown functions, e.g. WFS1.

Connexin 26, GJB2 (gap junction β 2)
- Accounts for 50% of autosomal recessive non-syndromic hearing loss.
- It was the first non-syndromic sensori-neural deafness gene to be discovered.
- GJB2 gene, on chromosome 13, encodes connexin 26.
- Expressed in stria vacularis, basement membrane, limbus, spiral prominence of the cochlea.
- It recycles potassium back into the endolymph following sensory hair cell stimulation.
- Most common mutation is 35delG, which has a high prevalence among Caucasians and has an available screening test.

A1555G mitochondrial mutation
- Maternally transmitted predisposition to aminoglycoside toxicity.
- Accounts for 15% of all aminoglycoside induced deafness.
- Caused by a A1555G mutation in the 12S ribosomal RNA.

Further reading
Hereditary Hearing Loss Homepage. http://webh01.ua.ac.be/hhh/
Online Mendelian Inheritance in Man (OMIM). http://www.ncbi.nlm.nih.gov/OMIM

Syndromes in paediatric ENT

Definitions

- A syndrome is a pattern of multiple anomalies believed to be pathogenetically related and not representing a sequence, e.g. Down syndrome.
- A sequence is a pattern of multiple anomalies that occur as a result of a single presumed structural anomaly, e.g. Pierre–Robin sequence.
- An association is a non-random occurrence of a group of anomlies in multiple individuals, not known to be a sequence or syndrome, e.g. Charge association.

Many syndromes, sequences and associations have anomalies that cause ENT problems. The main problems are:

- Ear abnormalities causing hearing problems and cosmetic deformity.
- Airway problems in particular obstructive sleep apnoea.
- Speech problems.

Below is a list of the most common conditions presenting to the ENT surgeon.

Down syndrome

- First described by Langdon Down in 1866.
- Caused by trisomy 21.
- 1 in 1000 births.
- Facial features:
  - Up-slanting palpebral fissures.
  - Epicanthic folds.
  - Hypertelorism.
  - Low nasal bridge, small nose.
  - Macroglossia.
  - Hypotonia.
  - Macroglossia.
  - Narrow pharynx and nasopharynx.
- Otological features:
  - Low-set small pinna.
  - Narrow external ear canals.
  - Conductive hearing loss and sensori-neural hearing loss.
  - Narrow Eustachian tube and muscular defects of tensor veli palatini.
  - Ossicular abnormalities, e.g. deformed stapes and thickened malleus.
  - Inner ear abnormalities, vestibulocochlear anomalies, wide 2nd genu of the facial nerve.
- Other features:
  - Mental retardation.
  - Short stature.
  - Hypotonia.
  - Atlantoaxial joint instability—beware extending neck if performing adenotonsillectomy.
  - Congenital subglottic stenosis caused by an ovoid cricoid ring.
  - Cardiac anomalies.

Treacher–Collins syndrome

Franceschetti syndrome.

- Mandibulofacial dysostosis due to 1st and 2nd branchial arch abnormalities.
- Autosomal dominant condition with incomplete penetrance and variable expression.
- 60% of cases are spontaneous new mutations.
- Defective gene is the TCOF1 gene (treacle gene); involved in nucleolar-cytoplasmic transport; its locus is 5q32-33.1.
- Facial features:
  - Down-sloping palpebral fissures.
  - Lower eyelid coloboma.
  - Depressed cheekbones secondary to maxillary hypoplasia.
  - Teleocanthus.
  - 'Parrot face' deformity.
  - Hypoplastic mandible.
  - Dental malocclusion.
  - Receding chin.
  - Large fish-like mouth.
- Otological features:
  - Microtia and canal atresia.
  - Hypoplastic middle-ear cavity.
  - Absent or dysplastic ossicles.
  - Occasional cochlear abnormalities.
- Other features:
  - Cleft palate.
  - Palatopharygeal incompetence.
  - Normal intelligence.
  - Absent parotid gland.
  - Cardiac and renal abnormalities have been reported.

Goldenhar syndrome

Oculo-auricularvertebral (OAV) syndrome.

- Most common syndrome occurring in approximately 1 in 10 000 live births.
- Caused by 1st and 2nd branchial arch abnormalities but vertebral, cardiac, and renal problems can also be associated.
- Majority of cases are sporadic in nature but occasional dominant families with incomplete penetrance have been described.
- Facial features:
  - Hemifacial microsomia.
  - Facial asymmetry.
  - Maxilla and temporal bones reduced and flattened.
  - Hypoplasia/aplasia of the mandible.
  - Epibulbar dermoid.
- Otological features:
  - Flattened helical rim.
  - Pre-auricular tags.
  - Microtia.
  - EAC stenosis/atresia.

- Ossicular malformations.
- Facial nerve weakness 10–20%.
- Rarely inner-ear abnormalities.
- Other features:
  - Vertebral abnormalities.
  - Cleft lip/palate.
  - Velopharyngeal insufficiency.
  - Mental retardation 15%.

Velo-cardio-facial syndrome

- Autosomal dominant condition caused by microdeletion of chromosome 22q11.
- Very variable presentation from complete normality to death *in utero*.
- Almost 200 different characteristics are known at present.
- Facial features:
  - Long hypotonic flaccid facies.
  - Prominent nose.
  - Long philtrum.
  - Narrow palpebral fissures.
  - Retrognathia.
- Otological features:
  - Minor ear anomalies.
  - Conductive hearing loss is usually due frequent infection secondary to immune deficiency and associated palatal anomalies.
- Other features:
  - Commonest cleft syndrome (5–8% of all cleft patients).
  - Cardiac anomalies.
  - Medialized internal carotid artery (beware in adenoidectomy).
  - Laryngeal web.
  - Laryngomalacia.
  - Thymus deficiency (Di George sequence in 10%).
  - Pierre–Robin Sequence.
  - Learning difficulties.
  - Skeletal disorders.

Pierre–Robin sequence

An initial micrognathia leads to a relative glossoptosis, which inhibits fusion of the palate hence a cleft palate deformity. The aetiology is likely to be some intra-uterine interference with mandibular growth. This commonly occurs in association with other abnormalities, e.g. Stickler syndrome (skeletal abnormalities and cataracts) and velocardiofacial syndrome. These patients often present with symptoms of OSA in early infancy, which tends to improve with mandibular growth and increasing muscular tone.

Charge association

This is a sporadic condition of unknown aetiology but occasional dominant families and siblings have been reported. The acronym stands for:
- Coloboma present in 80–90%.
- Congenital heart defects.
- Choanal atresia 50–60%.

- Retardation of growth and development 100%.
- Genitorenal anomalies.
- Ear 90% (may involve external, middle, and inner ear deformities).

Other features include:
- Cleft lip and palate.
- Tracheoesophageal fistula.
- Oral frenulae.

Craniosynostoses

Craniosynostoses is a term used to describe premature fusion of one or more cranial sutures *in utero*. This results in abnormalities of the skull. Syndromal craniosynostosis include Crouzon's, Apert's, and Pfieffer's syndromes. All three defects are thought to be caused by mutations in the fibroblast growth factor receptor gene (FGFR2), 10q25-26.

Crouzon's syndrome

- Commonest craniofacial syndrome.
- Autosomal dominant disorder with de novo mutations occurring in up to 50% of cases.
- Facial features:
  - Bilateral coronal craniosynostosis (brachycephaly).
  - lambdoid and sagittal sutures can also be involved resulting in clover leaf deformity.
  - Maxillary hypoplasia.
  - Relative mandibular prognathism.
  - Beak-like nose.
  - Exorbitism as a result of orbital deficiency, which can lead to exposure keratitis and blindness.
  - High-arch palate.
  - Cleft palate 3%.
  - Bifid uvula 10%.
- Otological features:
  - Stenosis/atresia of ear canals.
  - Ossicular abnormalities.
  - Glue ear.
- Other features:
  - OSA.
  - Cervical spine anomalies.
  - Stiff joints (especially elbows).
  - Normal intelligence.

Apert's syndrome

- Autosomal dominant disorder.
- Facial features:
  - Turribrachycephalic, bilateral coronal craniosynostosis with a wide gaping open anterior fontanelle.
  - High forehead, flattened occiput.
  - Marked midface hypoplasia.
  - Beak nose.
  - High-arched palate.

- Cleft palate 30%.
- Hypertelorism.
- Some proptosis.
- Otological features:
  - Glue ear.
  - Fixed footplate.
- Other features:
  - Syndactyly (2nd, 3rd and 4th digits).
  - OSA.
  - Mental retardation.
  - Ankylosis of elbow, shoulder and hip.

Pfeiffer's syndrome

- Caused by a mutation in FRGF 1 and 2.
- Facial features:
  - Bilateral coronal craniosynostosis with a very flat forehead and a tower shaped skull. Some have clover-leaf skull.
  - Proptosis.
  - Maxillary hypoplasia.
  - High arched palate.
- Otological features:
  - Low-set ears.
  - External and middle ear abnormalities.
- Other features:
  - Thumbs and great toes are broad and large with respect to the other digits.
  - Choanal atresia.
  - Often normal Intelligence.

Mucopolysaccharidoses

This is a group of conditions caused by defective lysosomal catabolism of glycosaminoglycans. This results in accumulation of specific glycosaminoglycans within the tissues, in particular the nasopharynx, oropharynx, hypopharynx, and larynx. This can lead to airway obstruction and glue ear. Patients also suffer from recurrent infections, e.g. otitis media and sinusitis.

Osteogenesis imperfecta

This comprises a complex group of disorders involving abnormalities in type 1 collagen. There are several types with different clinical manifestations. Deafness in osteogenesis imperfecta can be conductive, sensorineural, or mixed. The ossicular abnormality most commonly seen is a fixed or obliterated footplate. Other features that are often present are blue sclera and progressive skeletal deformities with short stature.

Paediatric neck masses

Paediatric neck masses can be broadly split into 4 categories (see Table 23.8). The likely diagnosis varies with age.

Congenital neck masses

Presentation

Congenital neck reminants can present as masses, sinuses, or fistulas. They are present at birth but may remain unnoticed until adulthood when they enlarge due to secondary infection. The anatomical location often gives some clue to the embryological origin.

Investigations

- Ultrasound is useful to identify size, shape, and relationship to surrounding structures. It can determine cystic/solid/complex structures. It is also useful in midline masses to determine whether there is a normal placed thyroid.
- CT and MRI can give more precise image definition but a small child may require sedation or even general anaesthetic.
- Fine-needle aspiraton cytology can be useful in older children to exclude malignant masses. Fine-needle aspirate cytology in branchial cysts yields pus-like aspirate rich in cholesterol crystals.

Table 23.8 Causes of neck masses

Most Likely	**Neonatal**	**Child/young adult**	**Adult**
↓	Congenital	Infective	Neoplastic
	Infective	Congenital	Infective
Least Likely	Neoplastic	Neoplastic	Congenital
		Rare Inflammatory	

Table 23.9 Origns of neck masses

Midline	Anterior Triangle	Posterior Triangle
Thyroglossal duct cyst	Branchial cyst	Vascular malformations
Ectopic cervical thyroid	Dermoid cyst	Haemangiomas
Dermoid cyst.	Branchial fistula	
Laryngocele	Hemangioma	
Laryngocele	Vascular malformations	
	Thymic cysts	
	Teratoma	

Thyroglossal cysts and sinuses

During the 4th week of embryological development, the thyroid develops between the 1st and 2nd pharyngeal pouches from the floor of the pharynx, between the tuberculum impar and the posterior 3rd of the tongue. This enlarges, becoming a bilobed diverticulum as it descends through the tissues of the neck to reach its final position overlying the trachea. As it moves down, it leaves a tract behind that normally atrophies and disappears between the 5th and 10th weeks, but the caudal attachment may remain as the pyramidal lobe of the thyroid. Thyroglossal cysts and sinuses arise from congenital abnormalities of this process.

Presentation

- It is the most common midline neck cyst.
- It is most common in children and adolescents.
- ♂ : ♀, 1 : 1.
- It represents 90% of asymptomatic midline neck swellings.
- It is usually at the level of the hyoid (75%) but can occur anywhere from tongue base to thyroid.
- They rise on tongue protusion.
- They can present as infection, abscess or secondary sinus (15%).
- There is a rare familial variant inherited as an autosomal dominant in prepubertal girls.

Investigation

Before excision, ensure that a normal functioning thyroid gland is present by performing the following tests:

- Thyroid function tests.
- Ultrasound.
- MRI/CT (an alternative to ultrasound giving good images of the cyst and thyroid).
- Radioactive iodine scan where there is doubt regarding normal functioning thyroid.

FNA can also be performed and typically shows mucoid material with benign squamous cells.

Treatment

Treat infected cysts with antibiotics and aspiration. Try to avoid incision as this may lead to fistula formation. Simple cyst excision is associated with up to 50% recurrence. For this reason in 1983 Schlange proposed the removal of the additional the central portion of the hyoid bone reducing the recurrence rate to 20%. In 1920, Sistrunk developed this technique further advocating excision of the core tissue to include hyoid and a wedge of tongue base (originally up to foramen caecum but this caused entry into oral cavity). For sinus tracts, an ellipse of tissue to include tract and core should be removed.

In recurrent tracts, an *en bloc* anterior neck dissection, clearing a core of straps down to pretracheal fascia, should be considered.

Operative notes

- Position patient with a head ring and shoulder bag allowing extension of the neck.

- After infiltration with local anaesthetic and adrenaline, perform a horizontal incision at lower edge of cyst (or ellipse of skin around fistulous tract if present).
- Raise subplatysmal flaps.
- Identify normal strap muscles either side of cyst.
- Dissect out a core of tissue including cyst/tract in a cephalad direction up to the level of the hyoid.
- Do not dissect the tract from the hyoid bone, remove the central portion/body of the hyoid bone (which is intimately associated with the tract) along with the main specimen.
- To remove the hyoid body, cut between the lesser horns bilaterally with mayo scissors or bone shears.
- Note by cutting medial to the lesser horns, there is minimal to the hypoglossal nerves.
- Now extend the dissection to include the raphe adjoining myoglossus and a 1cm core of genioglossus. To achieve this, the dissection must be angled upwards and backwards at an angle of 45 degrees. This can be aided by placing a finger in the mouth and pressing the tongue base upwards and forwards into the wound.
- The wound should be closed in layers with a suction drain inserted.

Complications
Haemorrhage, infection, recurrence, hypoglossal nerve damage.

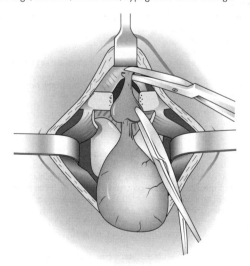

Fig. 23.10 Sistrunks operation to remove a thyroglossal cyst.

Thyroglossal cyst carcinoma

- This is rare but should be suspected if the cyst is hard, irregular, or has recently changed.
- It usually presents later in the 4th–6th decade with an equal ♂ : ♀ ratio.
- Histologically 85% are papillary thyroid carcinomas.
- Treatment is excision including total thyroidectomy followed by suppressive doses of iodine.
- Also consider adjuvant thyroidectomy and Iodine1–31 ablation.
- Prognosis is better than papillary carcinoma arising in the thyroid gland.

Dermoid cysts

Dermoid cysts form along lines of embryological fusion, including mid-dorsal fusion planes. There are three variants:

- Epidermoid cyst lined by squamous epithelium.
- True dermoid cyst lined by squamous epithelium and containing skin appendages.
- Teratoid cyst lined by squamous or respiratory epithelium and containing elements from ectoderm, endoderm, and mesoderm, nails teeth, brain, and glands.

They present as painless swellings. They do not move on tongue protrusion. Treatment is by simple excision but sometimes Sistrunks procedure is performed as those deep to the cervical strap muscles can be misdiagnosed and may infact be thyroglossal cysts.

Laryngocele

These are rare swellings caused by a distension of the saccule of the laryngeal ventricle. The saccule is a blind-ending sac arising from the anterior end of the laryngeal ventricle. 30% are external and expand through thyrohyoid membrane at the point of entry of superior thyroid vessels, 20% are internal presenting in the vallecula, and 50% are combined. There is a ♂ : ♀ ratio of 5 : 1. 1% are acquired laryngoceles and in these cases there is an association with laryngeal cancer of the saccule.

There is little evidence to support the supposition that this condition is more frequent in trumpet players and glass blowers.

Presentation

- Hoarseness.
- Respiratory distress.
- Soft compressible neck swelling that can increase on valsalva.
- Infection causing laryngopyocele.
- Air filled sac on imaging.

Management

- Asymptomatic laryngoceles especially in children do not absolutely require treatment.
- Symptomatic laryngoceles and infected laryngopyoceles should be excised.
- Suspected acquired laryngoceles should have examination and biopsy of the saccule to rule out carcinoma.

Operative notes
- After infiltration with local anaesthetic and adrenaline, make an horizontal incision over the thyroid cartilage.
- Locate the sac and follow in downwards to expose the neck.
- Elevate the perichondrium from the upper-half of the ipsilateral thyroid cartilage.
- Excise the upper-half of the thyroid cartilage to allow the sac to be removed at its origin from the saccule.
- Place remaining perichondrium over cartilage defect.
- Place a drain and close the wound in layers.

Branchial system anomalies

Branchial system anomalies comprise of:
- sinuses,
- fistulas, and
- cysts.

The anatomical origin of the anomaly reflects the presumed branchial cleft or pouch of origin. These anomalies are most commonly derived from the 2nd branchial system (65–90%) followed by the 1st (8–25%) and then more rarely the 3rd or 4th (2–10%). Occasionally these anomalies can occur as part of another condition such as Branchio-oto-renal syndrome or Digeorge Sequence. Asymptomatic branchial systems anomalies may not require treatment but, if repeated infections occur or the diagnosis is in doubt, complete excision is recommended.

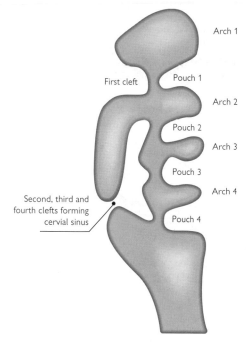

Fig. 23.11 Branchial system.

Branchial cysts

These account for up to 17% of all paediatric cervical masses. Branchial cysts are usually lined by stratified squamous epithelium and 80% have lymphoid tissue in the wall. There are 4 theories of origin:
- They originate from a remnant of the 2nd branchial cleft or pharyngeal pouch.
- They are the remains of the cervical sinus of His, which is formed from the 2nd branchial arch growing downwards to meet the 5th.
- The thymopharyngeal duct theory suggests that cysts are reminants of the original connection between the thymus and the 3rd branchial pouch.
- The Inclusion theory suggests that cysts are epithelial inclusions in the lymph nodes.

Presentation
- The ♂ : ♀ ratio is 3 : 2.
- The peak age is the 3rd decade.
- 2/3 are left-sided.
- 2/3 lie anterior to upper sternocleidomastoid.
- 80% present as persistent swelling, 20% are fluctuant.
- FNA—straw-coloured fluid containing cholesterol.
- 30% present with pain.
- 15% present with infection.
- 70% are clinically cystic; 30% feel solid.

Investigations
- FNA.
- U/S, MRI, or CT—can delineate extent of mass but cannot easily differentiate from a metastatic squamous cell carcinoma lymph node that has undergone cystic degeneration.

Differential diagnosis
- Benign lymph node.
- Metastatic lymph node.
- Branchiogenic carcinoma.

Management
Antibiotics and aspiration for infection. Try not to incise and drain as this can lead to sinus formation. Definitive treatment is surgical excision.

Operative notes
- Position patient with a head ring and shoulder bag, allowing extension and rotation of the neck.
- After infiltration with local anaesthetic and adrenaline, make a transverse incision below the swelling (at least 2 finger-widths below jaw to avoid marginal mandibular nerve).
- Raise subplatysmal flaps.
- Identify the anterior edge of sternocleidomastoid, taking care not to damage the greater auricular nerve.
- Identify the cyst and slowly dissect it out trying to avoid puncture.

- Free it anteriorly, inferiorly, posteriorly, and superiorly.
- Care should be taken in the deeper part of the dissection where dissection medially may expose the contents of the carotid sheath. The cyst may need careful dissecting off the jugular vein.
- It is important to be aware that some cysts can extend between the internal and external carotid arteries (see Fig. 23.12).
- The tail of parotid may need to be elevated.
- Watch out for accessory nerve as it crosses the internal jugular vein superiorly.
- Following removal of the cyst insert a suction drain.
- Close in layers and insert a drain.

In adults consider a panendoscopy prior to branchial cyst excision to avoid the misdiagnosis of squamous cell carcinoma from an upper aerodigestive tract malignancy.

Complications
- Bleeding.
- Infection.
- Nerve damage; marginal mandibular nerve (if initial incision is too high) vagus, hypoglossal, accessory and greater auricular nerve.

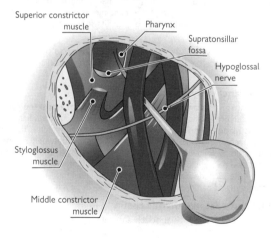

Superior constrictor muscle
Pharynx
Supratonsillar fossa
Hypoglossal nerve
Styloglossus muscle
Middle constrictor muscle

Fig. 23.12 Removal of branchial cyst.

Branchial fistula/sinus

- Most commonly a 2nd branchial system anomaly with persistence of both cleft and pouch.
- Most common presentation is an external opening along the anterior border of sternocleidomastoid, usually below the hyoid, which discharges intermittently.
- The internal opening, if it is a fistula is usually located in the tonsillar fossa.

Operative notes

Take an ellipse of skin around the tract and start dissecting in a cephalad direction. Then perform further stepladder incisions to follow the tract, taking care that it may course over the hypoglossal and glossopharyngeal nerves, and between the internal and external carotid vessels. Tonsillectomy may be required for internal tract closure.

1st Branchial system anomalies

- Type I: a cyst or sinus tract paralleling the external auditory canal running medial, inferior, or posterior to the conchal cartilage and pinna.
- Type II: a cyst or external opening in the neck superior to the hyoid bone coursing over the angle of the mandible through the parotid gland, terminating at or near the bony cartilaginous junction of the EAC.

These anomalies have a close and variable relationship to the facial nerve, so it is recommended that excision should be via a superficial parotidectomy approach.

3rd/4th Branchial system anomalies

These are rare and usually present as internal openings within the pyriform sinus. They can present as recurrent neck abscesses or suppurative thyroiditis. Diagnosis is made by barium swallow or endoscopy. A standard thyroidectomy approach allows access for excision. Distinction between 3rd or 4th pouch is made by following the tract. If it pierces thyrohyoid membrane, a 3rd pouch anomaly is suspected. A tract in the cricothyroid region would suggest a 4thpouch derivative. Care must be taken not to damage the recurrent laryngeal nerve, especially with the fourth pouch derivative.

Thymic cysts/ectopic thymic tissue

These represent 3rd branchial pouch anomalies. They tend to present in 1st decade of life as a mass in the left paramedian position.

Treatment is surgical excision in similar fashion as 3rd/4th branchial system anomalies.

Congenital vascular anomalies of the head and neck

In 1982, Glowacki and Mulliken[1] classified congenital vascular anomalies into two distinct types, haemangiomas and vascular malformations, based on their endothelial cell turnover.

Haemangiomas
- Hemangiomas are the most common tumours of infancy.
- They are most prevalent in the head and neck region.

Histology
They are made up of endothelial cells, which undergo three specific phases of development:
- Proliferating phase—made up of plump hyperplastic endothelial cells.
- Involuting phase.
- Involuted phase.

Presentation
- They are usually not present at birth but start to appear at around 2 weeks.
- They may be superficial or deep.
- Superficial haemangiomas are raised firm and crimson coloured.
- Deep haemangiomas are bluish, with less raised skin that feels warm.
- Risk factors include Caucasian, female, prematurity, history of prenatal chorionic villus sampling.
- 80% are single and 20% multiple and likely to involve extracutaneous organs.
- 10% of cutaneous lesions are associated with a subglottic hemangioma.
- They rapidly increase in size up to 1 year then start to regress/involute.
- Most are fully involuted by 7–12 years.
- They can leave residual scarring, skin atrophy, wrinkling, telangiectasis, hypopigmentation, or fibrofatty residuum.
- Intervention may be required if there is risk of complications. These include:
  - Ulceration.
  - Airway obstruction.
  - Visual impairment.
  - High output cardiac failure.
  - Kasabach–Merrit syndrome.
  - Psychosocial problems associated with the cosmetic appearance of the lesion.

Investigation
The history, examination, and pattern of growth may be enough to make the diagnosis. Imaging can supplement this:
- CT: lobulated appearance enhancing with contrast.

1 Classification of pediatric vascular lesions. *Plast. Reconstructive Surg.* 1982; Jul (70)1: 120–1.

- MRI: the proliferation phase is characterized by solid tissue of intermediate intensity on T1W image and moderate hyperintensity on T2W image with prominent flow voids. The involuting stage shows fewer flow voids and feeding vessels and increased lobularity and fatty tissue.

Treatment

For most lesions, the natural history is involution ∴ no treatment is necessary unless complications or failure to show signs of involution by the age of 5.

Subglottic haemangioma treatment is discussed separately on 📖 p. 698. If intervention is required the options are:

- Oral steroids are thought to decrease the size of haemangiomas by blocking estradiol-induced-growth or modifying capillary vasoconstriction. The risks of growth retardation and immunosuppression associated with long-term steroid use have to be taken into consideration.
- Intralesional injection with steroids has been described with some success.
- Interferon can slow the proliferation phase but there are some complications with long term use.
- Laser–flashlamp pumped dye can be used for superficial lesions.
- Surgical excision/debulking is often the treatment of choice if steroids fail.

Vascular malformations

Vascular malformations are localized or diffuse abnormalities in normal vasculogenesis leading to anomalous capillary, lymphatic venous, arterial, or mixed vascular channels. Unlike haemagiomas, they display normal endothelial cell turnover. They are:

- Present at birth.
- Never proliferate.
- Never involute.
- Tend to grow with the child.
- Can be subject to periods of rapid enlargement due to hormonal changes, infection of trauma.

Capillary malformations (CMs)

Historically known as port-wine stains.

- They can be extensive but are rarely mulitiple.
- They present as pink-red flat lesions that darken and are prone to fibrovascular overgrowth in adulthood.
- They are often associated with hypertrophy of the underlying facial soft tissues.
- They can be associated with underlying structural abnormalities, such as encephalocoeles or vascular anomalies of the choroid plexus and leptomeninges as in Sturge–Weber syndrome.

Histology

Histologically they are characterized by flat, normally-appearing endothelial cells with abnormal capillary channels in the dermis, which dilate and develop nodular ectasias.

Investigations

These lesions are superficial and do not require imaging though leptomeningial capillary anomalies can be seen as pial vascular enhancement on MR imaging.

Natural history

- These lesions do not regress and continue to cause disfigurement throughout life.
- Orbital CMs can cause retinal detachment, glaucoma, and blindness.
- Leptommeningeal anomalies can cause seizures and neurological problems.

Treatment

- Depends on the location and the extent of the lesion.
- Supportive therapy is commonly chosen.
- Laser photocoagulation with the tunable flashlamp pulse-dyed laser can produce significant lightning in 70% of patients.
- Underlying soft tissue hypertrophy may need surgery.

Venous malformations (VMs)

Previously called cavernous hemangiomas.

Presentation

- They often present as a bluish soft tissue mass within the skin subcutaneous tissues, compressible, distending on valsalva.
- Most common sites are muscles of mastication, periorbital region, and deep neck spaces.
- They gradually increase in size.
- Sudden pain and swelling can occur due to localised thrombophlebitis.

Histology

They are characterized by thin-walled dilated sponge-like vessels with disorganised arrangement of smooth muscle and variable dilatation and stagnant flow. Microscopy shows phleboliths in as young as 2-year-olds.

Imaging

- Phleboliths are seen on CT images.
- MRI is the chosen modality. Intermediate signal is seen on T1W images, slightly more intense than adjacent tissues. Lesions show increased signal on T2W images. There is contrast enhancement of the contents of the vascular spaces which is not seen with lymphatic malformations (LMs). Lack of flow voids differentiate LMs from arteriovenous malformations (AVMs) and proliferating hemangiomas.
- Ultrasound imaging reveals hyperechoic spaces that are compressible and slow venous flow with Doppler.

Treatment

Main indications for treatment are pain, cosmesis, and function. Main options are:

- Nd:YAG laser or copper vapour laser for superficial lesions.
- Sclerotherapy using saline, sodium tetradecyl sulphate or ethibloc.
- Surgical resection.

Lymphatic malformations (LMs)

Presentation

- These lesions exist at birth but are most evident by 2 years.
- 10% appear in adulthood.
- 90% in the cervical region.
- They can be macrocystic, microcystic, or mixed. Mixed lesions contain macro, micro, and angiomatous components.
- Macrocystic lesions were previously called cystic hygromas and can be detected by pre-natal ultrasound.
- Microcystic lymphangiomas develop later and are more diffuse and infiltrative.
- The clinical picture varies from lymphoedema to localized sponge-like lesions to huge swellings causing massive distorsion and overgrowth of the normal surrounding anatomy.
- Diffuse lymphangiomatosis is incompatible with life.
- Overlying skin is normal but it may be bluish.
- Tethering or dimpling of the skin suggests dermal involvement.
- These lesion can be associated with other conditions such as Turner's, Noonan's, and foetal-alcohol syndrome.

Histology

Differing sizes of dilated lymphatic spaces can be seen, lined by a single layer of flat endothelium surrounded by walls of abnormally smooth and skeletal muscle elements. There are vascular spaces with protein rich eosinophilic fluid.

Imaging
- CT shows a sharply demarcated low attenuation mass with no visible wall.
- MRI: hyperintense lesions on T2W due to high water content. They do not enhance with contrast. There are no flow voids.

Natural history
- LMs grow steady with the child, some causing massive disfigurement, orbital and airway complications due to local gigantism.
- They tend to fluctuate in size due to systemic bacterial and viral infections.
- The incidence of cervico-facial lesions is reported to be 17%. Spontaneous haemorrhage and local infection are the most common complications, causing the LM to suddenly enlarge and become painful.

Treatment
- Resection is the only potential cure for LMs.
- Aspiration, antibiotics, pain management, and rest only provides temporary relief during acute exacerbations.
- Often staged excision is necessary and total excision is sometimes impossible.
- Recurrence rate is 17–40%.
- Percutaneous sclerotherapy with substances such as ethanol, sodium teradecyl sulphate, or OK432 can shrink lesions.
- The role of interferon is also under investigation.

Arteriovenous malformations (AVMs)

- These lesions arise from abnormal communications between arteries and veins. They include arterio-malformations and fistula, and are characterized radiologically as high-flow lesions.
- Most are intracranial but some exist in the head and neck.
- The overlying skin at birth is usually noted to have a blush stain or feel warm.
- During childhood their fast flow becomes more evident but they often do not change until trauma or hormonal changes, such as puberty or pregnancy, cause their expansion.
- On expansion they deepen in colour and mass may appear. Superficial AVMS may be associated with a palpable thrill or bruit.

Histology

AVMs result from the abnormal development of arterial, capillary, and/or venous components. Flat, normal-looking endothelial cells and abnormal dilated vascular channels of variable mural thickness are seen histologically.

Imaging

- MRI imaging demonstates multiple flow voids and large vessels.
- Doppler ultrasound analysis best demonstrates the high-flow state with arterial and venous components. Arterialized waveforms of a draining vein due to arteriovenous shunting may also be seen.
- Angiography has a role in treatment as well as diagnosis, evaluating the presence of contra-lateral vessel formation between branches of the external carotid and the vertebral artery or internal carotid artery during endovascular procedures.

Natural history

AVMs persist in a quiescent state during childhood (stage I), then sudden expansion can occur making them become more clinically evident (stage II). Persistent high-flow state can lead to pain and destructive complications, such as dystrophic skin changes, ulceration, tissue necrosis (stage III), and eventual decompensation and high-output cardiac failure (stage IV).

Treatment

Some advocate resection at stage I, but most delay surgery until there are signs of endangering complications (stages II–IV). Wherever possible the lesion is embolized prior to surgical excision. Complete resection of the nidus is necessary to prevent recurrence. This is more successful for well-localised lesions, diffuse lesions are usually palliated with embolization.

Paediatric cervical lymphadenopathy

Up to 50% of children aged 6 months to 6 years will have palpable cervical lymphadenopathy. The majority of these lymph nodes are reactive and serious pathology is rare, unlike in adults where palpable lymphadenopathy raises the suspicion of malignancy.

The main aim of the consultation is to find an infective/inflammatory cause for the lymphadenopathy and confidently exclude malignancy.

History

Table 23.10 Aid to differentiating benign and malignant paediatric cervical lymphadenopathy

	History	Examination
Factors suggesting benign pathology	• Recent URTI/tonsillitis. • Fluctuating size with infections. • Skin condition affecting the scalp. • Exposure to toxoplasmosis, cat scratch. • Travel abroad/TB exposures.	• Multiple nodes. • Soft consistency. • Mobile. • Tender. • Local Infective cause found. • Skin discolouration.
Factors suggesting malignant pathology	• No precipitating infection. • Onset in neonatal period. • Progressive increase in size. • Weight loss, night sweats, and fever. • History of previous malignancy.	• Large firm/rubbery nodes (>1cm in children <1y, >3cm in children >1y). • Irregular shape. • Solitary. • Supraclavicular.

Investigations
- FBC and differential.
- Serological tests.
  - Epstein–Barr virus.
  - Cytomegalovirus.
  - Bartonella.
  - Toxoplasma.
- CXR.

Node imaging
- Ultrasound—in experienced hands can be used to determine whether the mass is a lymph node or other lesion. It can be used to distinguish the normal architecture of reactive lymphadopathy from more sinister

lesions, such as lymphoma. It has the advantage over other imaging in that it does not involve irradiation and does not require sedation or general anaesthetic.
- MRI/CT may be indicated for staging purposes if sinister pathology is suspected.

Fine-needle aspirate cytology (FNAC)

FNAC is good in diagnosing carcinoma in adults but its role is controversial in children for several reasons:
- Paediatric tumours are difficult to diagnose on FNAC.
- The most common malignancy is lymphoma; an FNAC is inadequate for subtyping.
- It is an invasive procedure that often requires general anaesthetic ∴ definitive formal biopsy may as well be performed.

In most circumstances the history, examination, and initial investigations provide enough evidence to support benign pathology but if diagnosis is still doubt then excision biopsy may be necessary.

Causes of cervical lymphadenopathy

Infection

Most common cause of lymphadenopathy is reactive hyperplasia secondary to upper respiratory tract infection/tonsillitis.

Viral

Cervical lymphadenopathy is a common feature of infection with Epstein–Barr virus (EBV, glandular fever) and cytomegalovirus (CMV). The picture varies from multiple, shotty nodes in the posterior triangle to huge widespread nodes leading to the description of ' bull neck'. Acute/recent infection with EBV in adults can be diagnosed by the monosopt test but this test is often unreliable in the early stages of infection and in younger children. A more sensitive test is IgM anti-viral capsid antigen (VCA). IgG anti-VCA can also be used to test for acute or recent exposure to EBV. Treatment is supportive; steroids can be helpful with acute glandular fever.

The clinical picture for cmV is similar but often milder than EBV.

Cervical lymphadenopathy can also be a presenting symptom of HIV infection.

Acute bacterial

The most common organisms are *Staphylococcus aureus* and group B streptococci. The clinical history often reveals a recent sore throat or cough, while physical findings include impetigo, pharyngitis, tonsillitis, or acute otitis media. The primary sites involved include the submandibular, upper cervical, submental, occipital, and lower cervical nodal regions. The treatment involves administration of β-lactamase–resistant antibiotics and drainage of purulence when fluctuation is present.

Suppuration of nodes within the neck can lead to neck-space infections. The most common neck-space infections in children are retropharyngeal and parapharyngeal abscesses.

Mycobacterium tuberculosis

Lymph node involvement with *Mycobacterium tuberculosis* is commonly referred to as scrofula. It was previously a well-known manifestation of extra pulmonary tuberculosis; however, as tuberculosis has declined, so has the incidence of scrofula. Nonetheless, it is still prevalent in much of the world; patients with scrofula present with cervical-node enlargement, most often in the paratracheal nodes or the supraclavicular nodes. Abnormal findings are observed on chest radiography in most but not all cases. Clinical features are not helpful in distinguishing tuberculous from atypical tuberculous mycobacterial infections. Nodal enlargement is usually painless; nodes are likely to suppurate and form sinuses. Performing a tuberculin test is usually helpful. Treatment involves administration of rifampicin and isoniazid.

Atypical mycobacterium

Infections with non-tuberculous mycobacteria such as *Mycobacterium avium*, *Mycobatcerium scrofulaeceum*, usually present with cervical lymphadenopathy in children. These organisms are often found in soil and it is thought that they are transmitted by ingestion. These infections are commonly seen in 2–5-year-olds. They usually present with a mass often in the submandibular region that has been present for several weeks. It often has a red-blush appearance. Its presentation is more indolent than an acute suppurative node. Its chronic nature may suggest TB but the chest X-ray is usually clear and tuberculin PPD testing is usually negative. Histologically both infections share the same histological features of caseous necrosis but the diagnosis can be established by culturing the mycobacterium responsible. If left untreated, the natural history of atypical mycobacterium infection is eventual resolution over several months. However, suppuration may occur leading to scarring and an unsightly discharging sinus. The recommended treatment is excision before the suppuration occurs. Incision and drainage should be avoided as it increases the risk of sinus formation. Depending on the site of the lesion, there may be a risk of damage to underlying nerves, such as the marginal mandibular nerve in the submandibular region or to the facial nerve in the parotid region. Therefore, a conservative approach may be advocated in some cases. Such studies have shown effective treatment with aminoglycosides, such as clarithromycin and azithromycin.

Catscratch disease
Catscratch disease is a zoonotic infection that originates from animal scratches, most likely cat or kitten scratches. The primary inoculation of the skin, eye, or mucosal membrane leaves a small papule that may or may not be evident on examination. Indeed, the papule may resolve before the lymphadenitis appears. Patients usually have accompanying constitutional symptoms, such as fever, malaise, and fatigue. The causative agent is Bartonella henselae, a Gram-negative rickettsial organism. The disease is usually self-limiting and requires only supportive treatment.

Toxoplasmosis
Toxoplasmosis is an infection caused Toxoplasmosis gondii. This single-celled parasite is usually transmitted by exposure to soil containing cat faeces, contaminated water, or raw meats. In the immunocompetent individual, acute infection may go unnoticed or a 'flu-like illness with cervical lymphadenopathy' may develop. Symptoms are often self-limiting and pass without any treatment. In immunocompromised individuals, neonates, and pregnant women, severe infection requires urgent antimicrobial treatment, as it can lead to ophthalmological, otological, and neurological damage.

Inflammatory disorders
Kawasaki's disease
This condition has also been termed mucocutaneous lymph-node syndrome. It has been classified as a vasculitis because of its occasionally lethal vascular complications. It is a disease affecting infants and children, although adult cases have been reported. There is fever, non-exudative conjunctivitis, cervical lymphadenopathy, oropharyngeal inflammation, erythematous rash with oedema, and erythema of the palms of the hands and feet, thrombocytosis, and vasculitis. The vasculitis may involve the coronary arteries, which may lead to aneurysm or thrombosis in 20% of cases.

In 1% of cases, this may be fatal. There may be epidemic outbreaks suggesting an infectious vector.

The skin findings are prominent and include an erythematous rash with oedema and erythema of the palms and soles. A combination of aspirin and intravenous gamma globulin has been used successfully to treat patients, dramatically reducing the incidence of coronary artery thrombosis.

Rosai dorfman disease

Also known as sinus histiocytosis with massive lymphadenopathy, it commonly presents as massive, painless, bilateral lymph-node enlargement in the neck with fevers. Most cases occur in the 1st or 2nd decade, more common in Afro-Carribeans. Rarely sites other than the lymph nodes are involved, including the central nervous system, eyes, upper respiratory tract, skin, and head and neck region. Interestingly, the spleen and bone marrow are spared. Half of the patients have at least one site of extra-nodal disease.

The cause is unknown although viral aetiology suspected. Some cases have responded to chemotherapy but many times the disease undergoes spontaneous resolution. In others, an insidious course develops for years or decades.

Neoplasic

See 📖 p. 760.

Paediatric neoplasia

Although rare, neoplastic lesions must be suspected in children once congenital, infective, and inflammatory causes have been excluded.

Benign neoplasms

There are a small number of benign neoplasms occurring in children including:

- Lipomas.
- Papillomas.
- Schwannomas.
- Neurofibromas.
- Adenoma and pleomorphic adenomas.
- Pilomatrixomas.

These also occur in adults and most have been discussed in other chapters.

Sternocleidomastoid tumour of infancy

This is a cervical mass seen in neonates. A firm mass arises in the sternocleidomastoid around birth. There may be associated torticollis. The cause is thought to be haemorrhage into the muscle with a subsequent inflammatory response followed by fibrosis. There is often no clear history of birth trauma. If the diagnosis is in doubt, it can usually be clinically confirmed by ultrasound or CT scanning. Most cases resolve spontaneously over several weeks to months with physiotherapy. Where there is incomplete resolution after 8 months (10–20%), a distal sternocleidomastoid muscle release to prevent permanent torticollis and subsequent craniofacial asymmetry may be required.

Table 23.11 Paediatric head and neck malignancies

Type of malignancy	Proportion of total malignancies in paediatric head and neck
Lymphomas	50%
Rhabdomyosarcoma	20%*
Neuroblastoma	6%*
Nasopharyngeal carcinoma	6%
Thyroid Carcinoma	4%
Rare tumours (other soft tissue sarcomas, salivary malignancies)	14%

* Rhabdomyosarcomas and neuroblastomas are the commonest malignancies in the <2 age-group.

Lymphoma

The two types are Hodgkins and non-Hodgkins lymphoma. Overall non-Hodgkins accounts for 2/3 of childhood lymphomas but, in the head and neck region, the two diseases occur with equal frequency.

Hodgkin's lymphoma
- Most common in adolescents and young adults.
- ♂ : ♀, 2 : 1.

Presentation
- Enlarged non-tender nodes.
- Especially in supraclavicular region.
- Up to 1/3 have associated with fever, night sweats, weight loss, pruritis.

Investigation
- CT neck/chest/pelvis.
- Excision/incision biopsy.

Classification
- Ann Arbor Classification System Stage I–IV.

Treatment
- ENT role limited to diagnostic biopsy.
- Referral to haematologist/oncologist.
- Treatment usually involves multi-agent chemotherapy and/or radiotherapy.
- Prognosis is excellent (90% 5y remission/cure) for stage I decreasing to 35% for advanced disease.

Non-Hodgkin's lymphoma
- Most common lymphoma in 2–12 year olds.
- ♂ : ♀, 2 : 1.

Presentation
- Disease often more widespread than Hodgkin's lymphoma.
- Enlarged non-tender nodes.
- Involvement of Waldeyer's ring.
- Fever, night sweats, weight loss, pruritis.

Classification
- St. Jude's staging system I–IV.

Investigation and Management
These are the same as for Hodgkin's lymphoma.
- Immunotyping of the biopsy allows subtyping into B-cell and T-cell categories.
- Combination chemotherapy is the mainstay of treatment.
- Prognosis is poorer than for Hodgkin's lymphoma; however, early stage, low-grade disease is associated with 80% 5y survival.

Rhabdomyosarcoma
- Most common soft-tissue malignancy in children (50–70% of all childhood sarcomas).
- 43% are younger than 5y, 70% younger than 12y. Four times more common in Caucasians than any other race.

Histological types
- Embryonal (60%).
- Alveolar (20%).
- Undifferentiated (20%).

Site

Head and neck is most frequent site. Subdivided according to site of origin.

- Orbital.
- Non-orbital parameningeal, e.g. nasopharynx, paranasal sinuses, middle-ear cleft, infratemporal region.
- Non-orbital/non-parameningeal, e.g. mouth, neck, face, scalp, larynx.

Presentation

- Usually as a painless mass, can cause obstruction locally.
- Direct extension to skull, brain or meninges from parameningeal site is common.
- Metastasis via lymph and blood vessels.

Classification system

- Intergroup Rhabdomyosarcoma Study Clinical Grouping System I–IV.

Investigations

- Biopsy.
- CT/MRI to delineate lesion and look for nodal metastasis.

Management

- Multimodality treatment recommended.
- Surgical excision of primary lesion if imposes no functional disability.
- Radiotherapy for incomplete excision/regional disease.
- Chemotherapy.
- No neck—chemotherapy.
- N+ neck—chemotherapy and neck dissection ± radiotherapy.
- Prognosis is excellent (90% 5 y survival) for group I decreasing to 37% for group IV.

Neuroblastoma

- Most common malignancy in infants <1y.
- Embryological tumour derived from neural crest cells destined to form the peripheral sympathetic chain.
- Most arise in abdomen but 5% are cervical.

Presentation

- Firm, fixed cervical mass.
- Non-tender.
- Ipsilateral Horner's syndrome.
- Heterochromia.
- Compression symptoms, e.g. stridor, dysphagia, cranial nerve palsies.
- Metastasises to nodes, bone, bone marrow, and liver.

Investigation

- MRI/CT define extent of disease and associated lymphadenopathy.
- Urine homovanillic acid (HVA) and vanillylmandelic acid (VMA) (raised in 90% of neuroblastomas).
- Bone scan.
- Bone marrow biopsy.
- MIBG scan to define metastatic spread.
- Biopsy, preferably excision.

Classification system
- International Staging System for Neuroblastoma (1–4).

Management
- Surgical excision for localized lesions.
- Chemotherapy for unresectable/metastatic disease.
- Cervical neuroblastoma has better prognosis than other sites attributable to earlier presentation. Prognosis is 100% for stage 1 to 20–30% for stage 4. Infants <1 have a high chance of cure regardless of the extent of disease.

Nasopharyngeal carcinoma
See also Chapter 20 📖 p. 556.
- Rare in children.
- Mainly occurring in black adolescents.
- Most common type is undifferentiated lymphoepithelioma.
- Strong correlation between the tumour and raised Epstein—Barr virus antibody titres.
- The presentation, investigation, and subsequent management is the same as for adults, although the differential diagnoses of a PNS mass in children are rhabdomyosarcoma and non-Hodgkins lymphoma.
- The overall 5y survival in children is 40%.

Salivary gland tumours
The investigation and management of salivary neoplasms are essentially the same as for adults (see Chapter 7). There are, however, a few facts worth noting.
- At least 2/3 of salivary gland swellings in children are not neoplastic. The most common lesions are mucoceles, followed by sialadenitis.
- Salivary gland neoplasms are uncommon in children, <5% occurring in <16y.
- The types of tumours occurring in children and adults are the same but they occur at different frequencies.
- Benign lesions in children are more likely to represent haemangiomas/vascular malformations than adenomas.
- Rapid enlargement of a salivary mass without evidence of infection suggests malignancy.
- A solitary salivary lesion in a child is more likely to represent a malignant tumour (>50%) than in an adult (25%).
- Both benign and malignant neoplasms affect the parotid more than the submandibular gland.
- Mucoepidermoid carcinomas are the most common tumours (50%) followed by acinic cell carcinomas (15—20%).
- High-grade malignancies tend to occur in younger children.
- Some reports suggest that there is an overall higher rate of local recurrence and cervical node metastasis in children compared to adults with the same tumour.

Paediatric nasal obstruction

The causes and effect of nasal obstruction depend on the age of the child. Neonates are obligate nasal breathers until 3 months old ∴ bilateral nasal obstruction in this age group can present as an emergency at birth.

Bilateral nasal obstruction in older children is unlikely to cause a life-threatening problem unless it is associated with obstructive sleep apnoea or the obstructing cause is neoplastic.

Table 23.12 lists the causes of paediatric nasal obstruction.

History
Neonate
Complete nasal blockage in the neonate can present as an emergency airway obstruction at birth requiring the immediate insertion and securing of an oral airway or orotracheal intubation.

Snuffly babies with rhinorrhoea is a common, often harmless scenario but if there is a significant disturbance of airway, sleep, feeding, and/or growth then further investigation is necessary.

Symptoms
- Struggling to breath, often eased by crying.
- Inability to settle.
- Poor sleep.
- Apnoeas.
- Cyanotic attacks.
- Feeding difficulties.
- Gasping for air during feeds.
- Colic due to air swallowing.
- Chronic nasal obstruction leading to failure to thrive.

Child
Rarely would nasal obstruction represent acute airway emergency in an older child but chronic nasal blockage causes symptoms ranging from mild stuffiness to failure to thrive.

Symptoms
Symptoms suggesting significant pathology include:
- Nasal infections.
- Persistent rhinorrhea, unilateral or bilateral.
- Significant obstructive symptoms, including sleep apnoea and poor feeding, usually suggest a combination of nasopharyngeal and oropharyngeal obstruction usually adenotonsillar hypertrophy.
- History of atopy.
- Family history of atopy.
- Exposure to URTI in particular at nursery.

Table 23.12 Causes of paediatric nasal obstruction

Causes	Baby	Older child
Congenital		
Nasal malformation/agenesis/stenosis	+	
Choanal atresia	+	
Dermoid cyst	+	
Nasal glioma	+	
Meningoencephalocoele	+	
Haemangioma	+	+
Acquired		
Infective rhinitis	+	++
Allergic rhinitis	+	+++
Adenoidal hypertrophy		+++
Foreign body		+
Angiofibroma		+
Rhabdomyosarcoma		+
Idiopathic	+	+++
Rhinitis	++	+
Associated with systemic disease		
Cystic fibrosis		+
Immotile cilia syndrome		+

Physical examination

- Assess for signs of upper airway obstruction (mainly in neonates).
  - Laboured breathing at rest.
  - Stertor.
  - Soft-tissue recession.
  - Use of accessory muscles.
- Examine external nose for depressed nasal bridge, pits, or masses.
- Test nasal airflow using either wisps of cotton wool or place a metal tongue depressor under the nose to detect the mist of exhaled air (mist test).
- In a neonate, use gentle suction to clear secretions and see if airway improves. Suction mucus from nose, if necessary. Saline drops may be administrated to facilitate suctioning, while 0.25% phenylephridrine will allow comparison of congested and decongested mucosa.
- In neonates, assessment of nasal patency should also include passage of a soft nasal catheter (5–6FR) to at least 32mm to exclude choanal atresia. Trauma to nose may make airway worse ∴ ensure support (e.g. nurse, suction, access to oxygen, resus trolley) is available.

- Perform anterior rhinoscopy by using a thumb to lift up the tip of the nose and head light for illumination or gently insert an otoscope with a large speculum.
- Examine oropharynx and perform posterior rhinoscopy using angled mirror if child is cooperative.
- Examine the ears looking for evidence of malformation or glue ear.
- Complete the head and neck examination by looking for signs of other craniofacial disorders/syndromes associated with nasal obstruction.
- Look for signs of adenoidal facies (see 📖 p. 774).
- Consider general paediatric disease, which can have manefestations in the nose (see 📖 p. 781).

Investigations

A good history and examination are often sufficient but certain diagnoses can be helped by the use of the following investigations.

Nasendoscopy

This can be performed using flexible nasendoscope or 2.7mm Stortz-Hopkins rigid scope and local decongestant/anaesthetic spray. It allows examination of entire nasal passages and post-nasal space. It is an extremely useful if the child will tolerate an invasive procedure. Neoates with significant nasal obstruction and airway compromise may need this perfomed in theatre with anaesthetic backup, as trauma or blockage to the airway may result in respiratory compromise.

Imaging

Imaging can be helpful in selected cases:
- X-ray PNS can be used to assess the size of adenoids, although accuracy is doubtful.
- CT scanning provides high-definition scan of sino-nasal passages and can detect bony abnormalities, such as choanal atresia, piriform aperture stenosis, dermoids, gliomas, and other nasal and paranasal tumours. There is a high false-positive rate for rhinosinusistis, with 40% of asymptomatic children having coincidental CT changes suggestive of sinusitis. Therefore imaging of the sinuses should be reserved for selected cases, in particular where there is evidence of major structural abnormalities, complications or neoplastic pathology.
- MRI is helpful in the assessment of nasal lesions with possible intracranial extensions.

Skin tests

Skin testing plays an important role in determining allergic rhinitis from other causes of rhinitis and identifying the particular allergens responsible but may not be tolerated in younger children.

The alternative is a radioallergoabsorbent test (RAST), which looks for the presence of serum IgE to specific allergens. This tends to be less sensitive than skin testing.

Blood tests

Useful blood tests include:

- A full blood count looking for infection, esosinophilia.
- Thyroid-function tests (congenital hyperthyroidism may manifest as bilateral nasal obstruction).
- RAST to detect inhaled (grasses, house dust mite, cat hair) and ingested (wheat, milk, soya, egg white) allergens.
- An immunoglobulin screen looking for G subclass or specific Ig A immunodeficiencies.
- Haemophilus influenzae and streptococcus pneumoniae antibodies following immunization against these common 'URTI' causing organisms.

Nasal swabs/smears

These can be performed looking for evidence of infection or eosinophilia suggestive of allergic rhinosinusitis.

Nasal brushings

Can be performed to test cilliary function. Children >6 may cooperative with saccharine transport tests.

Sleep study

May be performed if sleep apnoea suspected.

Management of specific nasal conditions

Idiopathic neonatal rhinitis

Some neonates suffer from rhinitis causing nasal obstruction and discharge. In the absence of any bacterial, viral, or allergic cause, it is thought that faulty autonomic control or gastro-oesophageal reflux is to blame. Most patients benefit from simple extraction of the mucus using a nasal mucus-sucker aided by saline or topical steroid drops.

Choanal atresia

Choanal atresia is thought to be due to either failure of breakdown of the buccopharyngeal membrane or the persistence of epithelial rest cells, which proliferate in the nasal cavities during the 6th–8th week of intra-uterine development (Fig. 23.13). It occurs in 1 in 8000 births and is twice as common in girls. The atretic plate can be predominantly bony (90%) or membranous (10%).

Choanal atresia can occur in isolation or associated with other congenital abnormalities (70%), most commonly Charge association (30%) (see ☐ p. 734). A non-syndromic type can be autosomal recessive.

Presentation
- Bilateral atresia causes respiratory distress in the newborn, which improves when the baby cries.
- Unilateral usually presents later as unilateral obstruction or discharge.
- Suspected by failure to pass catheter more than 32mm past the anterior nares.
- Diagnosis confirmed by CT scan showing extent of bony and soft tissue involvement.

Treatment
- Urgent stabilization of airway is required in bilateral cases. The obstruction can temporarily be managed by taping in place an oral airway or orotracheal intubation. An orogastric feeding tube is also inserted.
- Surgical repair can be transnasal or transpalatal. The transnasal route is the preferred route initially and has been made much simpler by endoscopic techniques.
- Surgery can be deferred until child is older in unilateral cases where there is no airway compromise.

Operative notes

Transnasal approach
- Boyle–Davis gag and 120-degree endoscope are placed to inspect post nasal space.
- Decongestant drops are inserted into the nasal cavities followed by gentle suction and inspection with 0-degree Hopkins' rod.
- Once the diagnosis is confirmed the atretic plate, if predominantly membranous or thin bone, can be punctured and sequentially dilated using female urethral dilators passed through the nostril into the nasopharynx.

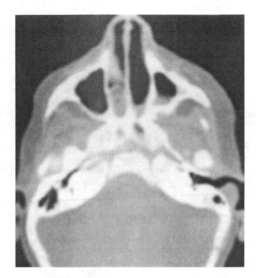

Fig. 23.13 Axial of nasal cavities demonstrating choanal atresia.

- The initial puncture should be endoscopically directed through the thinnest point of the atretic plate which is usually at the junction of the floor of the nose and posterior part of the nasal septum.
- Aim to dilate as large as possible (nostril size permitting) as a degree of restenosis is inevitable. Avoid forcing the dilators as this can result in basisphenoid fractures.
- Most atretic plates are predominantly bony and require drilling out.
- The posterior choanae are enlarged using a Choanal Atresia drill or combination of cutting and diamond burrs introduced transnasally and guided by visualization of the post-nasal space with the 120-degree scope. Laser ablation has also been used but most surgeons prefer cold steel methods.
- If using a burr, use an aural speculum to prevent damage to the alar margins. The oral surface of the palate must also be observed for mucosal blanching which is a sign of impending perforation through the palatal mucosa.
- Avoid excessive bone removal superiorly on the basisphenoid and beware of damaging the greater palatine and sphenopalatine arteries laterally. Also aim to remove the posterior end of the septum over a distance of 7mm.

Preventing restenosis

A degree of restenosis is inevitable. Some authors advocate trying to preserve a flap of mucosa covering the bony atretic plate, reflect it laterally whilst drilling, and then use it to cover the raw bony edges. This is very difficult to perform due to the small space within the posterior choanae.

Many surgeons recommend insertion of stents for 6 weeks. These can be made by cutting a size 3.5 portex tube (Fig. 23.14). The length of stent is then judged by introducing a portex tube into the nose until it is visible in the post-nasal space. A section of tube is then removed to allow non-traumatic positioning across the columnella and for insertion of catheters for later suctioning. The stent is then positioned in the nasal cavity and a catheter is passed into each stent lumen, into each nasal cavity, and introduced into the oropharynx, where they are attached to two ends of a 1.0 nylon suture thread. The catheters are then withdrawn nasally, pulling with them the suture that is tied over the columnella bridge of the stent. The stent is then assessed for excessive movement and pressure on the nares is avoided by close observation.

The patency of the stents is maintained by regular saline drops and suction. The stent is removed in outpatients and a short course of topical steroid drops given.

If nasal osbstruction develops, then a repeat procedure may be required. For repeated restenosis, mitomycin C has been used but the long-term effects of this are still unknown.

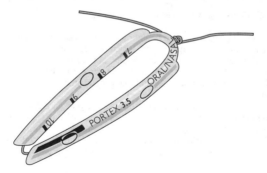

Fig. 23.14 Nasopharyngeal stents fashioned and secured with a suture.

Fig. 23.14 and 23.15 taken from chapter 28. Operative otorhinolaryngology. Bleach Milford & Van Hasselt. Blackwell Science.

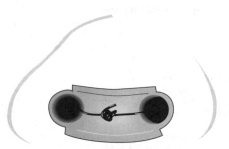

Fig. 23.15 Nasopharyngeal stents fashioned and secured with a suture - columnella view.

Transpalatal approach

Some feel that the transpalatal approach allows better visualization and is associated with a decreased risk of restenosis. It is a longer, more invasive procedure and often reserved for the older child.

- The Boyle–Davis gag is inserted.
- After infiltration, a curved incision is made starting level with the maxillary tuberosities, medial to the greater palatine foramen, coming anteriorly parallel to the alveolar ridge or gingivopalatal magin, if teeth are present.
- The mucoperisoteum is elevated to expose the bony margins of the palate.
- A diamond burr is then used to remove the bony atretic plate and posterior end of the septum.
- The mucoperiosteal flap is then repositioned and sutured.
- Transnasal stenting is performed as previously described.

Overall complications

Basishenoid fracture, spinal cord injury, palatal fistula, and alar/columnella necrosis secondary to stent use.

Piriform aperture stenosis

This is a rare condition caused by overgrowth of the medial aspect of the maxillae causing marked anterior nasal obstruction, which can significantly affect nasal airflow.

The classic finding is a shelf-like projection into the posterior nasal vestibule. The obstruction is confirmed on CT scanning. Nasal saline drops are the 1st-line treatment to keep the nasal passages patent, but if these fail, surgery may be required. This involves drilling open both sides of the pirifrom aperture via a sublabial incision. Temporary splints may applied for temporary swelling post operatively.

Bilateral congenital dacrocystoceles

This is a rare condition also know as congenital nasolacrimal duct cyst. It presents as a unilateral or bilateral nasal swelling, causing nasal obstruction and airway compromise in 50% of cases. Diagnosis can be confirmed in CT or MRI. Treatment involves marsupialization of the cysts.

Nasal malformations

Minor nasal deviations require no treatment and often improve with age. If the nasal septum is grossly deviated causing nasal obstruction and further deviation to the nasal tip as it grows, then a septoplasty may be performed. This is not to be considered lightly because disturbing the septal growth plate during septoplasty may also have a major impact on the resultant development of the nose.

Nasal malformations commonly occur in association with cleft lip. The nasal tip and septum can be distorted and deviated. Rhinoplasty may be required at the time of cleft lip repair. More severe deformities in association with other craniofacial malformations require a multidisciplinary team approach.

Nasal masses

Nasal masses in children are rare and should be treated with suspicion. Unlike adults, inflammatory nasal polyps are unusual in children and if present may raise the suspicion of a mucociliary clearance disorder, such as cystic fibrosis.

The most important true nasal masses to be aware of are gliomas, dermoids, and meningoencephalocoeles. It is essential that imaging is performed prior to considering any surgery to determine whether there is any intracranial extension. A CT scan will detect a bony defects suggesting intracranial extension, such as an enlarged foramen caecum and/or bifid crista galli, whereas MRI gives better soft-tissue definition and may demonstrate intracranial extension.

Nasal dermoids

Nasal dermoids can present as solid tumours, cysts, or sinuses containing hair, anywhere in the midline of the nose. They are formed as the result of sequestration of ectomesodermal elements following fusion of the medial nasal processes; consequently they may extend intra-cranially. The diagnosis can be delayed until adolescence or adulthood, and may only manifest if infection occurs.

Treatment is surgical excision, usually via some form of external nasal excision, including external rhinoplasty approach. The intracranial dermoids may require a combined intra and extracranial approach.

Nasal gliomas and meningoencephalocoeles

These congenital masses probably share a common origin, which is defective closure of the anterior neuropore, hence the anterior cranial fossa. Encephalocoeles or meningoencepphalocoeles retain their communication with the subarachnoid space, whereas gliomas become detached from the intracranial cavity by closure of skull sutures, although in some cases (15%) a connecting fibrous tract remains.

Nasal gliomas

These are solid masses that occur more frequently in males. They can occur entirely outside the nasal cavity (60%), entirely within the nasal cavity (30%), or both (10%). They are frequently associated with other congenital abnormalities. Most cases are diagnosed soon after birth, presenting as a mass or nasal obstruction that does not increase with straining or crying. These lesions tend to enlarge with age and treatment is by excision. Endoscopic debridement of the intranasal lesions with endoscopic repair of any small skull base defect is now becoming the favoured approach.

Meningoencephaloceles

These lesions represent herniation of the meninges with ectopic brain tissue that can extend over the nasal dorsum or intra-nasally or both. They can be differentiated from gliomas by Furstenberg's sign: an increase in the size of the mass with crying or jugular vein compression. Their intracranial connection means that they can present with CSF rhinorrhoea and meningitis. Treatment is by surgical excision. Traditionally this was approached by frontal craniotomy but more recently these lesions have been removed endoscopically combined with transnasal repair of the CSF leak.

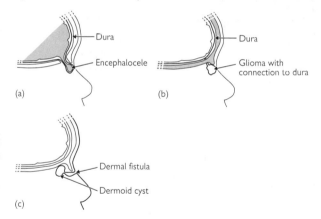

Fig. 23.16 a–c Differentiating features of encephalocele, glioma and dermoid cyst.

Childhood nasal obstruction

Adenoidal hypertrophy and allergic rhinitis are the most common causes of nasal obstruction in childhood.

Adenoidal hypertrophy

The adenoid (pharyngeal tonsil) is a triangular mass of lymphoid tissue located in the nasophaynx. It enlarges during early childhood as a response to various inhaled antigens and usually regresses by late childhood.

It has a role in mucocilliary clearance, antigen processing, and immune surveillance in childhood. Adenoidal hypertrophy is the most common cause of nasal obstruction in children age 3–7.

Adenoidal infection and hypertrophy can lead to complications:

- Stasis of mucocillary clearance, persistent rhinorrhoea and post-nasal drip.
- Nasal blockage.
- Obstructive sleep apnoea, usually combined with oropharygeal obstruction secondary to large tonsils.[*]
- Cor pulmonale secondary to the OSA.
- Recurrent AOM/glue ear.
- Hyponasal speech.
- Cough.
- Hallitosis.
- Failure to thrive.
- Poor orofacial development associated with nasal obstruction secondary to adenoidal hypertrophy causing child to adopt mouth open and head up position. This has been described as adenoidal facies and has the following features:
  - Thin dry upper lip.
  - Retrognathic mandible.
  - Narrowed maxilla.
  - Broad nasal arch.
  - Up-turned nose with visible nostrils.
  - Cervical spine complications.

Treatment of adenoiditis or hypertrophy is determined by the complications manifested.

Antibiotics

A trial of prophylactive antibiotics, e.g. directed towards betalactamase-producing organisms may help resolve adenoiditis associated with recurrent acute otitis media and otitis media with effusion, halitosis, post-nasal drip leading to halitosis, chronic tonsillitis and cough.

Nasal steroids

May help reduce adenoidal hyperplasia and will also treat any associated allergic rhinitis.

Adenoidectomy

The most common treatment for adenoidal problems is adenoidectomy.

---

[*] Tonsillar problems are discussed in chapter 6.

Indications for adenoidectomy
Obstruction
- Chronic nasal obstruction/mouth breathing.
- Obstructive sleep apnoea.
- Failure to thrive.

Infection
- Recurrent/chronic adenoiditis.
- Recurrent/chronic otitis media with effusion.
- Recurrent acute otitis media.

Neoplasia
- Suspected benign or malignant.

Operative notes
- Adenoidectomy is performed under general anaesthetic using an endotracheal tube or laryngeal mask.
- The child is positioned supine supported with a head ring and shoulder bag. Overextension of the neck should be avoided as this increases risk of pre-vertebral muscle damage and cervical spine injuries, this is particularly true in children with downs syndrome.
- A Boyle–Davis gag is inserted and the palate is palpated for a submucosal cleft (a notch felt in the back of the hard palate). This is a relative contraindication to adenoidectomy but in the case of severe OSA or glue ear, superior or lateral adenoids can be carefully removed.
- Two methods are now described. Many surgeons favour the latter in small children (<3y, <15kg) as there is lower risk of primary haemorrhage.

Cold-steel technique
- A finger is placed in the post-nasal space to confirm the presence of large adenoids.
- A curette is introduced through the mouth into the nasopharynx until it can be felt against posterior choanae.
- The curette is pressed down firmly onto adenoidal bed and swept down into oropharynx scraping the adenoidal tissue from the posterior nasal pharyngeal wall. Avoid curetting too laterally to prevent damaging the eustachian tube.
- A smaller curette can be swept around the Eustachian cushions.
- The post-nasal space is packed with gauze swabs for 5min to allow haemostasis.
- The packs are removed and residual clots are suctioned via nasal catheter and the head is tilted upwards to check residual bleeding has stopped.
- If bleeding continues, the adenoidal bed should be felt for residual adenoids, if present repeat the curettage and consider repacking with adrenalin soaked swabs (1 : 1000).
- If possible, bleeding areas should be identified with the mirror and diathermied.
- If bleeding persists a post-nasal pack should be inserted and child transfered to HDU post op as pack can compromise airway.

Suction diathermy technique

- This technique uses a combination of monopolar diathermy and suction to perform a controlled resection of the adenoids in a near bloodless field. A clear view of the entire resection is obtained with a mirror and a nasal catheter to retract the soft palate.
- A malleable suction diathermy instrument is angled to reach into the posterior choanae. Using a mirror, the instrument is stroked across the adenoidal pad vapourizing it away until the posterior choanae can be seen.
- The suction tip is used to clear smoke and blood.
- As it is performed under direct vision minor oozing can be dealt with immediately and no packing is necessary. Adenoids extending into the posterior choanae can be removed with ease.

Complications of adenoidectomy

These include:

- Primary haemorrhage <1%.
- Secondary haemorrhage 1.7–4.4 % depending on the technique.[1]
- Infection.
- Temporary smelly rhinorrhea and halitosis, particularly with suction diathermy technique.
- Inflammation/infection of cervical fascia and spinal ligaments.
- Torticollis.
- C-spine subluxation (particular care must be taken with Down syndrome children who are at risk of this complication).

Post-adenoidectomy haemorrhage

This is the main complication of adenoidectomy and failure to recognize and deal with this problem effectively can have life-threatening results. Post-operative bleeding can occur at any time within the first 2 weeks following the surgery. The child usually presents with epistaxis, spitting out, or swallowing blood. Minor bleeds with a history of minimal blood loss may settle with decongestant nose drops and antibiotics. It is important to remember that it may be difficult to estimate the amount of blood that has been swallowed. The child should be assessed for signs of hypovolaemia. Intravenous access, FBC, clotting, GandS ± cross match chould be performed. (See 📖 p. 674 for the management of haemorrhage in children.) If there are signs of ongoing active bleeding, then the child may need to return to theatre to stop the bleeding, using packing or diathermy as previously described.

---

1 (Walker 2001).

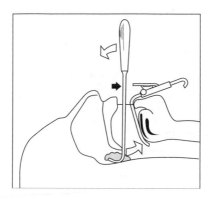

Fig. 23.17 Adenoidectomy curettage.

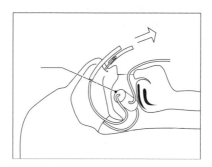

Fig. 23.18 Nasopharyngeal packing placement.

Rhinitis in children

Rhinitis is the most common cause of chronic nasal obstruction, particularly in older children. This topic has been extensively discussed in Chapter 20 but it is worth mentioning some factors about rhinitis that are predominantly related to children.

The most common cause of chronic rhinitis in children is allergic rhinitis. There may be a family history of atopy, including asthma and eczema. 75% of astmatics suffer from rhinitits, 20% of rhinitis sufferers have asthma. There is often also a strong family history of atopy. If there is one atopic parent, the risk of a child being atopic is 38–58%, this increases to 60–80% if both parents are atopic.

Causes of allergic rhinitis

In younger children the allergens tend to be perennial allergens such as house dust-mite. As a child gets older, grass pollen allergens become more common.

Food allergy rarely causes allergic rhinitis in isolation but can give rise to nasal symptoms as part of an allergic response, usually including eczema. If so, the response is usually rapid occurring within 15min of ingestion.

Allergy to milk protein has been associated increase in rhinitis and mucus production.

Presentation

The main nasal symptoms are:
- Bilateral nasal blockage.
- Rhinorrhoea.
- Sneezing.
- Itching of the palate and nose.
- Post-nasal drip.
- Anosmia.
- Symptoms of an ongoing cold.

These symptoms can be severe enough to impair quality of life, disturb sleep, and cause poor performance at school. On examination the following may suggest allergic rhinitis:
- Poor nasal air entry.
- Clear nasal discharge.
- Congested blue boggy or pale nasal mucosa.
- Hypertrophic inferior turbinates.

Other features characteritic of rhinitic include:
- Allergic 'shiners'—these are dark peri-orbital circles caused by chronic venous and lymphatic stasis in the peri-orbital region, secondary to chronic airway oedema.
- Dennie's line—this is a transverse nasal crease caused by rubbing the nose to relieve the pruritis.
- The hard palate may show petechail haemorrhages caused by negative pressures created by the tongue in an attempt to scratch to relieve palatal itching.

- There may be evidence of associated Eustachian-tube dysfunction, glue ears, or retracted tympanic membranes.
- There may also be other signs of atopy including eczema or asthma.

The differential diagnosis of allergic rhinitis includes the following:
- Vasomotor rhinitis.
- Adenoidal hypertrophy.
- Mucocillary disorders such as cystic fibrosis, immotile cilia should be suspected if nasal polyps are present.
- Structural abnormalities such as septal deviation, foreign bodies, unilateral choanal atresia should be considered if symptoms are predominantly unilateral.

Management

It is important in children to treat rhinitis for the following reasons:
- To improve symptom control, which may be affecting quality of life and leading to poor concentration at school or poor sleeping.
- It has been shown that early treatment of allergy may reduce development of worsening allergy in the future, probably as it has an effect on the developing immune system (T helper 1/T Helper 2 ratio) to cause a shift from allergy to tolerance.
- It may also prevent allergic rhinitis exacerbating bronchial hyperresponsiveness, as there is a suggestion that asthma may be a sequelae of continued antigen exposure.

A detailed discussion of the varying medications in allergic rhinitis is covered in Chapter 20 Here we focus on the drugs most commonly used among the paediatric population. These include:
- Antihistamines. Probably remain first drug of choice for children, as they can be taken orally. They help with the nasal itch and hypersecretion more so than the nasal mucosa oedema. The newer brands, such as loratidine and cetrizine, are known to be less sedating and do not cause cardiac arythmias.
- Corticosteroids. These are extremely effective in the treatment of allergic rhinitis. Some topical nasal sprays are now licensed for use in as young as 4 years old. They are sometimes even used down to 2 years old but compliance can be a problem. There are concerns about the systemic effects of topical steroids on growth but there is little evidence to support it in most of the sprays. However, it is worth monitoring growth in children on inhaled steroids for asthma too.
- Cromolyn. This mast-cell stabilizer is useful in the treatment of allergic rhinitis but it requires use up to 6 times daily.
- Decongestants have little place in chronic allergic rhinitis, as their prolonged use can lead to rhinitis medicamentosa.
- Immunotherapy is also called desensitization or hyposensitization. This is usually reserved for patients where the specific allergic allergen is known and is not controlled by optimum avoidance measures and other nasal sprays or antihistamines. The desensitization programme can take several years. It usually requires regular subcutaneous injections but sublingual therapy is now becoming available for some allergens such as grass.

Medical conditions associated with nasal symptoms

Cystic fibrosis

Nasal polyposis is one of the manifestations of cystic fibrosis. Nasal steroids can be used for the milder cases but most will require surgery for symptomatic relef at some stage. These cases can be difficult because the polyps tend to re-occur and extensive sinus surgery can prove difficult because of the grossly distorted nasal anatomy.

Immotile cilia syndrome

The poor functioning cilia predispose these patients to sinusitis, otitis media, and bronchiectasis. Medical treatment including nasal douching should be considered but endoscopic sinus surgery and turbinectomy may be necessary.

Juvenile angiofibromatosis

See Chapter 20.

Nasal tumours

- The most common benign growth affecting the nose is a haemangioma. Spontaneous involution may occur but if not, or there is evidence of complications, steroids, laser, or surgery may be required (for treatment of haemangiomas see 📖 p. 750).
- The most common malignant tumours are lymphomas and rhabdomyosarcomas. The treatment of both of these malignancies has been discussed in more detail.
- Nasopharyngeal carcinoma can present in young teenagers. The treatment is the same as for adults and is described in Chapter 20 on 📖 pp. 672–3.

Minor procedures in ENT

How to remove foreign bodies

You will need:
- A good light.
- A cooperative patient.
- Good equipment.

The first attempt will usually be the best-tolerated. If you are not confident that you will be able to remove the foreign body, refer to ENT for more experienced help.

Foreign bodies in the ear
Signs and symptoms
- Pain.
- Deafness.
- Unilateral discharge.
- Bleeding.
- May be symptomless.

Management
- Children will usually require a general anaesthetic unless they are remarkably cooperative.
- Insects may be drowned with olive oil.
- Syringing may be used, if you can be certain there is no trauma to the ear canal or drum.
- Use a head-lamp or mirror, an operating auroscope or an operating microscope.
- Soft foreign bodies, such as cottonwool, may be grasped with a pair of crocodile or Tilley's forceps.
- Solid foreign bodies, such as a bead, are best remove by passing a wax hook or Jobson–Horne probe beyond the foreign body and gently pulling towards you.

Refer to senior staff ± GA if
- Failed attempt.
- Uncooperative child.
- Suspected trauma to the drum.

Foreign bodies in the nose
Signs and symptoms
- Unilateral foul-smelling discharge.
- Unilateral nasal obstruction.
- Unilateral vestibulitis.
- Epistaxis.

Management
- An auroscope can easily be used to examine a child's nose.
- Ask the child to blow their nose if they are able.
- Solid foreign bodies, such as beads, are best removed by passing a wax hook or Jobson–Horne probe beyond the foreign body and gently pulling it towards you. Avoid grasping the object with a pair of forceps, since this may simply push it further back into the nose or airway.

- Soft foreign bodies may be grasped and removed with crocodile or Tilley's forceps.

Refer to senior staff if
- Failed removal.
- Uncooperative child.

Foreign bodies in the throat

The cause is often fish, chicken, or lamb bones.

Signs and symptoms
- Acute onset of symptoms (not days later).
- Constant pricking sensation on every swallow.
- Drooling.
- Dysphagia.
- Localized tenderness in the neck; if above the thyroid cartilage, then look carefully in the tongue base and tonsil regions.
- Pain on rocking the larynx from side to side.
- Soft tissue swelling.

Management
- Use a good light to examine the patient.
- Anaesthetize the throat using Xylocaine spray.
- Try feeling for a foreign body (FB), even if you cannot see one in the tonsil or tongue base.
- Flecks of calcification around the thyroid cartilage are common on X-ray.
- Perform an AP and lateral soft-tissue X-ray of the neck looking for foreign bodies at the common sites (see Fig. 24.1). Pay particular attention to the:
  - Tonsil.
  - Tongue base/vallecula.
  - Posterior pharyngeal wall.
- Tilley's forceps are best for removing foreign bodies in the mouth.
- McGill's intubating forceps may be useful for removing foreign bodies in the tongue base or pharynx.

Consider for endoscopy under GA in case of
- Airway compromise—**URGENT!**
- Failed removal.
- Good history but no FB seen.
- X-ray evidence of a FB.

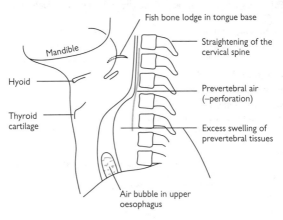

Fig. 24.1 Lateral soft tissues X-ray of the neck.

How to syringe an ear

See Fig. 24.2. Check that the patient has no previous history of TM perforation, grommet insertion, middle ear, or mastoid surgery.

Procedure
- Warm the water to body temperature.
- Pull the pinna up and back.
- Use a dedicated ear syringe.
- Aim the jet of water towards the roof of the ear canal.
- STOP if the patient complains of pain.

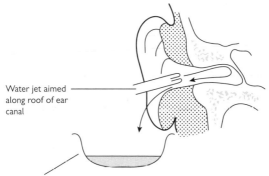

Water jet aimed
along roof of ear
canal

Basin to collect water, placed
under the ear.
Held in position by the patient

Fig. 24.2 How to syringe an ear.

How to dry mop an ear

A dry mop should be performed in any ear that is discharging, before topical antibiotics and steroid ear drops are instilled.

Procedure

- Tease out a clean piece of cottonwool into a flat sheet.
- Twist this onto a suitable carrier, such as an orange stick, a Jobson–Horne probe, or even a clean matchstick (see Fig. 24.3).
- Gently rotate the soft end of the mop in the outer ear canal.
- Discard the cottonwool and make a new mop—continue until the wool is returned clean.

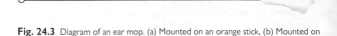

Fig. 24.3 Diagram of an ear mop. (a) Mounted on an orange stick, (b) Mounted on a Jobson Horne Probe.

How to instill ear drops

See Fig. 24.4.

Procedure
- Lie the patient down with the affected ear uppermost.
- Straighten the ear canal by pulling the pinna up and back.
- Squeeze in the appropriate number of drops.
- Use a gentle pumping motion of your finger in the outer ear canal. This will encourage the drops to penetrate into the deep ear canal.

Consider using an 'otowick'. This is like a preformed sponge and it acts as a reservoir, helping to prevent the drops leaking out of the ear canal. An otowick is particularly useful in otitis externa.

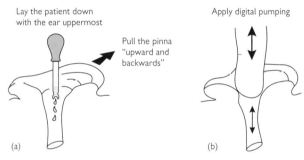

Lay the patient down
with the ear uppermost

Pull the pinna
"upward and
backwards"

Apply digital pumping

(a)   (b)

Fig. 24.4 How to instill ear drops.

How to drain a quinsy

Signs and symptoms
- Sore throat—worse on one side.
- Pyrexia.
- Trismus.
- Drooling.
- Fetor.
- Peritonsillar swelling.
- Displacement of the uvula away from the affected side (see Fig. 24.5).

Procedure
- This procedure usually requires admission.
- Re-hydrate with IV fluids.
- IV antibiotics.
- Spray the throat with xylocaine or inject lignocaine into the mucosa as shown.
- Lie the patient down.
- Get a good light and a sucker.
- Use a 5ml syringe and a large bore needle or IV cannula to perform 3-point aspiration (see Fig. 24.5).
- Send any pus obtained to microbiology.
- Reserve incision for those cases which recur or fail to resolve within 24h.

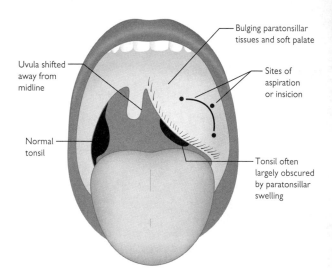

Fig. 24.5 Quinsy/incision/aspiration.

ENT numbers

Head and neck

Subject	Data
Salivary Gland Neoplasms	80% Parotid, of these 80% benign
	30% of SMG malignant
	50% of Minor salivary gland tumours malignant
Spilled pleomorphic in Parotid surgery	30% chance of recurrence without DXT
	5% chance of recurrence with DXT
	50% chance of Facial palsy in surgery for recurrence
	0.7% chance of DXT induced primary
Mucoepidermoids	90% low grade
	10% high grade = Malignant of these 40% 5y 40% N+
Malignant Parotid Tumours	1.2 : 100 000
	43% superficial lobe, 27% both, 10% deep
	20% Extra-glandular spread
	Ca Ex-pleomorphic 3% risk in 10y
Warthins Tumours	10% bilateral,
	7 : 1 M : F,
	>70y,
	7% of all salivary gland tumours
Paediatric Salivary Tumours	80% in parotid
	60% of all tumours are malignant
	50% of malignant tumours are mucoepidermoid
Minor salivary gland cancer	Adenoidcystic carcinoma 40%
	Adenocarcinoma 30%
	Mucoepidermoid cancer 20%
Radio-opaque stones	Submandibular gland 65%
	Parotid 35%
Some causes of bilateral parotid enlargement	Vitamin deficiency
	Malnutrition
	Diabetes
	Obesity
	Sjögrens syndrome
	Malabsorption
	Cirrhosis

(Contd.)	
Facial nerve involvement	20% of Adenocarcinoma
	20% of Adenoid cystic carcinoma
Malignancy in salivary gland tumours	Parotid 32%
	Submandibular 41%
	Minor 60%
Survival figures for salivary gland cancer. (5y survival)	Mucoepidermoid
	(low grade)–92%
	(High grade)–49%
	Adenoid cystic carcinoma–30%
	Squamous cell carcinoma–26%
Ways to identify the facial nerve	1. Identify posterior belly of digastric. Following back toward digastric ridge. Nerve lies just superior to digastric muscle at insertion and on the same sagittal plane
	2. Identify the tympano-mastoid suture line- nerve lies inferior and deep to this point
	3. Identify the buccal branch
	4. Identify the tragal pointer. One centime- tre deep and one cm inferior to this point
Sjögren's syndrome	10% chance of developing a Lymphoma
Lump in the throat	4% of all ENT referrals
Incidence of H&N cancer in primary care	150 consultations by GP: referral for ANY neoplasm
	Average British GP can expect 1 laryngeal Ca every 13 years
Nutrition in H&N cancer	Weight loss >10% has significant effects on local control rates
Undiagnosed Primary	50% will identify primary on ENT examination
	40% will identify primary on panendoscopy
Node +ve neck	N+ve neck reduces the 5y survival by half
N +ve	In the N+ve neck, 65% of nodes <3cm will have Extracapsular spread
Identification of Neck nodes	Palpation 20–30% false negative, 70% sensitive
	CT 85% sensitive
	MRI 81% sensitive (but more specific)
	USS & FNA >95% specific & 75% sensitive

(Contd.)

When to treat the N0 neck?	If the risk of metastases = 15% (which it is for most advanced H&N Ca's)
N1 neck & DXT	81% local control
DXT & the Neck	Palliative dose 45Gy
	Prophylactic dose 50Gy (eliminates 95% of micro mets)
	Curative dose 70Gy
Risk from Smoking in H&N Cancer	<10/day increases risk by 2.4
	>25/day increases risk by 16.4
Risk in Patterson-Brown/ Plummer Vinson Syndrome	90% Female
	Scandinavian descent
	Iron deficiency anaemia
	Upper oesophageal web
	Glossitis
	Gastritis
	2–15% risk of developing post-cricoid Ca
	10% of post-cricoid Cas have a web
Hypopharyngeal Ca	<1 : 100 000
	60% Pyiform fossa
	30% Post-cricoid
	10% Posterior wall
	Skip lesions in 10%
	60% N+ve, of these 60% bilateral
	60% die within 1 year
	25–30% 5 year survival
Glomus Tumours	5% Malignant
	10% Multiple
	10% Secrete
	Otoscopy Abnormal in 50% of tympanicums, & 40% of Jugulares
	Fisch Classification
	A – middle ear
	B – Tympanomastoid
	C – Infralabrynthine
	D – Intracranial
Risk of Ca in Situ developing into invasive disease	Mid cord 17%
	Anterior commisure 92%
Carcinoma in situ	If treated with DXT –25% will later require laryngectomy
	If treated with cordectomy, 3% will need laryngectomy

(Contd.)	
Risk of SCC in VC dysplasia	Mild dysplasia – 2.5%
	Moderate Dysplasia – 13.5%
	Severe Dysplasia – 28.8%
	Risk of 2nd primary 21%
Stomal recurrence	Incidence 5–15%
	Classification
	1 – superior
	2 – posterior
	3 – inferior
	4 – lateral
	1&2 do better than 3&4
Settings for CO_2 laser	6W, 0.8mm, 0.1 sec pulsed for papillomata, etc.
	10W, 0.6mm, continuous for arytenoidectomy, etc.
Vocal cord paralysis	25% malignant
	25% iatrogenic
	15% Idiopathic
	15% External trauma
Supraclavicular mets	60% SCC
	20% AdenoCa
	10% Undifferentiated
Sinonasal tumours	1 : 100 000
	66% maxillary most of the rest ethmoidal
	50% SCC
	10% lymphomas
	15% anaplastic
	5% Adenocarcinoma
	4% Adenoid-cystic
	Surgery or DXT 20% 5y
	Surgery & DXT 45% 5y

(Contd.)	
Inverted papilloma	<2%chance of malignant transformation
	5% of all sinonasal tumours
	0.4 : 100 000
	HPV 6,11,16, identified in 40%
	(HPV 16 increased risk of SCC)
	EBV DNA identified in 60%
	7% synchronous SCC
	2.5% metacranous SCC
	10–30% multicentric
	overall recurrence rate 30%
	60% conservative resection
	16% med maxillectomy
Recurrent respiratory papillomatosis	1 : 100 000
	bimodal distribution @5 & 20y
	10% progress to involve bronchus
	1% pulmonary
Laryngeal tumours	95% malignant
	5% Benign
	55% Glottic
	40% Supraglottic
T3 Larynx presentation	50% in fact T4 on final stagnig
Tongue base tumours	65% N+ve, of these 25% bilateral
	20% of patients with undiagnosed primary will have tongue base Ca
	20% die from recurrent primary
	10% die from neck disease
	10% die from distant mets
	30% of survivors develop 2nd Primary & 66% of these die from it
Oropharyngeal Ca	0.8 : 100 000 UK
	6 : 100 000 USA
	90% SCC, 8% lymphoma
	2% minor salivary tumour
	SCC 60% lateral wall
	25% tongue base
	10% soft palate
	5% posterior wall
	30% chance of 2nd primary (cf. 15%risk in other sites)
	8% distant mets
	90% of lymphomas affect the tongue base
	If thickness <2mm – Death is unusual

(Contd.)	
NPC	20% of all Hong-Kong Malignancies
	80% of all H&N Ca in Hong-Kong
	12.4 : 100 000 in Hong-Kong
	0.5 : 100 000 in UK
	20% present with nodes
	small tumours 80% 5y
	large tumours 0–20% 5y
P53 & tumour margins	52% of histologically clear margins are +ve with p53
	38% of those with p53 +ve margins recurr, cf. 0% if clear
	(Critics say p53 only 70% reliable)
SCC lip	0.8 : 100 000
SCC ear	1 : 100 000
Malignant melanoma	Familial dysplastic nevus syndrome-risk is 400 times higher
	Critical Breslow level = 1.7mm
Adjuvant radiotherapy in H+N SCC	Indications are:
	T greater than 4 centimetre,
	In to bone,
	Beyond primary site
	Multiple positive neck nodes
	Extra Capsular nodal extension
	Positive resection margins
	Recurrent disease
Side-effects of radiotherapy	Xerostomia whenever the salivary plans are exposed to more than 2000 cG
	Alopecia in regions treated with greater than 6000 cG
The veterans Affairs laryngeal cancer study group	RCT with 332 patients
	Either laryngectomy plus radiotherapy or
	Chemotherapy and radiotherapy
	64 per cent preserved the larynx
Risks for sinonasal malignancy	nickel = 800 times
	Wood dust
	Leather working
	Inverted papilloma = 10 to 15%

(*Contd.*)

Survival in laryngeal cancer	T1 – T2 = 95%
	T3 = 50–80% with surgery alone
	T4 = 50% for combined treatment
Risks of second primary	Laryngeal cancer = 5 to 10%
	2nd primary rate 4% per year to year five
Horizontal supraglottic laryngectomy - must have	Normal pulmonary function
	Under 65 years
	5mm anterior commissure clearance
	Normal vocal cord mobility
	No cartilage invasion
	No tongue extension within 5mms of the circumvallate papillae
	No extension to post-cricoid, the arytenoid
	<N3
Oesophageal dysmotility in systemic disease	Polymyositis 30%
	Scleroderma 52% (histopath 72%)
	SLE
	Raynauds
	Dermatomyositis
	DM
	Alcoholism
	Chagas
Lingual thyoids	10% of population
	70–80% it is the only functioning thyoid
	15% of these patients are hypothyoid
Leukoplakia	SCC in 8%
	Epithelial hyperplasia in 80% dysplasia 30%
	SCC *in situ* 2%
Lichen planus	Malignant transformation rate 4%
ELSOC classification of Endolaryngeal Resection	1 – Submucosal
	2 – Subligamental
	3 – Transmuscular
	4 – Complete cordectomy
	5 – Extended cordectomy
	a – other cord
	b – False cord
	c – Subglottis

(Contd.)	
Resection Margins in endolaryngeal resection	2mm acceptable
Erythroplakia	15 to 20% SCC
Human papilloma virus Sub types	Types 6 and 11 = benign papillary tumours Types 16 and 18 = malignant degeneration
Facial nerve anatomy	Frontal branch and mandibular branch-only in 15% of cases is there crossover communication between these branches and adjacent branches The crossover in the rest of the face is 70%
Lymph node levels	Level 1 - Submental & Submandibular Level 2 - Upper IJ chain Skull base to hyoid/carotid bifurcation Level 3 - Middle IJ chain Hyoid to omohyoid/cricothyoid Notch Level 4 - Lower IJ chain Omohyoid to clavicle Level 5 - Posterior Triangle Level 6 - Anterior Group Level 7 - Paratracheal
Anatomic divisions of the neck in trauma	Zone 1-sternal notch - cricoid, cartilage Zone 2-cricoid to mandible angle Zone three-angle of mandible to base of skull
Barrets Oesophagus	Adenocarcinoma 15% Reflux induced
Breaks in DXT	1.5–6% reduction in local control per day of DXT suspended
Pre v post op DXT	Pre op DXT 31% recurrence Post op DXT 18% recurrence
When not to treat the N0 neck	Early lip T1 oral cavity & if thin Floor of mouth <2cm T1 & T2 glottis
Orderly spread of H&N cancer?	15.8% of SCCs form oral cavity have skipped levels. i.e. levels 3&4 involved with no affected nodes in levels 1&2
Caustic Oesophageal Burns	20% will have oesophageal burn without oral burn

Thyroid

Thyroid Carcinoma	1.2 : 100 000
	2,500 new cases per year in UK
	Deaths 0.6 : 100 000 in USA
	2% mortality from thyoid Ca in UK
	5% chance of clinical "simple goitre" representing malignancy
	Papillary 50%
	Follicular 25%
	Anaplastic 20%
	Cold nodule – 30% malignant
	95% of malignancies are "Cold"
	5% warm nodules are malignant
	Solitary nodule in patients <30y – 15–30% malignant
	5–20% of nodules are malignant
Solitary nodules	Prevalence = 3–8% – half of these are solitary
	4 times more common in women
	5–10% risk of malignancy
	1000 new cases per year in England
	25% on clinically single nodules and in fact multiple
	26% of thyroid Cas have a cystic component
Risk of a solitary nodule being malignant	Solid on USS 50% risk
	Cold/warm 20% risk
	5–10% overall
	Hot <1% risk
USS & FNA Sensitivity	If USS & FNA suggestive of benign disease – then at 10y follow up only 0.1% actually found to be Malignant.
	Therefore if FNA and USS benign × 2 – safe to discharge the patient
	False –ve 2.4%
	False +ve 1.2%

(Contd.)

Thyroid Lumps	**Benign**
	Follicular 90%
	Hurtle Cell Adenoma 10%
	Malignant
	80% Papillary
	10% Follicular
	3% Hurtle Cell Ca
	5% Medullar Ca
	1% Anaplastic Ca
Papillary thyroid cancer (85%)	36% multifocal—but only 10% of these develop into frank malignancy
	80% of children will have palpable lymph nodes
	20% of adults will have lymph nodes
Follicular thyroid cancer (10%)	7% will have palpable lymph nodes
Medullary thyroid cancer (2–5%)	20% are familial
MEN I – (Wermer's syndrome)	Hyperparathyoidism
	Pancreatic islet cell tumours
	Pituitary tumours
	Gastric carcinoid
MEN 2 A (Sipple syndrome)	Medullary carcinoma
	Pheochromocytoma
	Hyperparathyoidism
MEN 2 B	Medullary carcinoma
	Pheochromocytoma
	Mucosal neuromas
Risk factors for malignancy in thyroid carcinoma	Less than 20 years
	Over 60 years
	Irradiation
	Male
	Family history of medullary carcinoma
Parathyroid gland	35 milligrams
	Tan colour
	Oval shape
	Sink in saline when adenomatous

Rhinology

Epistaxis	60% of population will experience epistaxis
	6% will seek medical attention for it
	Anterior ethmoidal artery absent in 14%
	Bilaterally so in 2.5%
Intra-orbital distances from anterior lachrymal crest	24mm to anterior ethmoidal artery
	12mm between anterior and posterior Arteries
	6mm between posterior artery and optic nerve
Sino-nasal distances	Nasal spine – sphenoid sinus = 7cm
Snoring and OSA	**Prevalence** 40%
	60% of men >60y snore
	10% of snorers have OSA = 6% of men
	Apnoea = cessation of respiration >10sec
	>30 apnoeas in 7hrs sleep = OSA
	Hypopnoea = >50% reduction in tidal volume despite respiratory effort
	Hypopnoea/Apnoea index (summed per hour)
	>5 = OSA Mild
	>10 = moderate
	>40 = severe
	Epworth score >8–12 = - OSA
	If H/A index >20, 37% chance of dying within the next 8years
	UPPP 80% successful for simple snoring
	Septal surgery (if indicated) reduces snoring in 50%)
Accessory ostia	Present in 25%
Concha bullosa	Present in 30%
Optic nerve dehiscence in Sphenoid sinus +?	6%
	14–17%
Carotid dehiscence in Sphenoid sinus +?	25% clinically dehiscent
Outcomes of FESS	85% very good benefit—Stamberger 1990
	85–95% symptomatic improvement Wigand 1990
	87% overall improvement Lund & MacKay 1994

(Contd.)			
Chronic sinusitis	8 weeks persistent or		
	4 acute infections, each lasting no less than 10 days in 1 year, with CT changes 4 weeks after medical therapy		
Staging of sinusitis on CT	0	1	2
0=Clear	Maxillary		
2=Opaque	Omu		X
	Anterior ethmoids		
	Posterior ethmoids		
	Sphenoid		
	Frontal		
	Stage left & right therefore		Maximum score 22
Radiation doses	Plain X-ray 0.26msv		
	CT coronal 45msv		
	CT coronal & Axial 73msv		
	Maximum permitted in radiosensitive areas 50msv		
Wegeners	>90% chronic rhinitis		
	85% renal involvement		
	40% middle ear		
	25% laryngeal		

(Contd.)	
Sinus development	*Frontal Sinus*
	birth = undeveloped
	Six years = just visible on x-ray
	12 years = developed
	Fully developed = late teens = 6–7ml
	Ethmoid Sinus
	Birth = 3–4 cells
	12 = adult size
	Average adult Sinus = 15 cells = 15ml
	Maxillary Sinus
	Birth = 4–7ml
	3 years = floor of sinus 4–5mm above the nasal floor
	Adolescence = floor of sinus 3–4mm below nasal floor
	Adult = floor of sinus = 5–10mm below nasal floor
	Sinus volume = 15ml
	Sphenoid Sinus
	Birth = not developed
	7 years = just developed
	12–15 years = 7–8ml
Saccharine Taste Test	Normal = 17min ± 5min
Ciliary beat frequency	12–15Hz
	inhibited by drying, drugs, excessive heat/cold, smoking, noxious fumes, anoxia
Prevalence of rhinosinusitis	1 in 6 (13%)
	30–60% have +ve skin tests
	75% of allergic asthma patients have rhinitis
	40% of non-allergic asthma patients have rhinitis
	20% of rhinitics have asthma
	8% of rhinitics have ASA triad
Mucosal thickening	Seen on CT in 25–40% of normal population
Resolution of rhinosinusitis in children	95% spontaneous
Septal & turbinate surgery	SMD 48% recurr within 2y
	TITs 20% recurr within 2y
	Septoplasty 84% satisfaction at 10y

(Contd.)	
Rhinoplasty	Nasal length = 1/3 of facial length
	Nasal width = intercanthal distance or 1/5 facial width
	Nasofrontal angle = 120 degrees
	Nasolabial angle 95–100 degrees
HHT	50% chance of affected adult having similarly affected child
Sinogenic brain abscess	15% mortality
Orbital complications classified	Group 1 – preseptal cellulites
	Group 2 – postseptal cellulitis
	Group 3 – subperiosteal abscess
	Group 4 – orbital abscess
	Group 5 – cavernous sinus thrombosis
Nasal septal perforation	Anterior 85%
	Posterior 15%
	77% < 2cm
	45% idiopathic
	39% traumatic
	8% inflammatory
	3% infections

Facial nerve

House -Brackman	I	Normal
	II	Mild weakness
	III	Weak but eye closes
	IV	Incomplete eye closure
	V	Flicker
	V	No movement
Dehiscent in middle ear	6–30%	
Facial nerve anatomy	Frontal branch and mandibular branch-only in 15% of cases is there crossover communication between these branches and adjacent branches	
	The crossover in the rest of the face is 70%	
Schirmers test	Difference of >25% significant	
	If less than 10mm after 5 minutes bilaterally also significant	
Ramsay Hunt	40% have SNHL	
	60% resolve	
	30% long term sequelae	
Facial nerve schwannoma	50% at CPA	
	50% intra-temporal	
	Not so – 80% arise in GG region	
Bells Palsy	Incidence: 15–40 cases per 100 000	
	Men = Women	
	14% +ve family history	
	60% viral prodrome	
	50% pain around the ear	
	50% change in taste	
	40% facial numbness	
	20% recurrent	
	8% bilateral	
	85% spontaneous recovery	
	66% have Diabetes or abnormal GTT	
	no visible weakness until 50% degeneration	
	4% long term sequelae	

(Contd.)	
Electroneuronography	Difference in the thresholds of <10% (i.e. 90% degeneration) is an indication for exploration of the nerve. Most reliable on 3rd–4th days
Facial nerve segment lengths	Meatal – 24mm
	IAM – 10mm
	Labyinthine – IAM to geniculate ganglion – 5mm
	Tympanic – gg to second genu – 13mm
	Mastoid – second genu to stylomastoid – 20mm
Congenital facial palsy	1 : 100 000
	43% have charge syndrome

Paediatrics

Choanal Atresia	70% bilateral
	30% unilateral
	70% bony
	30% CHARGE syndrome
	70% some other congenital abnormality
	84% success
Laryngeal Cleft	Classification
	1 – normal cricoid
	2 – into cricoid
	3 – all the way through cricoid
	4 – intrathoracic
	20% associated with TOF
Laryngomalacia	90% mild
	10% severe – aryepiglottoplasty
Tracheomalacia	<75% collapse – Watch
	>75% collapse – correct /stent with long T.tube
Subglottic Haemangioma	Grow for the 1st year - resolve by the age of 5
	50% also have cutaneous haemangioms
Speech development	6/12 babbles
	1y mamma/dadda, i.e. one word with meaning
	18/12 mum/dad & 18 other words
	2y "my mum" i.e. 2 words with meaning
	3y 3–4 word sentences
	5y name and address
Screening for hearing loss	Varies form region to region therefore check locally but in general
	All at risk kids = SCBU, family history, other congenital abnormality
	And
	6/52 – general check by health visitor parental concern noted
	6–8/12 – distraction testing by H.Visitor
	3–4y—pre-school check

(Contd.)		
Stridor	Laryngeal 60%	60% laryngomalacia
		20% Subglottic stenosis
	Tracheal 15%	45% Tracheomalacia
		45% Vascular compression
	Bronchial 5% Infection 5% Miscellaneous 15%	
Goldenhar syndrome	50% have facial palsy 10–20% absent facial nerve 50% Vertebral abnormalities	
Staging of subglottic stenosis	Grade 1 = 50% Grade 2 = 70% Grade 3 = 99% Grade 4 = No lumen	
Grading of Microtia	1 – malformed but recognisable as pinna 2 – Rudimentary bar 3 – malformed nodule Anotia	
Grading of congenital ear atresia	Grade 1 abnormal pinna or EAM only Grade 2 abnormal EAM and ossicles or VII Grade 3 abnormal middle and inner ears	
Congenital ear abnormalities	20 : 100 000 (all types) 10 : 100 000 Bilateral	
Cleft palate	8% syndromic Non affected parents with one child affected –4% risk of subsequent child developing the condition Repair within 6/12 for best speech & hearing results (but worse facial growth with early repair)	
Cleft lip	1% syndromic	
Branchial apparatus anomalies	Type 1 Cyst is inferior to the lobule; is a duplication anomaly of the EAC Type 2 First cleft and arch derivative May open in to SCM Or EAC	
Pre auricular abnormalities	1% syndromic 13% SNHL	

(Contd.)	
Tracheo-oesophageal fistula	One\3000
	87% upper oesophagus ends in blind pouch
	The lower oesophageal segments attached to the trachea
	Hydramnios in 16% of infants
	Clinical features drooling, coughing, distension, vomiting, poor feeding, inability to pass a catheter into the stomach
	60 to 70% survive
Strawberry Haemangioma	90% of Haemangioma
	80 per cent inviolate by five
Screening for hearing loss in children (UK)	840 new cases/y. in UK worse than 40dB of these 1/4 > 90dB
	Health Visitor Screening
	Distraction testing at 6/12
	88% sensitive in Nottingham (well motivated)
	26% sensitive in the UK as a whole
	Age at pick up = 20/12 (9/12 if profound loss)
	Cost £20 000/child fitted with H.aid
	(C.F. £8–10 000 for universal OAE screening)
	Universal neonatal OAE's
	Will detect 80% of affected children but
	Not all children born in hospital
	20% will develop h/loss after screen
	Targeted Screening (Syndromes/+ve FH/ SCBU)
	will test only 10% of popul'n but still
	picks up 50% of deaf children

(Contd.)	
At risk groups	Deaf parents
	Syndromic child
	Prem
	Meningitis
	Perinatal infection – Measles mumps, etc.
	Interuterine infection – CMV/Toxo/VDRL/Rubel
Congenital SNHL	1 : 100 000
	1 : 750 risk of child being born with worse than 40dB in better hearing ear
	50% genetic 90% of these are autosomal recessive
	Diagnosis = 1 ear <25dB

Otology

Meniere's	75% Idiopathic i.e. disease
	25% secondary
	Incidence 15 : 100 000
	Prevelance 200 : 100 000
	10% +ve family history
	Bilateral in 15% @ 2y
	40% @ 20y
	Canal paresis in 75%
	E.Cog. sp/ap ratio >30% & wide complex (>2ms)
	60–80% spontanous recovery
	Intra-tympanic Gent = 30mg per ml
	Non servicable hearing = >30dB and <70% SDS (some say >50dB and 50%)
	VIII nerve section 95% successful
	Gentamicin results
	95% complete or substantial results
	15% mild SNHL
	1–2% dead ear
AAO Criteria for Meniere's assessment	1. Assess for 6/12 pre Rx & 2y post Rx
	2. Vertigo Control =
	$$\frac{\text{No of attacks/month post Rx}}{\text{No of attacks/month pre Rx}} \times 100$$
	0 = perfect result, 100 = no change, >100 = worse after
	3. Disability Status = none – mild – mod— severe
	4. Hearing PTA avg. 0.5, 1, 2, 3K
	compare worst PTA + SDS in post Rx period with best in pre Rx period
Ototoxicity	Definition = >10dB reduction @ one or more frequency—Bilaterally
Gentisone HC	0.3% (wv) = 30mg in 10mls = one bottle = 1/3 of toxic dose
BAHA	Indicated if BC thresholds <50dB and >60% ODS
	10% Extrusion rate
	Skull thick enough at 2–3y

(Contd.)

Cochlear implants	Cost
	£20 000 first year
	£50 000/10y
	In children – 90% inserted for congenital deafness or meningitis
	Demand 1 : 100 000 = 850 per year in UK of these 1/3 are syndromic
	Neuronal plasticity
	Hair cells working at 18/40
	Tonotopic responses at 24/40
	By 6/12 child can recognise its own language
	Plasticity ends at age 5 – implant before
	Audiological criteria
	60dB aided or 105dB unaided thresholds
	Complications 22% minor
	10% major
	4% non users (2% in first year)
	Results in adults
	95% improves understanding with lip reading
	50% understand without lip reading
	35% can use the phone
	90% say improved quality of life
	95% of CI's are worn for 95% of waking life
Sudden onset SNHL	35dB in at least 3 frequencies in <3 days
	3–5% will have an acoustic neuroma
	15% of Acoustics present with SOSNHL
	8k affected = poor prognosis
	Overall 60% recover
	>90dB only 20% recover
	<70dB 85% recover
Presbycusis	33% of population >65y are affected

(Contd.)	
Noise Induced Hearing Loss (NIHL)	EAM resonates at 3kHz
	Maximal loss ½ octave above = 4kHz
	Temporary threshold shift 75–85dB
	Permanent Threshold Shift 140dB
	90dB for 8 hrs will give a hearing loss in 15%
	85dB for 8 hrs will give a hearing loss in 3%
	15 million workers at risk in Europe
	US military pays \$300million each year in compensation
	Leq8 = 84dB
	Calculate sum @ 1, 2, & 3 kHz for medico-legal reports
Acoustic Neuromas	Post mortem incidence 0.7%
	8% of brain tumours
	80% of CPA tumours
	5% bilateral (NF2)
	15% present with SOSNHL
	20% present with meniere's like symptoms
	<5% have normal hearing
	Growth rate 1–2mm/y. (18–40% no growth)
	(Meningioma 6% of CPA tumours)
	Hearing preservation in Most hands 5–10%
	(House Group claim 60–90%)
	Tumour <2cm 15% temporary facial palsy
	2–5% permanent
	Tumour >3cm 10% permanent
	Gamma knife 91% 5y tumour control
	17% Facial palsy
	45% SNHL
NF2	5% of Acoustics
	1 : 100 000

(Contd.)	
Asymmetric S N H L	= >10dB average. BC or > 20dB at one frequency
	Incidence = 0.7%
	2–5% of patients investigated for a asymmetric hearing loss will have an acoustic neuroma
	85% idiopathic
	10% vestibulopathies
	5% acoustics
	1% Ototoxicity (60% of aminoglycoside ototoxicity only affects one ear)
Audiological screening for AN	ABR hands acoustic reflexes require a threshold less than 70dB-this rules out 15% of patients screened

Acoustic neuromas screening		Sensitivity	
	Specificity		
	ABR	95%	64%
	ACoustic Reflexes	100%	37%
	Calorics	80%	50%

Chance of having an acoustic neuromas with Asymmetric hearing	1 : 700 to 1 : 1400 in general population
	2–5% of MRIs ordered for AN will be +ve
Acute S.N.H.L	60 per cent resolve
Non-organic hearing loss	B C testing: all patients should hear a sound 25dB above the BC threshold in the better ear
	AC testing: unmasked differences of greater than 60dB should raise the possibility. (only definite when greater than 80dB)
	When the PTA and acoustic reflex thresholds are within 20dB of each other
Grommets	Cost of grommets to NHS £30M per year
	Insertion rate 5 : 1000 children under 15y

(Contd.)	

Complications of Grommets	Otorrhoea
	  <72h = 20%
	  needing drops = 5%
	  Long Term = 2%
	Perforation
	  2%
	  25–50% with T tubes
	SNHL < 1 : 10 000
	Second set of G's required in 26%

Glue ear prevalence	2y = 40% 5y = 20% 7y = 6% 12y = 2% 50% of these will resolve within 3/12 5% of these will still have glue at 1 y Otoscopy & SOM 90% sensitive 75% specific Tymps; if type B or C2 then 97% chance of hearing 20dB or worse
Watchful waiting	50% of Glue ears will resolve within 3/12 Even with Long standing SOM, 40% resolve in 3/12 But if PTA >35dB, SOM much less likely to resolve
When not to wait	If hearing worse than 40dB AND Winter/autumn presentation AND Community referral (rather than parental concern) Then 83% of SOM will not resolve with watchful waiting
Meningitis and SNHL	5–30% SNHL 1–4% dead ear
Risk factors on glue ear	30% in allergic population c.f. 10% in Normal popul'n Male Social class 1 Parental smoking Affected sibs Race Feeding/Sleeping position Breast feeding? Play groups?

(Contd.)	
Otosclerosis	Fissula ante fenestrum 80%
	Clinical disease 0.5–2%
	Sub clinical disease −10%
	85% bilateral
	60% family history
	20% chance of affected child
	10% Schwartz sign
	Twice as common in females
	Osteogenesis imperfecta = 0.15% of otosclerotics
	Fluoride 2.2mg p/o OD
	If patient using HRT suggest oestrogen levels no higher than normal i.e. <80picograms /day
Stapedectomy	If at least 15dB conductive loss and 60% SDS
	Incus to footplate = 4–5mm
	Footplate dimensions = 1.75 × 3.2mm
	Piston should enter vestibule by 0.1–0.2mm
	Saccule 0.4mm beneath the foot plate
	Stapedotomy = 0.8mm
	Piston = 0.6mm
	Length of piston does not include loop
	Most = 4.25mm
	Closure of AB gap to with in 10dB >90%
	Causse 65–90% best of the rest
	Dead ear rate 4% in most hands
	21 year average benefit from successful surgery
	5–10% no appreciable benefit
	5% SNHL at 4K > 15dB
	30% Chorda Tympani damage
	Revision surgery <50% closure of AB gap to within 10dB, & 14% dead ear rate

(Contd.)

Barotrauma	90mmHg leads to ET locking
	500mmHg leads to TM rupture (= 5.5meters of sea water)
	−30mmHg for 15 min—transudate
	valsalva generates 20–40mmHg
Tympanoplasty Types	1. Ossicular Chain
	2. onto LPI
	3. onto Stapes head
	4. Fenestration
	5. Round window baffle
Staging of pars tensa retraction	1. Annular retraction
	2. TM touching LPI
	3. TM touching LPI and promontory
	4. TM adherent to promontory
Staging of pars flaccida retraction	1. attic dimple
	2. TM on to neck of malleus
	3. erosion of scutum
	4. non cleaning pocket
Retraction & SOM	Less that 10% of children with SOM have Sade ¾ retraction—and of these only 35% will still persist at 3/12 of watchful waiting—therefore retraction alone is not an indication for grommet insertion early on
	Flaccida retraction is even more likely to resolve
Buffer effect of mastoid	Middle ear volume = 0.5ml
	Mastoid volume = 1–30mls
	Therefore a change in volume of 20 micro-litres
	if mastoid/middle ear volume = 2ml—leads to pressure change of 100mm water
	If mastoid/middle ear volume = 20 mls – leads to pressure change of 10mm water

(Contd.)			
Middle ear Gasses		Air	Middle ear
	PCO_2	0	50
	PO_2	150	40
	PN_2	563	623
	Pressure	760	760
	1–2mls or air absorbed per day = 1–2microliters/min		
Acute otitis media	Everyone affected at least once in their life time		
	40% incidence in the first years of life		
	23% incidence in the first 12 months of life		
	60% viral		
	40% bacterial		
	50% will have glue ear for 3/12 after AOM		
	5% will have glue ear for 1year after AOM		
Complications of AOM	OME longer than three months = 33%		
	Facial palsy in 0.5–1.5%		
	Acute mastoiditis in 0.04%		
Perilymph fistula	60% oval window		
	20% round window		
	20% bilateral		
	In congenital types middle ear abnormality visible on CT in 85%		
Jahrsdoerfer grading of congenital EAC atresia (Page 347)	Total points = 10		
	Surgery considered if > 6 points		
Systemic Diseases with SNHL	Sickle Cell Disease 4% SNHL		
	Wegeners 20% mixed loss		
	AIDs: 8% SNHL		
	MS: 4% SNHL & 10% present with vertigo/imbalance		
	Also : SLE, PAN, R.A, DM, DIDMOAD		
Embryology & development	Pinna and middle ear formed at 20–28 days		
	Mastoid antrum present by age 1		

(Contd.)	
Cholesteatoma surgery	Canal wall up surgery – residual disease in 10–15%
	Facial palsy 1–2% in most series
	Dry ear in 70%
	Wet ear 20%
	Dead ear 2%
	Worse hearing 13%
	Better hearing 12% Mod rad (30% CAT)
	If AB gap <20dB then 65% chance that ISJ is intact
Ear + temporal bone anatomy	Petrous apex pneumatised in 30%
	IAM diameter <8mm
	Cochlear aqueduct 6.2mm
	TM diameter 9–10mm
	Surface area of TM 70–80mm^2
	Vibrating surface of TM 55mm^2
	Stapes footplate 1.75 x 3.2mm
	surface 4mm^2
	Effective surface ratio TM and footplate = 14 : 1
	Ossicular lever action = 1.3 times
	Total transformer ratio = 18 : 1
	Total middle ear transformer = 25dB
	65% of sound energy transferred to cochlear fluids
	A TM defect (perforation) = 30dB hearing loss
	A ossicular defect >40dB hearing loss
	EAM volume 2ml
	TM & ossicles most efficient between 0.5–3KHz
	Eustachian tube length = 36mm in adults. Lateral third bony (diameter 2mm), middle two-thirds fibrocartilaginous
	Facial nerve dehiscent in 6–30%
	Sclerotic mastoid in 20%
	In child <2 mastoid antrum 2mm deep cf. Adult = 10–15mm
	12 000 OHCs, if lost 60–70dB
	3,500 IHC's if lost >70dB
	VIII 30 000 fibres

(Contd.)	
Regions of Temporal bone pneumatisation	1. Middle ear
	2. Mastoid
	3. Perilabyinthine—Supra & infra lab
	4. Petrous Apex—Peritubal & apical
	5. Accessory—Zygomatic, Squamous, Occipital, Styloid
Temporal bone fractures	Longitudinal – 90% (30% bilateral)
	20% have facial nerve palsy
	90%% geniculate ganglion
	Transverse –10%
	50% have facial nerve palsy
	High incidence of SNHL
	And vestibular symptoms
	20% of temporal bone fractures have subsequent CSF leaks
Glycerol Dehydration Test	PTA/Ecog/Speech audio
	1–5ml/kg of glycerol orally
	sufficient to increase plasma osmolality > 10mos/kg
	Repeat PTA/Ecog/Speech Audio
Myingoplasty take rate	82.2% (1070 patients at 1 year)
	and 67% improved hearing
Speech listening disability	<20dB none
	20–35dB problems in background noise if not able to lip read
	35–55dB problems in background noise even with lip reading
	55–70dB Problems in quiet room if not able to lip read
	>70dB Problems in quiet room even if able to lip read
Wide vestibular aqueduct	On CT if >1.5mm at mid point of duct
	Normal duct 10mm long
	If wide assoc with SNHL, progressive and 60% have some other ear abnormality
Risk of otogenic i/c abscess	Annual risk 1 : 10 000
	3 x increased in males
	If age 30 then lifetime risk = 1 : 200
	5% of abscess occur immediately post op
	No evidence that surgery reduces the risk

(Contd.)	
Tinnitus	Intrusive in 0.5–3% of adults
	15–20% of adults will experience Tinnitus = 18dB avg.
Austin and Kartush classification of ossicular chain defects	Incus missing either totally or in part:
	Malleus handle and stapes superstructure present.
	Malleus handle present and stapes super-structure absent.
	Malleus handle absent and stapes superstructure present.
	Malleus handle and stapes superstructure absent.
	Rarely there is isolated erosion of:
	O. Malleus, incus and stapes all present.
	Ossicle head fixation with all ossicles present.
	Stapes fixation with all ossicles present.

Audiology

The range of normal hearing	20–20 000 Hz
	Realistically, 200–10 000 Hz
	Speech frequency = 300–3 000 Hz
	3dB = doubling of sound intensity
Hearing Aids	250–4000Hz
Noise levels	PTA booth = 30dB
	Classroom = 50dB
Hearing thresholds @ 1 meter	30dB soft whisper
	60dB conversational Voice
	90dB shouting
	discomfort at 120dB
Tuning fork tests	Weber lateralises @ 10–15dB
	Rinne becomes –ve @ 20–25dB
	only 50% accurate when AB gap >20dB, and 90% accurate when AB gap >40dB
	If –ve, AB gap of at least 10dB exists
	512 TF activation-70 to 90dB S. P. L.
Otoacoustic emissions	Evoked OAEs
	0.7–4KHz
	Present in threshold 40dB or better
	93% sensitive
	84% specific
Belfast 15/30 Rule of Thumb	Significant hearing improvement if the operated ear threshold is closed to 30dB, and no more than 15dB difference between the ears
Glasgow benefit plot	Take average thresholds at 0.5, 1, 2, 4K & plot-operated ear against non-operated ear.
	Aim to elevate the threshold of the operated ear to with in 10dB of the other ear
Calorics	Patient at 30 degrees
	250mls water @ 30 & 44°C
	water for 40s

(Contd.)	
Hearing loss	2% prevalence with hearing worse than 45dB
	Majority of patients seek a hearing aid only when their hearing is worse than 45dB.
	Patients benefit from a hearing aid when their worse hearing ear is worse than 25dB
Free field voice test	Spondees in children
	Numbers and Letters, etc. in adults
	Mask non test ear with tragal rubbing
	Start with a whisper at 2 t (60cm)
	– 50% of words correctly identified—hearing is 12dB or better
	– if 50% not correctly repeated—then
	Whisper at 6 inches (15cm) = 34dB
	Conversational voice—2ft (48dB) and then 6 inches (56dB)
	Loud voice -2ft (76dB) and then 6 inches
Masking	Paper rubbing—not loud enough
	Finger occlusion 10dB
	Tragal rub-50dB
	Barany box-100dB
	AC attenuation in PTA is 40dB i.e. if > 40dB between the AC left and right , need to mask
	AC attenuation across the skull = 15dB in free field testing i.e. the shadow effect of the head is 15dB
	BC attenuation across the skull = 0–5dB
	Compulsory if:
	Hearing on air conduction in the poorer ear is > 40dB worse than bone conduction hearing in the better ear
	Any conductive hearing loss
Rules of masking	1st rule = A/C "mask if >40dB difference between the AC" (i.e. o—x >40)
	2nd rule = B/C "mask if >10dB difference between A/C in the better ear and un-masked B/C" (i.e. o or x—^ > 10)
	3rd rule = A/C "mask if >40dB difference between the A/C in the better ear and the unmasked B/C" (i.e. o or x—^ >40)

(Contd.)

Hearing impairment Mean of .5,1,2,4 kHz	None < 20dB Mild 20–40dB Moderate 41–70dB Severe 71–95dB Profound > 95dB
Hearing impairment British MRC national study	2.6% inactive chronic otitis media 1.5% active chronic otitis media 2% otosclerosis
Ear plugs	Attenuation by ear defenders – 25dB Attenuation with ear plugs – 15 to 20dB
PTA	Vertical axis is indB HL Reproducibility/Sensitivity of PTA = 5dB
Sound Pressure LeveldB SPL	Equal amount of energy in dynes/cm2
Hearing level dB HL	International Standards Organisation 1964 The ear is not equally sensitive to all frequencies – 250Hz sound has to be raised to 25dB SPL before it is heard therefore HL scale was set up - 0dB HL - least intensity needed for a normal ear to hear the sound 50% of the time Normal hearing individuals would have 0dB HL at all frequencies
Weighted audiometry Used to measure environmental sound	dB A scale Background noise in a quiet room = 30dBA
Calibration	Every 6 months
ABG < 10dB	Treated with caution Significant test/retest error
Audiogram	Start with better hearing ear 1, 2, 4, 8, 0.25 and 0.5kHz AC difference of greater than 40dB—requires masking Unmasked BC at 1, 2, 4, 0.5, 0.25 kHz with the vibrator on the side of the better AC thresholds If the unmasked BC and AC difference is less than 10dB-no BC thresholds required If unmasked BC and AC difference is greater than 10dB—masking is required

(Contd.)	
Conductive hearing loss	ABG increases linearly with perforation size up to a maximum of 30dB
	A 40dB ABG in a patient with a perforated drum-almost certainly ossicular chain is affected
	2% of adult population have otosclerosis
	6% of adults have C S O M
Progressive bilateral SNHL	94% idiopathic
	5% noise induced
ERA	Slow vertex wave averaged over three approximates to within tendB of the PTA average
	Electrocochleography is required to measure BC thresholds
NHS aid	Bone anchored hearing aid-2000 pounds
	Cochlear implant-20 000 1st year
Definition of Hearing impairment	Conductive Loss
	0.5, 1,2, kHz average > 10dB AB gap
	Sensorineural
	0.5, 1, 2, 4, kHz average worse than 25–30dB
	Remember that 10dB = 50% attenuation of sound
	20dB = 75%, etc.
Severe or profound hearing loss	65% have a mixed hearing loss
Prevalence of hearing loss in children – congenital	133 per 100 000-impairment worse than 40dB in better hearing ear
	23% will have a profound hearing loss

(Contd.)	
Tympanometry	−600 to + 200mms water
	Type A +200 to −100
	Type C1 −100 to −200
	Type C2 −200 to −400
	Type C3 −400 to −600
	Type B > −600/flat
	If Types C2 or C3 or B then likely that avg. H/Loss
	> 25dB
	(98% sensitive & 37% specific)
Acoustic reflexes	Normally 70dB above pure tone threshold
	In recruiting ears, it can be as low as 10dB
Tymps in OME	If screen kids with tymps then assuming 25dB as cut off point
	If types B and C2 only tested with PTA, reduces the work load of PTA's by 69% but still picks up 95% of affected children
Acoustic reflex decay	A normal reflex should last 10 seconds before decaying to 50% of its starting value

Miscellaneous

Tonsillitis in UK	35 million school/work days lost each year due to sore throat
	Tonsillectomy rate 100: 100 000
	Adenoidectomy rate 40: 100 000
	Adenotonsillectomy rate 50: 100 000
	60 000 Tonsillectomies/year
	30 000 Adenotonsillectomies/year
	Re-admission rate 1.3%
	97% satisfied following tonsillectomy
	95% say less time off following tonsillectomy

Oesophagoscopy Distances from upper incisor teeth		Cricopharyngeus	Arch	Hiatus
	Adult	15cm	22cm	38cm
	3y	10cm	14cm	22cm

French Guage	French = Circumference – divide by 3 to convert to approximate diameter
	E.g. 15f = 5mm external diameter

Safe doses of L.A.	% to mg/ml (X by 10)
	e.g. 5% cocaine = 50mg/ml
	safe dose = <200mg = 4ml of 5%
	Lignocaine 3mg/kg
	Ligocaine + ad 7mg/kg
	Bupivicaine 2mg/kg
	1 : 200 000 Adrenaline – primary toxic effect is that of the anaesthetic
	1 : 80 000 toxic effect is that of the adrenaline
	1 : 80 000 = 12.5microg /ml
	1 : 80 000 no more than 8mls (4 cartridges) in 10 mins

Sjorgrens Syndrome	40% salivary glands affected
	10% develop lymphoma

(Contd.)

Lasers	*CO2 10 600nm*
	0.3mm penetration
	coagulates BV's <0.5mm
	(0.2 sec, 5watts, 0.8mm spot for laryngology)
	Nd-Yag 1064nm
	3mm penetration
	coagulates up to 2mm
	KTP 532nm
	1.5mm penetration
	Argon 500nm
	Most adsorbed by blood
	Diode 810nm
Genetics.	Autosomal dominant 2% of children are affected.
	Autosomal recessive-25% of bilateral carrier
	X—linked recessive-
	Carrier females:
	50% of sons affected
	50% of daughters become carriers
	Affected males:
	50% of daughters become carriers
	No sons affected
Middle ear mechanics	Area of vibrating TM: surface area of foot plate = 17 : 1
	Length of handle: length of short process = 1. 3 : 1
	Combined effect = 22 : 1 = 25dB
Nystagmus	grade 1-eyes in direction of fast phase
	grade 2-eyes ahead and in direction of fast phase
	grade 3-even when eyes deviated away from fast phase
Pressure	Sea-level pressure is doubled at ten meters depth
	Every ten meters of descent causes a pressure increase of one atmosphere
	Air pressure at 18 thousandft = one half of that at sea level
Blood volume	75mls per Kg
	Transfuse if 20–25% of blood vol lost

(Contd.)

Blood Loss	Class 1–15%
	Class 2–15 to 30%
	Class 3–30 to 40%
	Class 4 greater than 40%
Parasympathetic ganglia	
Otic	ISN to the tympanic plexus by IX Jacobson's nerve to lesser petrosal nerve
	To the auriculotemporal nerve and from there to the parotid gland
Pterygopalatine	SSN to VII to greater superficial petrosal nerve
	Nerve of pterygoid canal to deep petrosal nerve
	From here to the Pterygopalatine fossa
	Via zygomatic nerve to the lacrimal nerve to lacrimal gland
Submandibular	SSN to brain stem to VII to chorda tympani to lingual nerve to submandibular ganglion
ENT conditions that may affect safe driving	• Sudden attacks of unprovoked or unprecipitated disabling giddiness: Cease driving on diagnosis, until symptoms controlled at least for one year for LGV licences
	• OSA: (Cease driving until symptoms controlled and confirmed medically)
Notification to DVLA	GMC guidelines:
	The DVLA is legally responsible to decide if a person is medically unfit for driving
	Explain to the patient he/she has the legal duty to inform the DVLA
	If patient refuses advice suggest seek a second opinion and advice not to drive until then
	If patient continues to drive, make every reasonable effort to persuade them to stop. Talk to their next of kin
	If you find evidence the patient continues to drive, inform the patient (also in written) that you are going to disclose the medical information to the DVLA and then contact the medical adviser at the DVLA
Consultants in the UK	600 consultants
	each covers about 80–120 000
	UK popul'n 60 million

Glossary

Acoustic neuroma (vestibular schwannoma): A benign tumour of the eighth cranial nerve.

ANCA: Anti nuclear cytoplasmic antibody: +ve in Wegeners granulomatosis.

Anosmia: Loss of the sense of smell.

Antrostomy: An artificially created opening between the maxillary sinus and the nasal cavity.

A's: Adenoids/adenoidectomy.

BAWO: Bilateral antral washouts.

BINA: Bilateral intranasal antrostomy.

BINP: Bilateral intranasal polypectomy.

BNF: British National Formulary.

BOR: Branchial-oto-renal.

BPPV: Benign paroxysmal positional vertigo.

BSER: Brainstem evoked response—an objective test of hearing.

Cachosmia: The sensation of an unpleasant odour.

Caloric tests: Tests of labyrinthine function.

CAT: Combined approach tympanoplasty. A type of mastoid surgery, usually performed for cholesteatoma in which the posterior canal wall is left intact, unlike a modified radical mastoidectomy.

CHL: Conductive hearing lose.

CJD: Creutzfeldt–Jakob disease.

CSOM: Chronic suppurative otitis media.

CT: Computerized tomography.

CXR: Chest X-ray.

Dohlman's operation: an endoscopic operation on a pharyngeal pouch.

DL: Direct laryngoscopy.

DO: Direct oesophagoscopy.

DP: Direct pharyngoscopy.

EAC: External auditory canal.

EAM: External auditory meatus.

ENG: Electronystagmography.

ENT: Ear, nose, and throat.

ESR: Erythrocyte sedimentation rate.

EUA: Examination under (general) anaesthesia.

EUM: Examination under the microscope—usually of the ears.

FBC: Full blood count.

FESS: Functional endoscopic sinus surgery.

FNAC: Fine needle aspiration cytology.

FOSIT: Medical shorthand for a feeling of something in the throat.

Free flap: The movement of a piece of tissue (skin ± muscle ± bone) with a supplying artery and vein from one site in the body to another. The blood supply is connected to local blood vessels via a micro vascular anastomsis. This is most frequently performed in reconstructing surgical defects following resection of head and neck malignancies.

Freys syndrome: Gustatory sweating, a complication of parotidectomy.

GA: General anaesthetic.

GORD: Gastro-oesophageal reflux disease.

Globus: A sensation of a lump in the throat, when on examination no lump can be found. (see also FOSIT).

Glottis: Another name for the vocal cords.

Glue ear: A common cause of conductive hearing loss, due to Eustachian tube dysfunction. The middle ear fills with thick sticky fluid, hence its name. Also known as otitis media with effusion (OME) and secretory otitis media (SOM).

Grommet: A ventilation tube placed in the eardrum in the treatment of glue ear also known as 'G's', 'tympanostomy tubes' or 'vent tubes'.

HHT: Haemorrhagic telangiectasia.

HIB: Haemophyllus influenzae type B.

HME: Heat and moisture exchanges.

HPV: Human papilloma virus.

IJV: Internal jugular vein.

IV: Intravenous.

Ludwigs's angina: Infection of the submandibular space.

MDT: Multi disciplinary team.

MLB: A diagnostic endoscopy. Microlaryngoscopy and bronchoscopy.

ML/Microlaryngoscopy: Microscopic surgical examination of the larynx using a suspended rigid laryngoscopy and a microscope.

MMA: Middle meatal antrostomy. A surgical enlargement of the natural maxillary sinus ostium. See FESS.

MOFIT: Multiple out fracture of the inferior turbinate. See also SMD and TITs.

MRI: Magnetic resonance imaging.

MRM: Modified radical mastoidectomy. Mastoid surgery performed for cholesteatoma.

MRND: Modifed radical neck dissection.

MUA: Manipulation under anaesthetic.

NARES: Non-allergic rhinitis with eosinophilia.

NIHL: Noise induced hearing loss.

od: Once daily.

OME: See glue ear.

OSA: Obstructive sleep apnoea.

Ostiomeatal complex (OMC): The area between the middle turbinate and the lateral nasal wall. The maxillary, frontal and anterior ethmoid sinuses drain into this area—the final common pathway.

Otorrhea: Ear discharge.

Panendoscopy (Pan): Full ENT examination performed under general anaesthetic in order to evaluate/exclude a malignancy of the upper aerodigestive tract.

Pec. major: Pectoralis major myocutaneous flap. Frequently used to reconstruct surgical defects in the head and neck region.

PEG: Percutaneous endoscopic gastrostomy.

PCU: Paediatric tensive care unit

PND: Post nasal drip.

po: Per oral.

post-op: Post-operative.

PPI: Proton pump inhibitor.

pre-op: Pre-operative.

Presbycusis: The common hearing loss of old age, high frequency, bilateral and sensorineural in type.

PSCC: Posterior semi circular canal.

Quinsy: Paratonsillar abscess.

Ramsay Hunt Syndrome: Herpes zoster infection of the facial nerve.

Reinkes oedema: Benign oedema of the vocal cords caused by smoking.

Rhinorrhoea: Nasal discharge.

SALT: Speech and language therapist.

SCBU: Special care baby unit

SCC: Squamous cell carcinoma.

Second look: A planned staged operation to ensure that cholesteatoma has not recurred in the mastoid after CAT.

Secretory otitis media (SOM): Glue ear.

SHO: Senior House Officer.

SMR: Sub mucus reception.

SMD: Submucus diathermy to the inferior turbinates, performed to reduce the nasal obstruction associated with inferior turbinate hypertrophy.

SNHL: Sensorineural hearing loss.

SOHND: Supra omohyoid neck dissection. A type of selective neck dissection.

SPR: Specialist Registrar.

STIR: Short tau inversion recovery.

T's: Tonsils/tonsillectomy.

tds: Three times daily.

tfts: Thyroid function tests

TITs: Trimming of the inferior turbinates. A surgical procedure performed to reduce the nasal obstruction associated with inferior turbinate hypertrophy, sometimes associated with spectacular heamorrhage!

TM: Tympanic membrane.

TMJ: Temporo mandibular joint.

TSH: Thyroid stimulating hormone.

T-tube: Long term grommet.

TTS: Temporary threshold shift.

Tympanometry: The indirect measurement of the middle ear pressure or compliance of the ear drum.

Tympanostomy tube: A grommet.

URT: Upper respiratory tract.

URTI: Upper respiratory tract infection.

VOR: Vestibulo-ocular reflux.

WS: Waardenburg's syndrome.

Index